Breast Cancer - Evolving Challenges and Next Frontiers

Edited by Mani T. Valarmathi

Published in London, United Kingdom

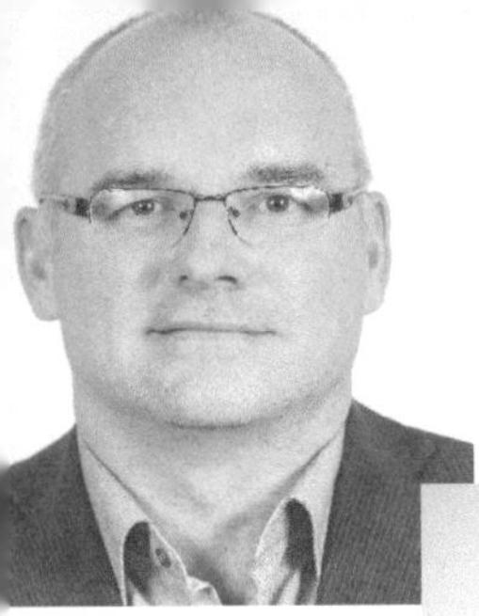
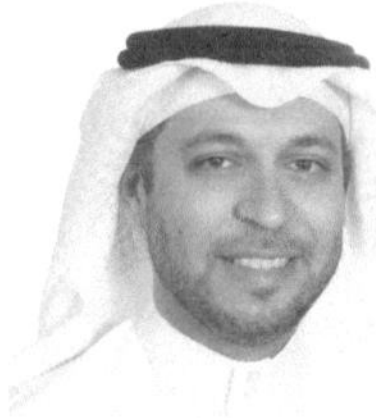
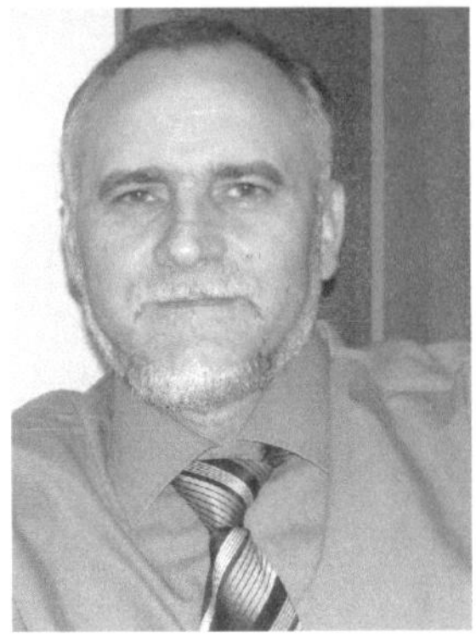
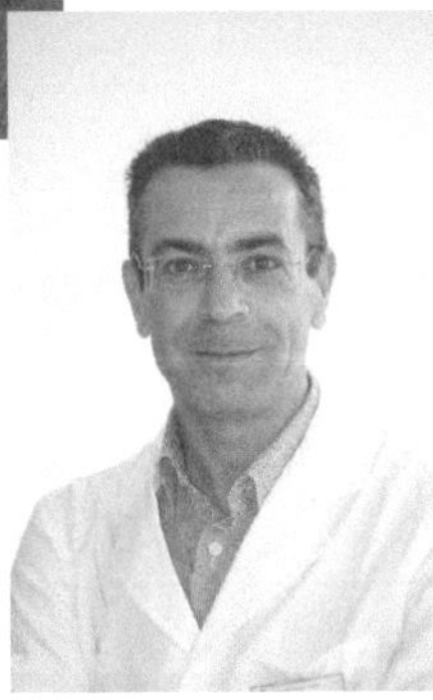
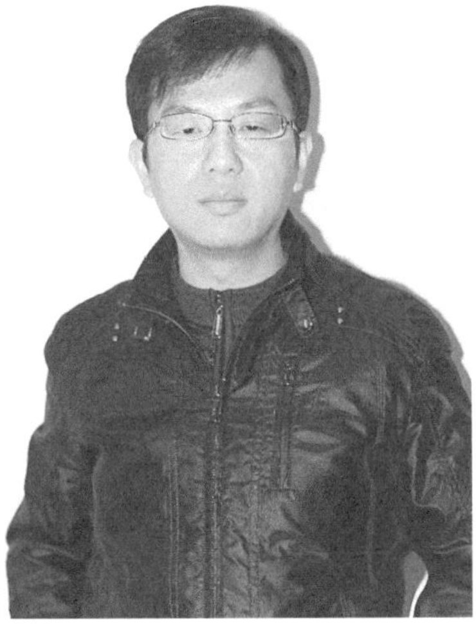
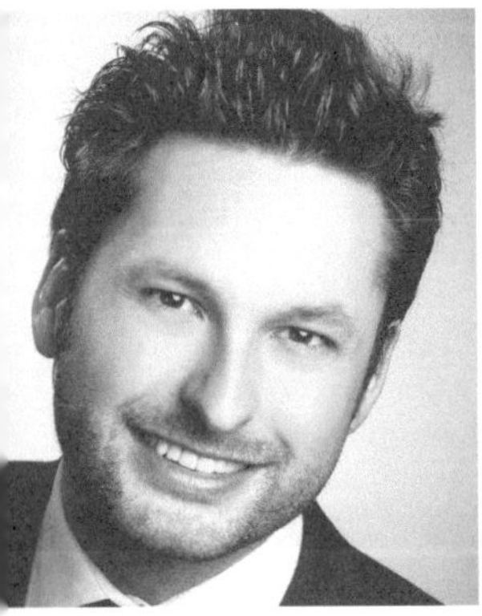
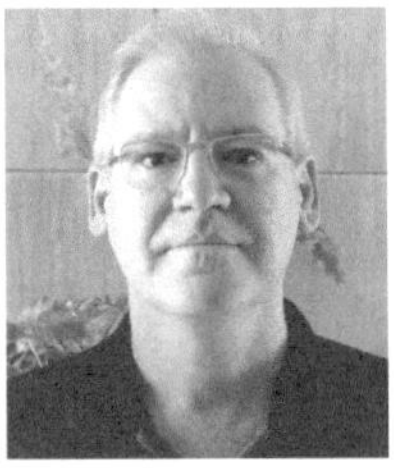

IntechOpen

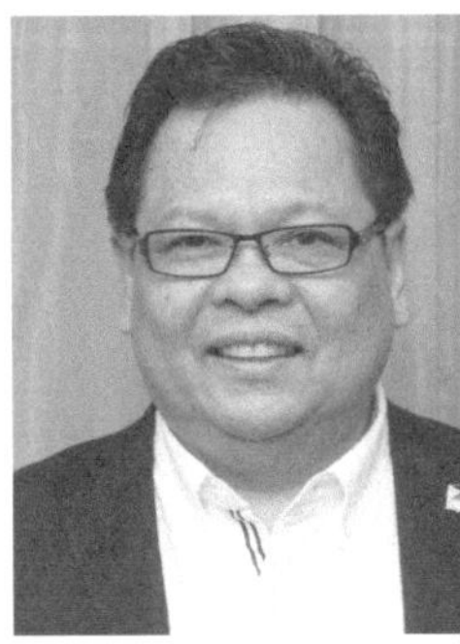
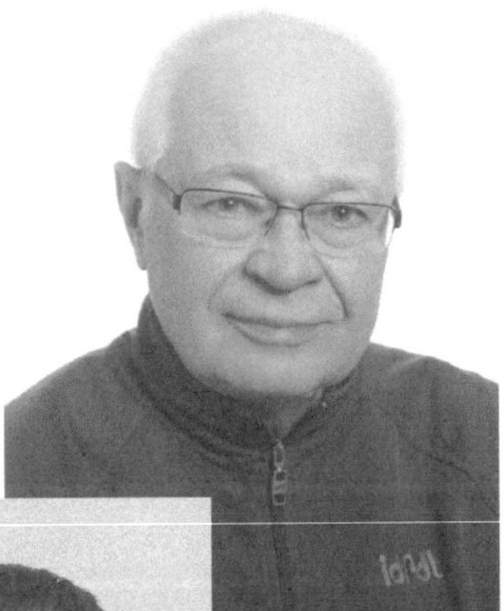
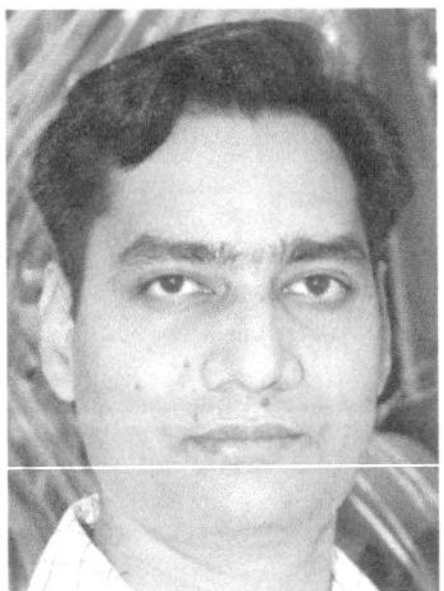
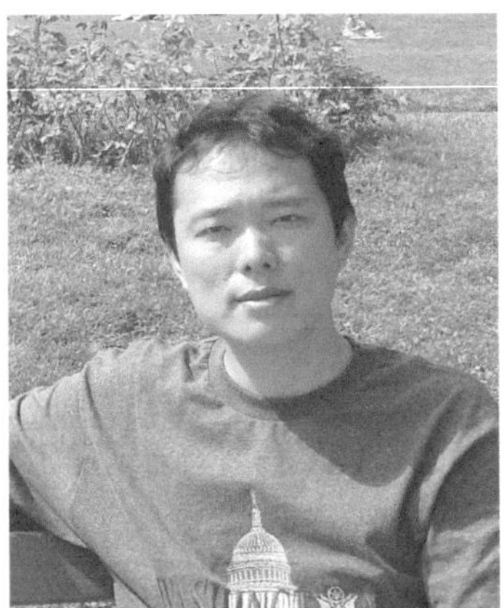
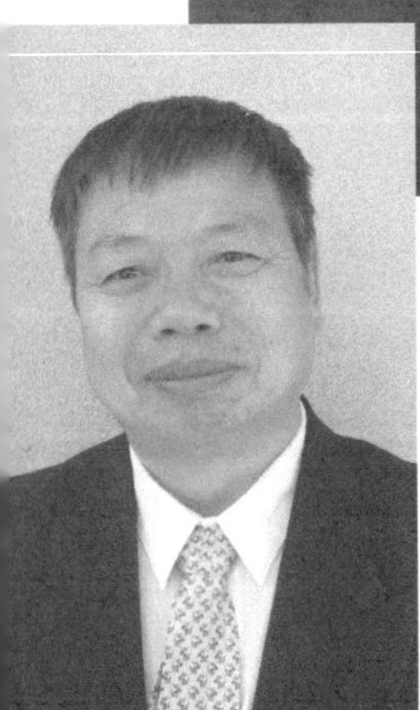
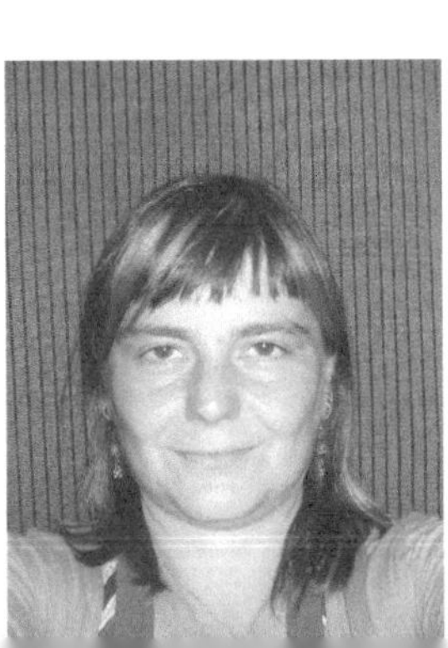

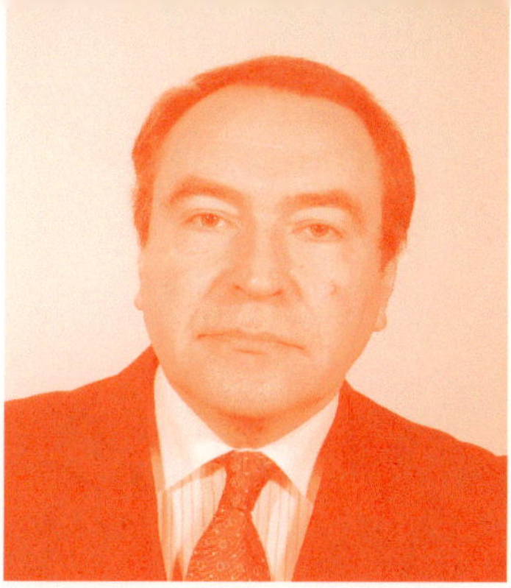
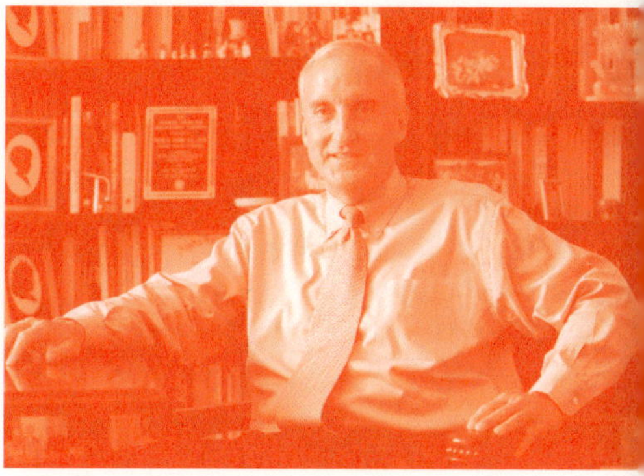
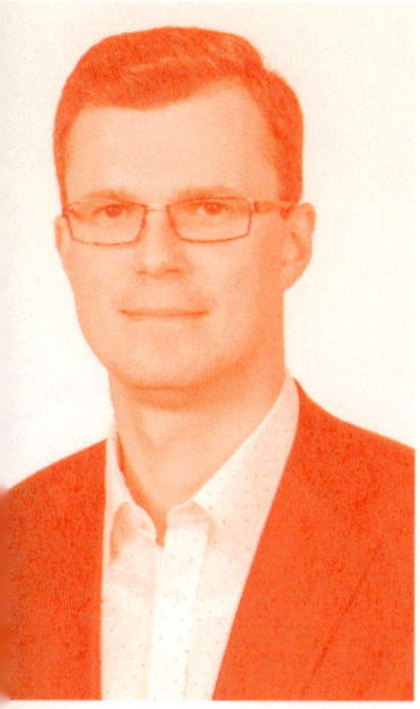
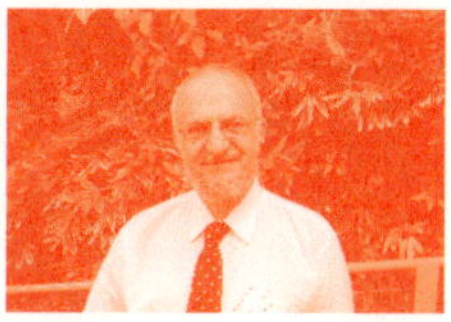
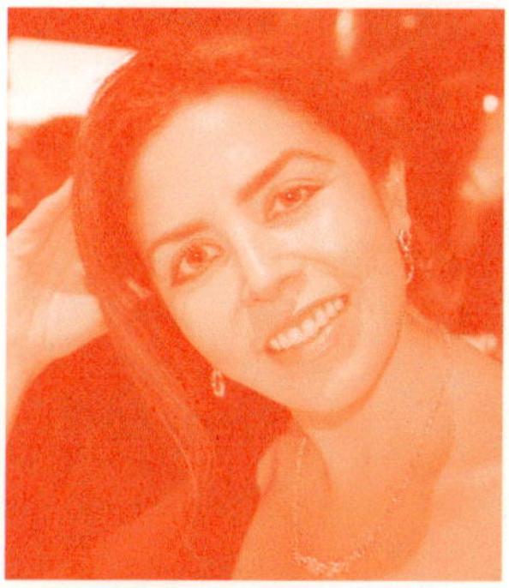

Supporting open minds since 2005

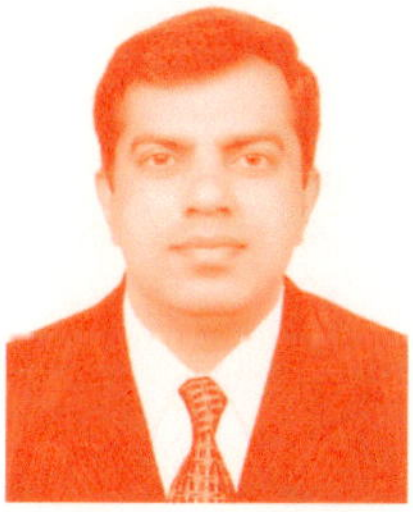
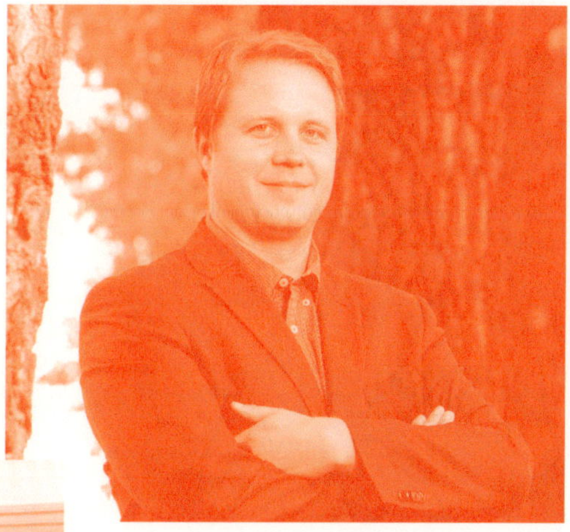
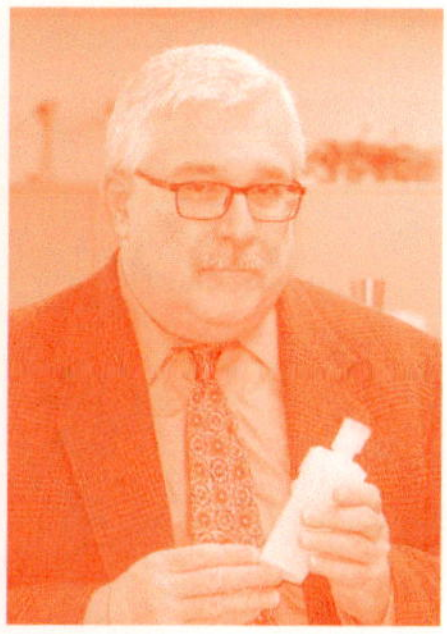
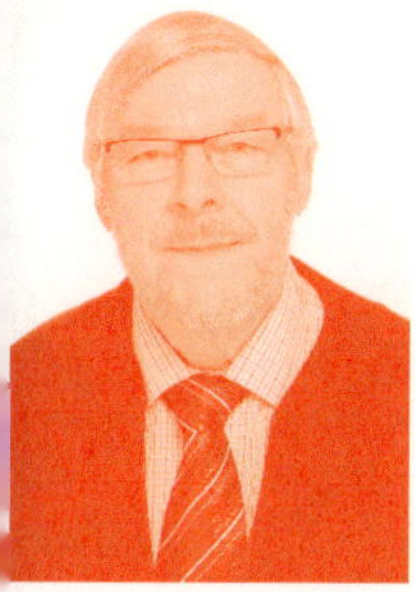
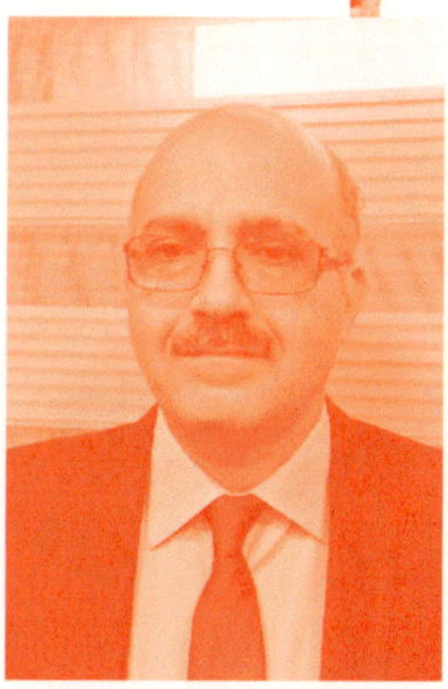
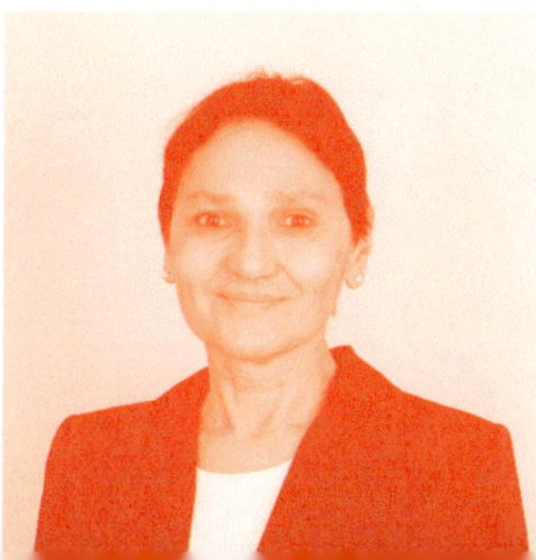
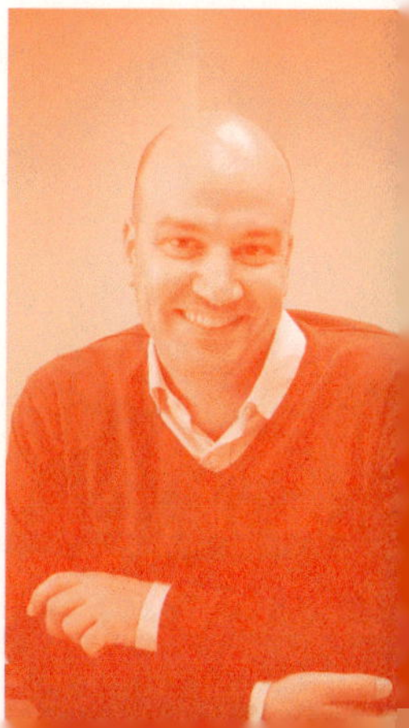

Breast Cancer - Evolving Challenges and Next Frontiers
http://dx.doi.org/10.5772/intechopen.91486
Edited by Mani T. Valarmathi

Contributors
Isadora De Fátima Braga Magalhães, Kátia Da Silva Calabrese, Ana Letícia Marinho Figueirêdo, Ana Lucia Abreu-Silva, Fernando Almeida De Souza, Hidetoshi Tahara, Yuki Yamamoto, Susmita Sahoo, Sabrina La Salvia, Mohammed Tareq Mutar, Mustafa Majid Hameed, Aqeel Shakir Mahmood, Mohammed Saleh Goyani, Abo-Alhasan Hamid Obaid, Yoshihiko kuwahara, Maribella Domenech, Heizel Rosado, Lyanne M. Suarez Torres, Marketa Koleckova, Zdenek Kolar, Katherine Vomackova, Ivan Ilić, Martiniano Bello, Miguel Ángel Vargas Mejía, Sachin Sahni, James Khan

First published in London, United Kingdom, 2021 by IntechOpen
IntechOpen is the global imprint of INTECHOPEN LIMITED, registered in England and Wales, registration number: 11086078, 5 Princes Gate Court, London, SW7 2QJ, United Kingdom
Printed in Croatia

British Library Cataloguing-in-Publication Data
A catalogue record for this book is available from the British Library

Additional hard and PDF copies can be obtained from orders@intechopen.com

Breast Cancer - Evolving Challenges and Next Frontiers
Edited by Mani T. Valarmathi
p. cm.
Print ISBN 978-1-83969-202-4
Online ISBN 978-1-83969-203-1
eBook (PDF) ISBN 978-1-83969-204-8

Meet the editor

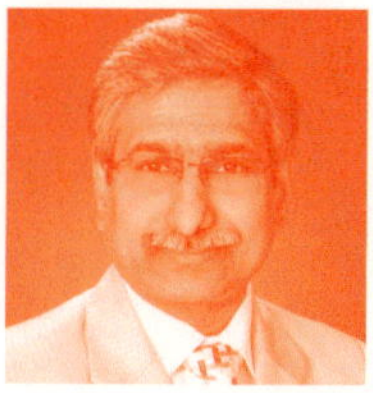

Mani T. Valarmathi is currently Director of Research and Development at Religen Inc., a life science company in Pennsylvania, USA. He began his scientific career as a cancer geneticist but soon became captivated with the emerging and translational fields of stem cell biology, tissue engineering, and regenerative medicine. After obtaining a bachelor's degree in Chemistry from the University of Madras, Chennai, Tamil Nadu, India, he obtained an MBBS in Medicine and Surgery and an MD in Pathology from the same university. Dr. Valarmathi also holds a Ph.D. in Medical Biotechnology from the All-India Institute of Medical Sciences, New Delhi, India. Over the past two decades, he has had extensive experience in research on various types of stem cells, and his research work has been focused on creating bioengineered human 3D vascularized tissues constructs for implantation purposes. At present, much of his research is directed towards developing innovative molecular genetic testing for precision and genetic medicine. He is a member of many prestigious national and international professional societies and scientific organizations, including the International Society for Stem Cell Research (ISSCR), Tissue Engineering and Regenerative Medicine International Society (TERMIS), American Association for Cancer Research (AACR), American Society for Investigative Pathology (ASIP), American Society for Clinical Pathology (ASCP), American Chemical Society (ACS), European Society of Cardiology (ESC), International Society for Heart Research (ISHR), American Society of Gene & Cell Therapy (ASGCT), and American Heart Association (AHA).

Contents

Preface XI

Section 1
Breast Cancer Pathobiology 1

Chapter 1 3
Multifocality, Multicentricity, and Bilaterality of Breast Cancer
by Ivan Ilić

Section 2
Breast Cancer Biomarkers 27

Chapter 2 29
Potential Biomarkers for Therapeutic Monitoring and Clinical Outcome in Breast Cancer
by Yuki Yamamoto, Sabrina La Salvia, Sahoo Susmita and Hidetoshi Tahara

Chapter 3 47
Molecular Prognostic and Predictive Markers in Triple - Negative Breast Cancer
by Marketa Koleckova, Katherine Vomackova and Zdenek Kolar

Section 3
Breast Cancer *In vitro* Models 63

Chapter 4 65
In vitro Approaches to Model Breast Tumor Complexity
by Heizel Rosado-Galindo, Lyanne Suarez and Maribella Domenech

Section 4
Breast Cancer Pharmacotherapy 85

Chapter 5 87
The Use of Plants' Natural Products in Breast Cancer: Have We Already Found the New Anticancer Drug?
by Isadora de Fátima Braga Magalhães, Kátia da Silva Calabrese, Ana Letícia Marinho Figueirêdo, Ana Lucia Abreu-Silva and Fernando Almeida-Souza

Chapter 6 107
Structural Insight of the Anticancer Properties of Doxazosin on Overexpressing EGFR/HER2 Cell Lines
by Martiniano Bello and Miguel Ángel Vargas Mejía

Section 5
Breast Cancer Screening and Management 121

Chapter 7 123
Persistent Breast Cancer Pain
by Sachin Sahni and James Khan

Chapter 8 145
Breast Cancer Screening
by Mohammed Tareq Mutar, Mustafa Majid Hameed, Mohammed Saleh Goyani, Aqeel Shakir Mahmood and Abo-Alhasan Hammed Obaid

Section 6
Breast Cancer Diagnostic Imaging 163

Chapter 9 165
Microwave Imaging for Breast Cancer Detection
by Yoshihiko Kuwahara

Preface

Breast cancer is the most frequent invasive cancer among women worldwide, impacting more than two million women each year. It is also the number one cause of cancer-related deaths among women. The incidence of breast cancer varies greatly around the world. While breast cancer rates are higher among women in more developed regions, rates are increasing in nearly every region globally. Researchers and clinicians around the world are working to find better ways to prevent, detect, and treat breast cancer, and to improve the quality of life of patients and survivors.

In recent years, there has been substantial development in breast cancer research and its clinical applications, for example, breast cancer biology and genomics; epidemiology and prevention; early detection and screening; as well as diagnosis and treatment. In addition, the advent of various emerging technologies, such as stem cell technology, genome editing technology, and bionanotechnology, as well as tissue engineering and regenerative medicine, have enhanced our understanding of breast cancer and produced novel insights that could lead to the development and deployment of newer clinical and/or therapeutic interventions.

Against this backdrop, this book examines recent advances in breast cancer biology and therapeutics. Chapters cover a broad spectrum of interrelated topics, presenting information in a comprehensible way to a greater scientific and clinical audience as well as patients, caregivers, and drug and device manufacturers to support breast cancer product development.

Written by leading experts in basic science and clinical care, this book consists of nine chapters over six sections. The first section introduces the pathobiology of breast cancer, emphasizing the current challenges and future perspectives of multifocal, multicentric, and bilateral synchronous aspects of breast cancer. The second section deals with selected biomarkers of breast cancer, such as non-coding RNAs, and highlights the potential significance of diagnostic and prognostic biomarkers as well as novel therapeutic targets. A chapter in this section examines the potential role of various molecular prognostic and predictive markers, such as p53, EGFR, Fas, miRNA, PD-1, androgen receptors, and more, in the case of triple-negative breast cancer.

The third section discusses in vitro breast tumor models focusing on their biomimetic capabilities, advantages, disadvantages, and specific applications. The fourth section explores recent developments in pharmacotherapy of breast cancer, particularly plant-based natural compounds that can be potentially harnessed as novel anticancer drugs. A chapter in this section delves into the structural insights of the anticancer properties of doxazosin, a selective alpha-1 adrenergic receptor antagonist, on overexpressing EGFR/HER2 cell lines.

The fifth section reflects on advances in breast cancer screening and management, for example, the pathophysiology of persistent pain after breast cancer surgery, including a review of pertinent risk factors, clinical features, and various treatment options. A chapter in this section synthesizes the knowledge and current perspectives of breast cancer screening. The final section of the book explores various aspects of diagnostic imaging, centering around microwave imaging for breast cancer detection.

This book is a valuable resource not only for medical and allied health students but also for researchers and clinicians in cancer biology, pathology, oncology, stem cell biology, tissue engineering, regenerative medicine, and precision medicine. This quick reference will benefit anyone desiring a thorough knowledge pertaining to recent advances in breast cancer and current and evolving diagnostic and therapeutic challenges.

I would like to thank the team at IntechOpen, including Commissioning Editors Sandra Bakic and Iva Simcic, and Author Service Manager Mia Vulovic, for excellent support throughout the preparation of this book; they were remarkably patient and persistent. Finally, I dedicate this to my beloved niece and nephew, Vidhya and Vignesh, the future.

Mani T. Valarmathi, MD, Ph.D.
Clinical Molecular Diagnostic Laboratory,
Religen Inc. | A Life Science Company,
Plymouth Meeting, Pennsylvania, USA

Section 1

Breast Cancer Pathobiology

Chapter 1

Multifocality, Multicentricity, and Bilaterality of Breast Cancer

Ivan Ilić

Abstract

Multifocal, multicentric, and bilateral breast tumours are either benign, precursor lesions or malignant neoplasms. A multidisciplinary review of these entities can offer clinicians a practical guidance for diagnostic and treatment procedures. Multiple synchronous (multifocal or multicentric) ipsilateral breast cancers (MSIBC) with heterogeneous histopathology require particular attention, since MSIBC tends toward more aggressive biology and higher rates of nodal positivity. Being independent of laterality, domination of the invasive carcinoma was observed in the bilateral and multifocal disease type. The TNM staging system for breast cancer does not include multifocality and multiplicity. Only the tumour with the largest diameter is considered for the pT category, neglecting the secondary foci which can make the treatment decision more difficult. MSIBC has a similar prognosis to unifocal cancers, but sometimes they might be negative prognostic parameters. Likewise, in comparison with unifocal breast cancer, MSIBC presents a different genetic pathway.

Keywords: Multiple synchronous tumour, multifocal, multicentric, bilateral, breast cancer

1. Introduction

The multifocal, multicentric, and bilateral aspects of breast cancer (BC) are the eternal dilemma in the scientific literature. Breast cancer is the most common tumour disease and the second leading cause of death in American women, with 268,600 new cases and 41,760 deaths in 2019 [1]. The second most common malignancy in patients with breast cancer is contralateral breast cancer [2]. Presence of another focus of breast cancer, far away from the dominant mass, was described as early as 1920 by Cheatle [3]. The appearance of such non-dominant lesions in multiple ducts of a single quadrant (multifocal), or in two or more quadrants (multicentric) was further elaborated in 1957 by Qualheim and Gall [4]. Multifocal/multicentric (MF/MC) breast cancer is occurring frequently, however, its genesis is not fully understood [5].

Previous studies evaluated histological and immunohistochemical characteristics [6, 7], revealing that most multicentric breast cancers share similar features in terms of histology and immunohistochemistry, suggesting that early-stage synchronous tumours develop from one breast cancer [6]. The heterogeneity of the focus of multiple cancers [8] is understudied in the literature, with a number of studies which have evaluated histological and immunohistochemical characteristics of tumour foci in multiple cancers arriving at contradictory results and different conclusions [7, 9].

Multiple synchronous ipsilateral breast cancer (MSIBC) with heterogeneous histopathology is a controversial condition in a clinical context, which has been discussed and studied extensively in the literature, but lacking international consensus on itsdefinition and clinical treatment options. Current incidence of MSIBC is unknown, but, owing to improved sensitivity of medical imaging methods and the use of magnetic resonance imaging (MRI) for BC screening and staging, is showing increased occurrence. This heterogeneous disease requires special attention during treatment, given the fact that MSIBC is a much more aggressive condition which produces metastases in lymph nodes more frequently [10].

Based on current therapies for breast cancer, the treatment of this heterogeneous disease calls for joint decision making in a multidisciplinary team and in collaboration with an oncology council, where the pathologist, working with the other members of the team, influences the new concept of individual approach to treatment of MC/MF breast cancer patients with their data and explanations obtained through testing. A new rigorous view on genetic patterns of heterogeneity in each individual focus would present a more specific approach to treating MSIBC [11].

2. Terminology and classification of multifocal, multicentric, and bilateral breast cancers

Multiple synchronous tumour foci in one breast are referred to as multifocal and multicentric, but without a consensus on terminology [12]. MF/MC cancer may occur due to intramammary proliferation of a single primary BC or multiple synchronous, independent primary breast cancers [5, 13]. Recently, the definition of multifocal cancer was changed. Previous definition of multiple synchronous lesions of breast cancer stated that these could be either MF or MC, depending on where the lesion was located (in the same or different quadrants). The use of breast quadrants to define and classify cancers is now considered inappropriate, since quadrants are not part of convention which correspond to the breast anatomy [14]. Pathologists define multiple simultaneous primary lesions when there are two or more tumour foci without malignant tissue between them [15].

Multifocality is usually determined microscopically, when a greater number of morphological cancer development centres are present, which is the same micromorphological unit or lobe in the breast. Radiologists do not have a more precise definition, but tumours are usually considered multifocal when the distance between the tumour masses is less than or equal to 5 cm, and multicentric when this distance is greater than 5 cm (**Figure 1**) [16, 17]. Given that a standardised definition is not established, multifocal and multicentric breast cancers are often grouped together as multifocal/multicentric breast cancers [18]. In histological terms, BC is defined as multiple cancer when it consists of more than one clearly distinguishable tumour foci which are separated by normal and benign breast tissue or ductal carcinoma in situ (DCIS) [19].

Various time intervals are used to define bilateral synchronous breast cancer (BSBC). In 1921, Kilgore defined BSBC as breast cancer where both tumours are diagnosed simultaneously [20]. Since 1921, various time intervals were introduced, ranging from one to five years [21]. A broadly accepted definition of BSBC is the one given by Hartman and co-authors in 2007 as a tumour diagnosed within 90 days after the initial mass has occurred. Although the reported time intervals vary, bilateral BCs are considered to be synchronous when contralateral BC is diagnosed within a period of three months, and as metachronous bilateral cancers (BMBC)

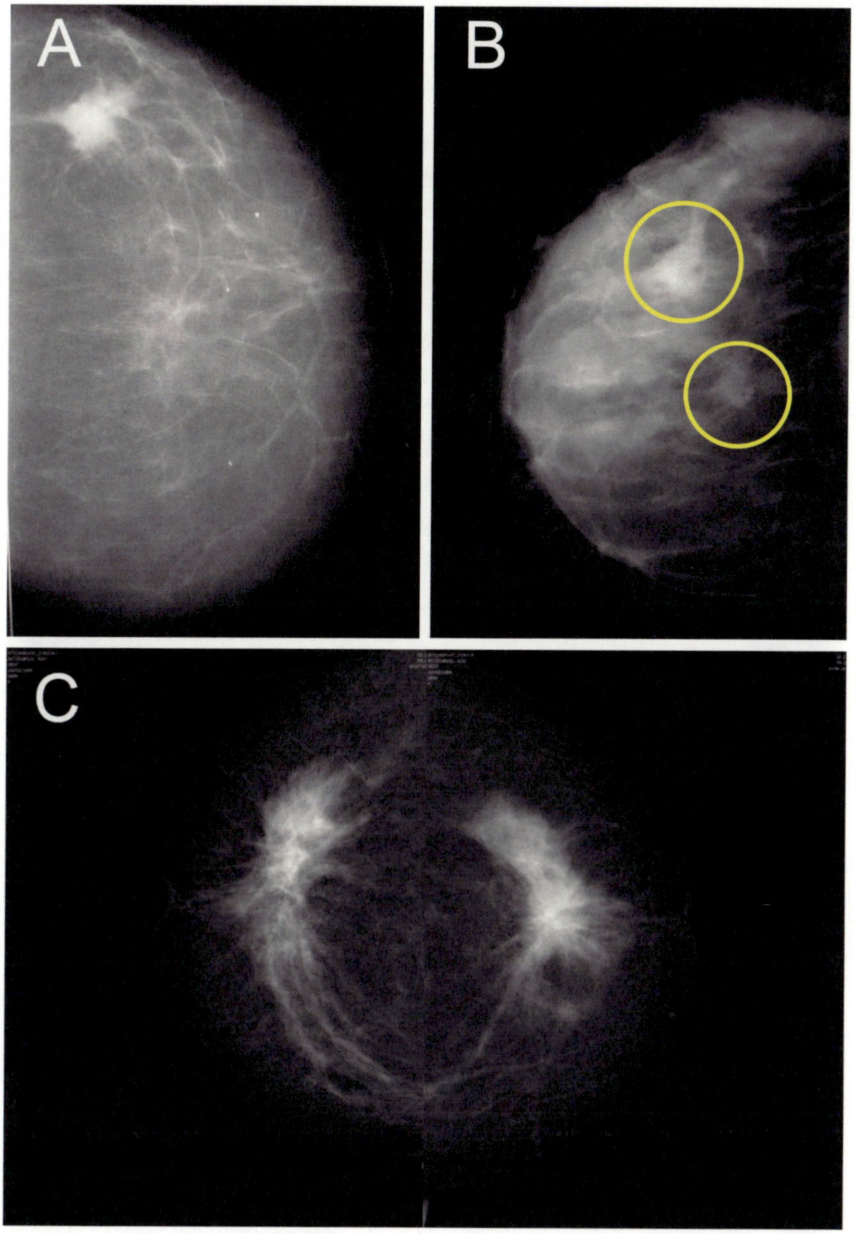

Figure 1.
Images from mammograms of ILC from three different patients: (A) stellate tumour shadow of unifocal ILC from the 58 years old patient; (B) multicentric (bicentric) ILC from the 53 years old patient; (C) bilateral synchronous ILC from the 32 years old patient. In reference [16] (the figure was taken from article; permission obtained from the copyright owner).

when diagnosed more than three months after the first diagnosis [22]. Limit values used in the literature to differentiate between BSBC and BMBC range from 1 to 12 months [23]. Before a bilateral breast cancer diagnosis is confirmed, metastatic contralateral breast cancer has to be ruled out [24].

The definitions of multifocality, multicentricity, and bilaterality refer primarily to the two most common types of breast cancer (ductal and lobular), but can also refer to certain lesions which occur less frequently in the breast. In terms of multifocality, between 10 and 20% of tubular carcinomas may present as multifocal [25, 26], and the identical frequency of multifocality is observed in cribriform cancers [27, 28]. A thorough sampling of large areas with high DCIS grade should be performed in order not to miss the foci of the carcinoma microinvasions (or invasions). Some reports suggested that when a microinvasive carcinoma occurs, it is likely to be multifocal [29].

Certain benign lesions, such as papilloma, are rarely multiple in nature (**Figure 2**). Breast lesions which often present as bilateral are DCIS [30], Paget's disease of the nipple, radial scars and complex sclerosinglesions, gynecomastia, Burkitt lymphoma [31], while bilateral breast cancer also frequently occurs in patients with Cowden syndrome and heterozygous ATM mutation carriers (ataxia telangiectasia), as a result of submitting patients suffering from Louis–Bar syndrome to radiotherapy [31–33]. Other types of potentially bilateral-onset breast lesions are atypical ductal hyperplasia [31], phyllodes tumour [32, 34], myofibroblastoma [33], desmoidfibromatosis [35], male breast cancer [36], angiosarcoma [37, 38], liposarcoma [31], lymphoma (about 10% of the cases), pseudoangiomatous stromal

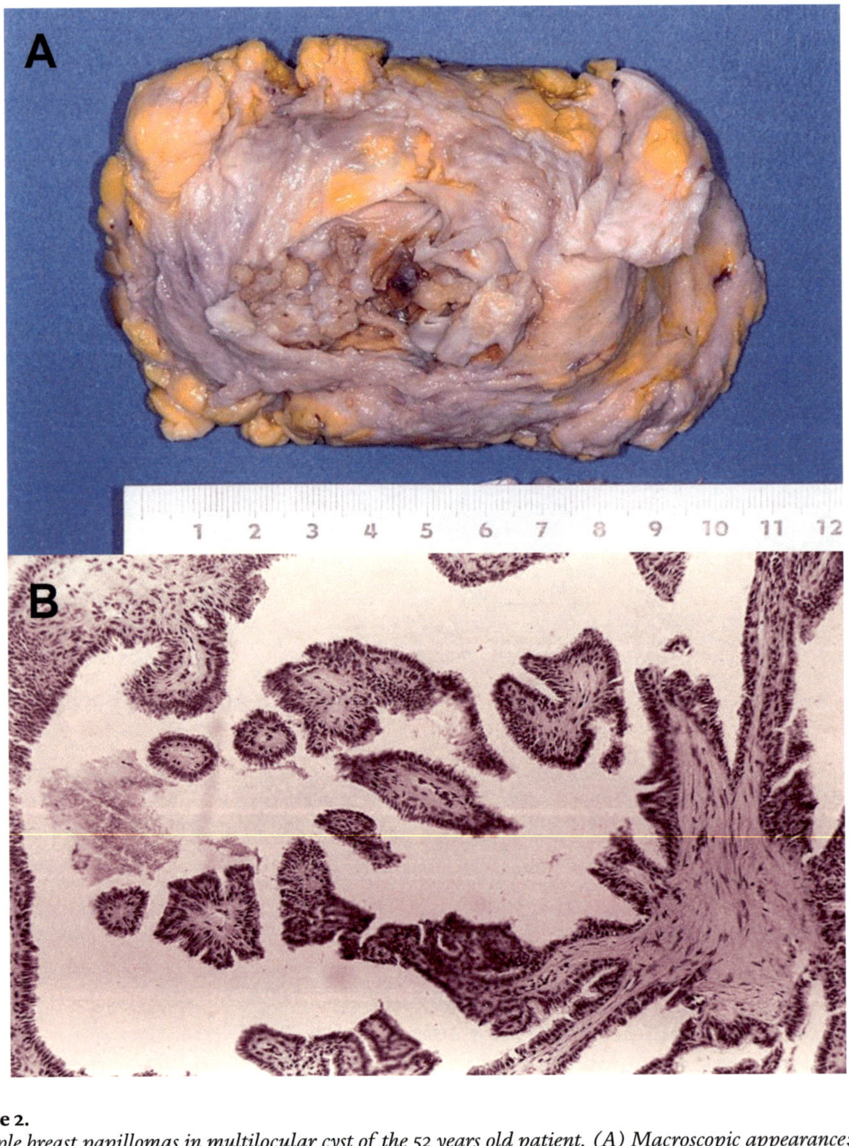

Figure 2.
Multiple breast papillomas in multilocular cyst of the 52 years old patient. (A) Macroscopic appearance; (B) microscopic appearance of breast papilloma (HE x 100) (image was taken from author's own lab).

hyperplasia [39], ductal adenoma in patients with Carney syndrome [40]. There are also lesions with unidentified bilaterality, some of which are ALK-negative anaplastic large cell lymphoma [31], mucosa associated lymphoid tissue lymphoma [41] and granular cell tumour [42]. Most patients with diffuse large B-cell lymphoma develop a unilateral condition, but there is a risk of relapse in the contralateral breast [43].

3. Epidemiology and risk factors

Based on data from the literature, there is no consensus on the factors relating to the development of multicentric carcinomas [44]. MF/MC BC incidence ranges from 6 to 77% [14]. Bilateral breast cancers are responsible for 2 to 6% of all breast carcinomas [22]. Earlier studies have shown that one of the most important risk factors for MCBC is if the first occurrence is an invasive lobular carcinoma (ILC) [45]. Low-grade invasive ductal carcinomas (IDC) are not linked with the number of tumour masses in the contralateral breast. All of these observations contradict the fact that ILC is more common among patients with bilateral and multifocal BC solely due to slower growth rates [46].

There are no differences when it comes to patient age, tumour stage, or the presence of multifocal, multicentric, and bilateral ILCs [47]. Contralateral tumour incidence, in particular synchronous ILCs, is in the 5 to 19% range, which is more than invasive ductal carcinoma of no special type [45, 48, 49]. BSBC is a rare entity with an incidence between 1 and 3%. Surprisingly, there has not been an increase in the BSBC incidence since 1980. A lower incidence of metachronous bilateral breast cancer was observed, likely due to the introduction of systemic adjuvant therapy. In the study on incidence of bilateral breast cancers in Sweden, conducted by Hartman and co-authors reported that the incidence of BSBC was approximately 100 times greater than what can be explained as coincidence or a cumulative effect of exogenous carcinogens [22],

Women with MF/MC breast cancers are often of younger age at the time of diagnosis and with positive oestrogen (ER) receptors expression than women with a unifocal condition [50]. Patients with MF/MC tumours are prevalently premenopausal and with a lower body mass index [51]. Women already suffering from BC are at two to six times greater risk of developing contralateral BC compared to the risk of other women developing their first primary BC, with the risk being inversely proportional to their age at the time of initial diagnosis [45, 52]. Average time between the diagnosis of the first BC and metachronous contralateral breast cancer varies from 3.9 to 7.7 years [22, 52].

Histological subtype of invasive carcinoma did not prove to be a predictive multicentricity factor, particularly in ILC subtypes [16, 47]. Earlier studies suggest that ILCs are much more prone to multicentric growth; but when lobular carcinoma in situ (LCIS) is excluded, multicentricity is not that common [44, 53]. When compared to IDCs, ILCs are ER and progesterone (PR) positive to a larger extent, but show lower HER2 positivity with the exception of pleomorphic lobular carcinoma [31]. Women diagnosed with MF/MC BC proportionally more frequently have positive ER receptors and lower prevalence of triple-negative tumour masses. Numerous studies documented significantly higher positivity levels of ER receptors among the BRCA2 mutation carriers in comparison to BRCA1 mutation carriers. Therefore, it is highly unlikely that ER signalisation leads to MF/MC disease [54]. An extensive meta-analysis found no connection between the ER status and sporadic MF/MC breast cancers, suggesting that the ER status does not play a part in the specific development of MF/MC disease [55]. The risk of other contralateral primary breast cancers varies depending on the status of hormone receptors of the first tumour, age, race, and/or ethnic origin [56].

A certain number of earlier studies discovered a strong correlation with the lobular histology in the first primary breast carcinoma and the occurrence of bilateral breast cancer [57]. Women with primary breast cancer who have positive hormone receptors show twice the risk of developing contralateral BC, while women who have cancers with negative hormone receptors are at almost four times higher risk as compared to general population with regard to age and race. Women with primary tumours who have negative hormone receptors more frequently develop secondary tumours which have negative hormone receptors, especially if the initial diagnosis is confirmed before the age of thirty [56].

Women who have next of kin with BC are at 50% higher relative risk of developing bilateral breast cancer than women without family history of this condition [22]. When compared to non-carriers, women with BRCA1 mutations are at 4.5 times greater risk and with BRCA2 mutations at 3.4 times greater risk of bilateral breast cancer [58]. On the other hand, carriers of similar ATM gene variants have a lower risk of developing contralateral breast cancer [59]. Family history of breast carcinoma, younger age at the time of initial diagnosis, or mutation of BRCA1 and BRCA2 genes are linked to a higher risk of developing contralateral tumours, placing them in the higher risk group [45]. Higher prevalence of multifocality/multicentricity than expected occurs in women diagnosed with cancer who are BRCA2 mutation carriers [50].

4. Radiodiagnostics

Mammography and ultrasound are complementary methods for evaluating the size, spread, and the presence of multifocality in BC (**Figure 1**) [16, 31]. However, not all MF/MC cases will necessarily be found using these imaging modalities [60]. Radiologic BC characteristics can vary significantly. These differences often depend on the tumour grade and histological subtype. Therefore, variations in the radiologic presentation can sometimes predict the differences in the morphology and biology of the tumour. ILC often invades normal tissue without causing desmoplastic stromal response which is usually found in IDC. For this reason, ILC density is often similar to the surrounding normal fibrous and glandular tissue of the breast, which makes it inconspicuous in mammographic screening [61, 62], particularly since non-desmoplastic ILC produces metastases in axillary lymph nodes more frequently [63].

Due to the limited use of mammography in diagnosing ILC and the risks of obtaining false negative results, other methods such as sonography and MRI are used to assess the tumour dissemination [64]. Magnetic resonance imaging is more useful for diagnosing ILC, in particular multifocal lesions, although this imaging procedure may produce false positive results or overestimate the tumour stage [65, 66]. Recent literature on the role of imaging modalities in the BSBC diagnosis suggests that family history of BC, multifocal BC, or the presence of an ILC should serve as recommendations to perform an MRI with the purpose of eliminating contralateral malignancy [67].

5. Pathology report

In recent decades, pathohistology has made a huge step forward from the typical traditional documentation to the ability to modify the histochemical and immunohistochemical methods [68], which has shed new light on some patho-histological parameters and consequently led to a new approach when it comes to recognising the criteria for classifying and grading tumours. Tot et al. support that there can be two different types of multifocal invasive carcinoma: one with multiple individual invasive foci which develop from *in-situ* lesions in different parts of the same lobe either at the same or at a different time, and one where individual foci are *in-transit* metastases of the primary focus and are not connected to the *in-situ* component [69].

When compared to unilateral BC, bilateral breast cancer is associated with significantly lower rate of the ductal type, with a higher histologic grade, HER2 positivity and metastases in lymph nodes, without differences relating to age, race, ER and PR status, or pathologic stage of the tumour disease (**Figures 3** and **4**). Synchronous breast cancer is associated with a higher rate of consistency with the ER, PR, and HER2 statuses (**Figure 4**) as compared to metachronous bilateral breast cancer, but without any difference regarding the histologic type or grade [70]. A high-grade malignancy and multifocal contralateral breast disease are inversely proportional [46], which is why patients with BSBC often develop slow-growing and low-grade carcinomas [71].

Greater size of the tumour masses and a larger number of the lymph nodes affected are also linked with multifocal carcinoma, both in unilateral and bilateral

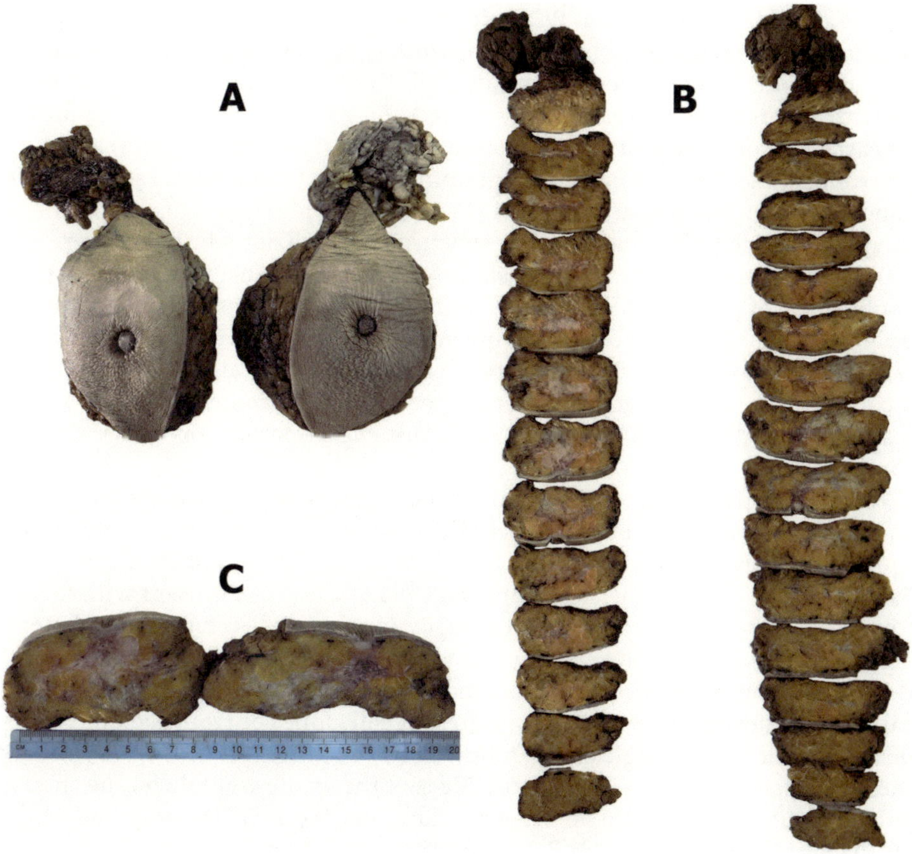

Figure 3.
Macroscopic appearance of BSBC from the 36 years old patient in stage IIIA and IIB: (A) mastectomies of both breasts with associated axillary adipose tissue; (B) macroscopic examination of the tumour infiltration zone by transverse serial sections; (C) foci of the largest tumour infiltration zones and their distance from the resection margins. (image was taken from author's own lab).

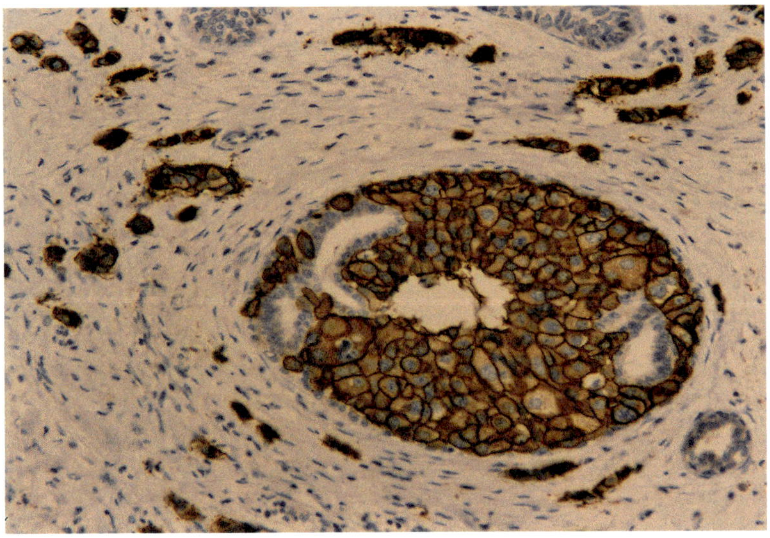

Figure 4.
Microscopic appearance of BSBC from the 36 years old patient in stage IIIA and IIB. Strong membranous expression of HER2 in invasive and "in situ" component of classical subtype of ILC (LSAB x 200). (image was taken from author's own lab).

breast cancers [46]. In unilateral BC patients with a multifocal disease, 40% present with tumour foci that have different histopathology [5, 13, 72]. Studies analysing clonal origin of the tumour focus in multifocal BC show that at least 50 to 70% of cases with different foci are genetically related [73–75], arguing that most multifocal breast carcinomas in patients with unilateral BC originated from the same precursor cell, therefore being an intramammary spread of metastases or an *in-situ* carcinoma with numerous invasive foci [14, 73].

Some studies revealed that multiple synchronous ipsilateral breast cancer (MSIBC) correlates with the known risk factors, suggesting aggressive biology, such as younger age of patients, higher grade, hormone receptor status, HER2 status, lymphovascular invasion and node involvement [76, 77]. Other factors can also play a part, such as the loss of E-cadherins, causing a loss of cell-to-cell adhesion and contributing to metastatic potential. A recent study demonstrated that MSIBC had a significant downregulation of E-cadherine expression as opposed to unifocal lesions [78].

While desmoplastic stromal response is not associated with higher frequency of metastases in axillary lymph nodes [63], there is a positive correlation between the presence of metastases in axillary lymph nodes and the number of tumour foci [77]. In multiple carcinomas, between 3 and 7% of cases can present with different histologic tumour types and/or histologic tumour grades (intratumor heterogeneity) [19, 77]. Using androgen receptor tests, it was discovered that some DCIS and LCIS develop from different cell clones [79]. If we assume that pure DCIS obtains its phenotypic diversity from different cell clones or from accumulated genetic alterations of a single clone, followed by the progression of the dominant clones to invasive carcinomas, it is possible that these represent different phenotypes in multifocal/multicentric BC with a heterogeneous DCIS component [5].

If the multifocal/multicentricBC in question develops as a consequence of lymphovascular invasion, a higher risk of further metastases is probable. Higher frequencies of lymph node involvement and higher relapse rates in MF/MC BC than in other unifocal BCs support the idea that they can occur as a result of lymphovascular invasion, although a high incidence of metastases in lymph nodes in MF/MC breast carcinomas is also associated with larger tumours [80, 81]. When the tumour (T) stage is determined with the diameter of the largest lesion, multifocality and multicentricity can act as independent predictors of axillary lymph node involvement.

6. Heterogeneity of tumour foci

Heterogeneity is a well-known trait of malignancies. It can be observed in individual tumours or among primary BCs and synchronous metastases in lymph nodes. This should be particularly emphasised in the case of MSIBC with different biology and positive lymph nodes in the diagnosis. The status of axillary lymph nodes is the most important individual prognostic factor for BC patients; an accurate histological characterisation of nodal metastases can help clinicians select the most appropriate .treatment [11].

Studies suggest that the tumour foci in MF and MC carcinomas may manifest clonal and behavioural heterogeneity [76], irrespective of the distance between the lesions [7], that ipsilateral foci usually have identical clonality while bilateral breast cancers vary [82], and that 25% of MC carcinomas is polyclonal [83]. The studyof Nortonand co-authors focusing on multifocal ILCs, numerous genetic copies between the foci are consistent to a high degree, suggesting clonal connection between the foci on the one side, while genetic heterogeneity was observed between the foci in patients on the other side [84]. Phenotypic differences are more common in foci (**Figure 5**) that are homogeneous in terms of tumour type and grade [76]. Actually, all tumour foci are considered to have the same phenotype, although genetic or phenotypic alterations may occur during the progression of the tumour [5].

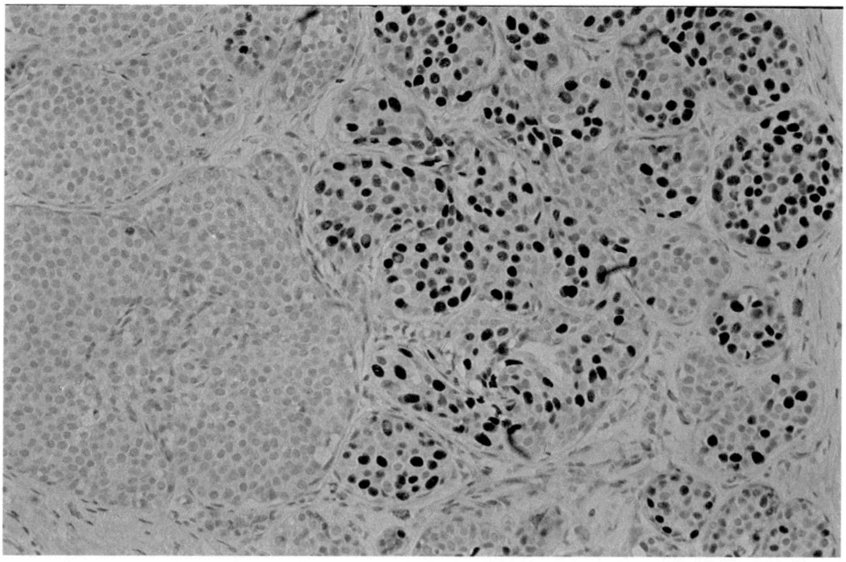

Figure 5.
Phenotypic differences in ER expression (positive nuclear staining on the right side and negative nuclear staining on the left side of tumour focus) may indicate clonal and behavioural heterogeneity of LCIS (LSAB x 200). (image was taken from author's own lab).

7. Molecular and genetic testing

It is not clear whether multifocal/multicentric BCs with different phenotypes are of independent origin due to the fact that phenotypic changes may occur during the tumour progression and dissemination [85]. A few studies, using various molecular methods, showed that bilateral breast cancers are most likely not genetically identical [86, 87]. While the presence of a different phenotype is a clear indicator of separate synchronous primary tumours, over 70% of invasive BCs classified as IDC have identical morphology, meaning that the tumours are clonally related. Using targeted gene sequencing in patients with multiple invasive ductal carcinomas of the same grade and hormone receptor status, it was determined that one third of the cases shows identical mutation profile, one third shares mutations with individual mutations in different foci suggesting identical clonal origin, and one third exhibits no common mutations. Despite common mutations not being present, common changes in copies among the lesions were found, which requires more detailed examinations with methods such as sequencing the entire genome, which would reveal common subclones with a clonal distinction in a larger number of cases [73].

The 21 gene recurrence score assay is a commercially available prognostic and predictive test that measures gene expression levels (16 cancer-related and 5 reference genes) using RT-PCR. The test generates a numeric RS on a scale of 0 to 100 to predict a ten-year risk of a distant metastasis as well as the benefit of chemotherapy in patients with an early-stage ER positive, HER2 negative breast cancer. This RS divides the patients into three risk categories: low (RS < 18), medium (RS 18 to 30), and high (RS ≥ 31). Adjuvant chemotherapy is added to endocrine therapy in patients with high RS; it is estimated that the benefit is low enough to outweigh the consequences in low RS patients [88]. The importance of genome testing for classification by risk category was recognised in the eighth edition of the AJCC Cancer Staging Manual [89], which integrates RC into BC staging. This study examines the consistency of RS in multiple synchronous ipsilateral BCs of similar histology [90].

Tsuda and Hirohashi [91]. investigated the loss of heterozygosity at 16q chromosome in multiple breast cancers and have decided to define multicentric carcinomas as those which are not related through the DCIS component and are not showing satellite nodules and can appear independently. On the other hand, Teixera et al [82], using cytogenetic analyses, concluded that the dominant origin of multiple BCs is intramammary spread from a single primary tumour, despite the fact that some cases develop as unrelated pathogenetic processes. Recently, Brommesson and co-authors compared genome similarities between synchronous multiple invasive breast cancers by means of a comparative microarray-based genome hybridisation and discovered that 5 out of 10 unilateral tumour pairs showed similar genome profiles, suggesting that some synchronous unilateral multiple tumours may have a common origin, while other develop independently [74].

8. Staging of multifocal/MulticentricTumours

Tumour classification as unifocal, MF, or MC is determined in accordance with the pathology reports. The size of the tumour is obtained from the pathology reports. In patients with MF/MC tumours, T stage is determined using two methods: diameter of the largest tumour focus (T_{max}) and by adding up the largest diameters of all tumour foci that are present in the pathological sample (T_{sum}) [51]. AJCC TNM classification defines tumour size as a measure of the largest individual focus of MSIBC [92]. BSBC should be classified independently to permit separation of cases by histological type. (**Figures 3** and **4**). Some authors support the hypothesis that MSIBCs can be best described as summarised dimensions which reclassify tumours to higher stages [93].

According to the College of American Pathologists' recommendations, when multiple synchronous ipsilateral invasive cancers of the same histology are present, the largest invasive carcinoma is used for classification and receptor evaluation [94]. The largest tumour focus is ranked as index or first-rank tumour, and other foci as second to n-rank of additional foci by descending diameter size. The number of lymph nodes affected with macrometastases (larger than 2 mm) or micrometastases (with a diameter between 2 and 0.2 mm) is also reported, as well as the total number of lymph nodes analysed [8]. When the T stage is determined based on the diameter of the largest lesion, multifocality and multicentricity are an independent predictor of axillary lymph node involvement. However, redetermining the T stage based on the sum of diameters of all foci compensates for their difference, leaving the proportion of lymph node metastases between the MC/MF and UF tumours equal [93]. These findings suggest that the increase in the lymph node involvement (or any other relation with unfavourable outcomes) is not a consequence of the common nature of the MC and MF tumours, but rather the result of underestimating the spread of the disease using current staging systems [95].

Some investigationssuggest that the sum of the largest diameters is actually greater than the overall size of the tumour mass and that a better criterion for assessing the tendency of metastasis formation is the total volume and surface area of the tumour [81]. After reclassifying the tumours according to this model, MF/MC tumours still show increased level of lymph node involvement, suggesting that the difference is not the result of the lower stage, but rather the basically more aggressive tumour biology [95].

9. Therapeutic modalities and prognosis

Breast-conserving therapy is now an established alternative to radical mastectomy. When it comes to tumours with more than one lesion, suggested treatments are changing at the moment. Many authors continue to support breast-conserving surgery for MC/MF tumours [96]. Furthermore, when breast-conserving surgery is proposed as a treatment option for patients who carry BRCA2 mutations and have ER positive receptor status, the surgeons should bear in mind the increased incidence of multifocality and plan the surgical procedure accordingly, ensure that the complete excision is performed in one procedure, as well as minimise the consequences related to repeated surgery due to marginal involvement [50]. Oncoplastic surgery enables a more precise resection of the tumour mass and free resection margin as compared to standard quadrantectomy or lumpectomy [97].

Considering that the effect of partial breast radiation therapy is limited to the index quadrant, it is of paramount importance that patients with low risk of occult microscopic disease in the remaining breast tissue are selected, meaning that local control is not less important than whole-breast radiation [11]. It has been proven that whole-breast radiation after a breast-conserving surgery is more efficient against microscopic foci of BC, which is demonstrated by the fact that leaving it out increases local recurrence rate to 39.2% [98]. Patients under 45 who have BC and were treated with post-lumpectomy tangential field radiotherapy are at higher risk of developing contralateral breast cancer, in particular women with family history of BC [52, 99]. Adjuvant chemotherapy is also associated with reduced incidence (up to 20%) of contralateral breast cancer in women under 50, but not in female patients of and above this age [100]. Moreover, chemotherapy is also related with a lower risk of contralateral breast cancer for a period of up to 10 years after the initial BC diagnosis [101].

It was reported that adjuvant systemic hormone ER positive therapy reduces the incidence of contralateral breast cancer by 39 to 55%, depending on the menopausal status [100], which is why detecting limit values for the ER receptor positivity is important [102]. The analysis of the study results revealed that adjuvant chemotherapy is not effective in patients with RS < 25 and above fifty years of age. However, women under 50 with BC who have RS in the medium range between 16 and 25 can still derive some benefit from chemotherapy [103].

Certain data supports the claim that multifocality/multicentricity is not an independent prognostic factor for BC. Although it is suggested that MF/MC can predict the outcome, it is a fact that the size of the tumour bears greater significance in these patients, rather than the presence of multifocality/multicentricity itself [50]. There is controversy in the literature relating to MF/MC prognosis. The rate of locoregional recurrence has increased in some studies [104], while others found no differences [95]. A 2.75 times higher risk of cancer-related death was reported in patients with MF breast cancer, irrespective of the molecular subtype [19]. In an extensive retrospective study, Weissenbacher et al. reported a lower median global survival (OS) in MF/MC patients as compared to unifocal tumours [104]. One earlier study showed that MC disease is related to higher local recurrence rates, but not MF disease (37 and 17% respectively) [105].

Histologic grade is a well-known prognostic factor for BC, with numerous studies demonstrating a strong connection with survival rates [31, 106]. The size of the tumour has been identified long ago as an independent indicator of lower global survival [107]. Two studies monitored the relation between different methods for T staging and survival. It was discovered that MF and MC tumours larger than 2 cm are accompanied by lower global survival when compared with unifocal carcinoma, but this difference vanishes if the sum of the tumour diameters is used in staging [93]. In patients with MF/MC disease, calculating the sum of diameters of multiple foci does not add any prognostic information apart from the conventionally determined T stage on the basis of the largest diameter of the largest focus [108]. A more intensive systemic chemotherapy could potentially mask an accurate prognosis which is determined by measuring the size of the tumour. The prognosis for patients with MF/MC tumours is similar to that for patients with unifocal tumours. In higher stages, the presence of lymph node positivity and distant metastases provides more significant prognostic information, while the T-stage effect on the prognosis is of little importance [51]. Most studies found increased frequency of metastases in multiple carcinomas when compared to unifocal carcinomas [77, 104], explaining the unfavourable outcome in MSIBC patients [109].

It is difficult to assess the prognosis of bilateral breast cancer, because the outcome may not be unevenly ascribed to either the first or the second carcinoma. The survival of BSBC patients seems to depend on tumours with poorer histological characteristics [110]. Women over the age of 50 with synchronous bilateral carcinoma or women who develop contralateral breast cancer within 5 years are at two- and four-times higher risk, respectively, of dying from cancer than women with unilateral carcinoma. The prognosis for women with bilateral breast cancer that was diagnosed after 10 years from the initial carcinoma is similar to that for women with unilateral BC [22]. There is no significant difference in survival for patients with bilateral BC compared to patients with unilateral tumours. However, synchronous tumours are accompanied by lower survival compared to metachronous tumours [111]. Conversely, global survival is not different in patients with bilateral BC and those with unilateral BC [112, 113].

There is a significantly higher risk of distant metastases being present in bilateral BCs [114]. Bilateral BC is associated with lower grade of the disease, patients show an absence of distant metastases prior to developing contralateral breast cancer; more importantly, no difference in the disease-specific survival (DSS) was noticed among patients with bilateral BC and unilateral BC. Bilateral BC is associated with shorter relapse-free survival (RFS), but similar DSS when compared to unilateral BC. Furthermore, BSBC is associated with favourable RFS, but has similar DSS when compared to BMBC with respect to other clinicopathologic parameters in patients with bilateral BC [70].

10. Limitations and future guidelines

The incidence of MF/MC breast cancer varies between 6 and 7%, depending on somewhat arbitrary definition of the MF/MC imaging method sensitivity and biopsy performed by the pathologist. The TNM stage does not include multifocality in the tumour classification [51]. As further progress is made in the pre-operative diagnostics, the number of identified MF and MC tumour is increasing [115]. and consequently better manuals are required for treating them [95], as well as standardised immunohistochemical procedures which would reduce the subjectivity and intralaboratory variations in the interpretation [102].

The National Comprehensive Cancer Network and American Society of Clinical Oncology recommended the use of RS as a manual for adjuvant systemic therapy in patients with ER positive, HER2 negative, lymph node-negative invasive BCs that are ≥0,5 cm in size [116, 117]. In some studies, the entity of focality was determined using histological parameters, while others use clinical and radiographic data only. Most authors do not differentiate between MF and MC tumours, and some almost universally analyse these groups together [95]. Not all patients underwent the same pre-operative radiologic assessment or surgical treatment, which may lead to inaccurate classification of the patients as having unifocal carcinomas when they actually had an unidentified MF or MC condition [76]. Oncological decisions in the systemic adjuvant therapy for BC are based on the histological criterion and immunohistochemical profile of the largest tumour focus, ignoring the smaller synchronous cancers [118, 119].

Histological characteristics of the metastases (type and grade) of axillary lymph nodes in multiple breast cancers correlate with the histological type with an unfavourable prognosis and/or highest histological grade, which may not necessarily correspond to the tumour focus of the largest diameter. For this reason, we accentuate the need to individually report on and assess every single tumour focus in multiple BCs [8]. A new classification may be required for bilateral BCs that would include the size of the tumour in both breasts [120]. TNM staging does not take the tumour biology (hormone receptor status, grade, Ki-67, genetic markers) into account. Additional studies are required about the advantage of using biomarkers to improve the accuracy of staging [51]. Despite the diameter of the largest focus being smaller than the volume of the entire tumour, the sum of diameters of all foci will be bigger than the actual tumour volume, since volume is proportional to one third of the diameter. However, using tumour diameter to assess the size is convenient in the sense of being easier to measure [81]. The use of T_{sum} in clinical practice may improve the current staging process and change the approach, in particular for patients with early stage of the disease [51].

There are certain limitations of the retrospective view of MF/MC breast cancer and information on macroscopic appearance which is no longer available. The status of ER/PR/HER2 is also not available for individual tumour foci, since in most cases it is not evaluated for all tumour foci, meaning that the morphological nature of the MF/MC condition in these patientscannot be reviewed. Tumour characteristics of the second largest lesion are usually not tested, since most medical centres do not routinely perform immunohistochemical staining of each focus. However, certain findings indicate that the biology of the second tumour may affect the prognosis [121], which is why it is recommended to assess tumour markers in each multiple focus [9]. For instance, if the second lesion was hormone-positive or HER2-positive and the main lesion was triple-negative, the chance to administer endocrine therapy or molecular targeted therapy may be missed. That being said, there is considerable controversy surrounding the assessment of Ki-67 in the literature and, despite the efforts to standardise it, a certain degree of subjectivity still remains. Likewise, its limit value is not generally accepted [8].

Future studies observing molecular profiles of separate tumour foci in the same breast could shed light on this matter and provide clinically relevant information for therapy manual-based decisions. Another limitation is the median monitoring of under 5 years [95] and the bias of multicentric studies [120]. Failure to factor in the heterogeneity of the focus of an additional tumour could prevent the patients from taking advantage of appropriate therapies [31, 89, 122]. Most studies are retrospective or incidental in nature, which neither compare breast-conserving surgery with mastectomy nor analyse locoregional recurrence as a primary goal in MSIBC [123].

Conflict of interest

The author declares no conflict of interest.

Author details

Ivan Ilić
Department of Pathology, Faculty of Medicine, University of Niš, Niš, Serbia

*Address all correspondence to: ilicko81@gmail.com

References

[1] Siegel RL, Miller KD, Jemal A. Cancer statistics, 2019. CA Cancer J Clin. 2019; 69: 7-34.DOI:10.3322/caac.21551

[2] Soerjomataram I, Louwman WJ, de Vries E. Primary malignancy after primary female breast cancer in the south of the Netherlands, 1972-2001. Breast Cancer Res Treat. 2005; 93: 91-5. DOI:10.1007/s10549-005-4016-2

[3] Cheatle G. Benign and malignant changes in duct epithelium of the breast. Br J Cancer. 1920; 8(31): 285-306. DOI:10.1002/bjs.1800083109

[4] Qualheim RE, Gall EA. Breast carcinoma with multiple sites of origin. Cancer. 1957; 10(3): 460-8. DOI:10.1002/1097-0142(195705/06)10:3

[5] Choi Y, Kim JE, Seol H. The hormone receptor, human epidermal growth factor receptor 2, and molecular subtype status of individual tumor foci in multifocal/multicentric invasive ductal carcinoma of breast. Hum Pathol. 2012;43(1):48-55.DOI: 10.1016/j.humpath.2010.08.026

[6] Middleton LP, Vlastos G, Mirza NQ. Multicentric mammary carcinoma: evidence of monoclonal proliferation. Cancer. 2002;94:1910-6.DOI: 10.1002/cncr.10452

[7] Dawson PJ, Baekey PA, Clark RA. Mechanisms of multifocal breast cancer: an immunocytochemical study. Hum Pathol. 1995;26:965-9.DOI: 10.1016/0046-8177(95)90085-3

[8] Boros M, Ilyes A, Boila NA. Morphologic and molecular subtype status of individual tumor foci in multiple breast carcinoma. A study of 155 cases with analysis of 463 tumor foci. Hum Pathol. 2014;45(2):409-16. DOI: 10.1016/j.humpath.2013.10.006

[9] Pekmezci M, Szpaderska A, Osipo C. Evaluation of biomarkers in multifocal/multicentric invasive breast carcinomas. Int J SurgPathol. 2013;21:126-32.DOI: 10.1177/1066896912467370

[10] Linshaw D, Tonneson J, Rosenkranz K. Surgical therapy for women with multiple synchronous ipsilateral breast cancer (MIBC): current evidence to guide clinical practice. Curr. Breast Cancer Rep. 2019;11(2): 67-73. DOI: 10.1007/s12609-019-0309-z

[11] Corso G, Magnoni F, Provenzano E. Multicentric breast cancer with heterogeneous histopathology: a multidisciplinary review. Future Oncol. 2020;16(8):395-412.DOI: 10.2217/fon-2019-0540

[12] Khan A: The many questions that surround multicentric and multifocal breast cancer. Breast J. 2010;16:219-221. DOI: 10.1111/j.1524-4741.2010.00929.x

[13] Buggi F, Folli S, Curcio A. Multicentric/multifocal breast cancer with a single histotype: is the biological characterization of all individual foci justified? Ann Oncol. 2012;23(8):2042-6.DOI: 10.1093/annonc/mdr570

[14] Salgado R, Aftimos P, Sotiriou C. Evolving paradigms in multifocal breast cancer. Semin Cancer Biol. 2015;31:111-8.DOI: 10.1016/j.semcancer.2014.07.002

[15] Rosen's Breast Pathology. 2nd edition. Philadelphia: Lippincott Williams & Wilkins; 2001.

[16] Ilić I, Petrović A, Živković V. Immunohistochemical features of multifocal and multicentric lobular breast carcinoma. Adv Med Sci. 2017;62(1):78-82.DOI: 10.1016/j.advms.2016.07.003

[17] Sardanelli F, Giuseppetti GM, Panizza P. Sensitivity of MRI versus

mammography for detecting foci of multifocal, multicentric breast cancer in fatty and dense breasts using the whole-breast pathologic examination as a gold standard. Am J Roentgenol. 2004;183:1149-1157.DOI: 10.2214/ajr.183.4.1831149

[18] Bozzini A, Renne G, Meneghetti L. Sensitivity of imaging for multifocal-multicentric breast carcinoma. BMC Cancer. 2008;8:275.DOI: 10.1186/1471-2407-8-275

[19] Pekar G, Gere M, Tarjan M. Molecular phenotype of the foci in multifocal invasive breast carcinomas: intertumoral heterogeneity is related to shorter survival and may influence the choice of therapy. Cancer. 2014;120(1): 26-34.DOI: 10.1002/cncr.28375

[20] Kilgore AR: The incidence of cancer in the second breast. JAMA. 1921;77:454-457.DOI:10.1001/jama.1921.02630320038011

[21] Haagensen CD. Diseases of the Breast. 2nd edition. Philadelphia: Saunders; 1971.DOI: 10.1002/bjs.1800590240

[22] Hartman M, Czene K, Reilly M. Genetic implications of bilateral breast cancer: a population based cohort study. Lancet Oncol.2005;6(6):377-382. DOI: 10.1016/s1470-2045(05)70174-1

[23] Pan B, Xu Y, Zhou YD. The prognostic comparison among unilateral, bilateral, synchronous bilateral, and metachronous bilateral breast cancer: a meta-analysis of studies from recent decade (2008-2018). Cancer Med. 2019;8:2908-18.DOI: 10.1002/cam4.2198

[24] Chaudary MA, Millis RR, Hoskins EO. Bilateral primary breast cancer: a prospective study of disease incidence. Br J Surg.1984;71:711-714. DOI: 10.1002/bjs.1800710924

[25] Green I, McCormick B, Cranor M. A comparative study of pure tubular and tubulolobular carcinoma of the breast. Am J Surg Pathol. 1997;21:653-657.DOI: 10.1097/00000478-199706000-00004

[26] Mitnick JS, Gianutsos R, Pollack AH. Tubular carcinoma of the breast: sensitivity of diagnostic techniques and correlation with histopathology. AJR Am J Roentgenol. 1999;172:319-323.DOI: 10.2214/ajr.172.2.9930775

[27] Marzullo F, Zito FA, Marzullo A. Infiltrating cribriform carcinoma of the breast. A clinico-pathologic and immunohistochemical study of 5 cases. Eur J Gynaecol Oncol. 1996;17:228-231. PMID: 8780923

[28] Page DL, Dixon JM, Anderson TJ. Invasive cribriform carcinoma of the breast. Histopathology.1983;7:525-536. DOI:10.1111/j.1365-2559.1983.tb02265.x

[29] Yang M, Moriya T, Oguma M. Microinvasive ductal carcinoma (T1mic) of the breast. The clinicopathological profile and immunohistochemical features of 28 cases. Pathol Int. 2003;53:422-428.DOI: 10.1046/j.1440-1827.2003.01498.x

[30] Ward BA, McKhann CF, Ravikumar TS. Ten-year follow-up of breast carcinoma in situ in Connecticut. Arch Surg. 1992;127:1392-1395. DOI:10.1001/archsurg.1992.01420120026004

[31] Lakhani S, Ellis IO, Schnitt SJ, Tan PH, et al. WHO Classification of Tumours of the Breast. 4th ed. IARC Press: Lyon; 2012. 10-71.

[32] Ilić I, Randjelović P, Ilić R. An approach to malignant mammary phyllodes tumors detection. Vojnosanit Pregl. 2009;66(4):277-282.DOI: 10.2298/vsp0904277i

[33] Hamele-Bena D, Cranor ML, Sciotto C. Uncommon presentation of mammary myofibroblastoma. Mod Pathol.1996;9:786-790.PMID: 8832563

[34] Tan PH, Jayabaskar T, Chuah KL. Phyllodestumors of the breast: the role of pathologic parameters. Am J Clin Pathol. 2005;123:529-540.DOI: 10.1309/u6dv-bfm8-1mlj-c1fn

[35] Rosen PP, Ernsberger D. Mammary fibromatosis. A benign spindle-cell tumor with significant risk for local recurrence. Cancer.1989;63:1363-1369. DOI: 10.1002/1097-0142(19890401)63:7

[36] Borgen PI, Wong GY, Vlamis V. Current management of male breast cancer. A review of 104 cases. Ann Surg.1992;215:451-457.DOI: 10.1097/00000658-199205000-00007

[37] Billings SD, McKenney JK, Folpe AL. Cutaneous angiosarcoma following breast-conserving surgery and radiation: an analysis of 27 cases. Am J SurgPathol.2004;28:781-788.DOI: 10.1097/01.pas.0000126055.33916.0b

[38] Brenn T, Fletcher CD. Radiationassociated cutaneous atypical vascular lesions and angiosarcoma: clinicopathologic analysis of 42 cases. Am J SurgPathol.2005;29:983-996. PMID: 16006792

[39] Prasad SN, Houserkova D, Svach I. Pseudoangiomatous stromal hyperplasia of breast: a case report. Biomed Pap Med FacUnivPalacky Olomouc Czech Repub.2008;152:117-120. DOI: 10.5507/bp.2008.018

[40] Carney JA, Stratakis CA. Ductal adenoma of the breast and the Carney complex. Am J SurgPathol.1996;20:1154-1155. DOI: 10.1097/00000478-199609000-00014

[41] Martinelli G, Ryan G, Seymour JF. Primary follicular and marginal-zone lymphoma of the breast: clinical features, prognostic factors and outcome: a study by the International Extranodal Lymphoma Study Group. Ann Oncol.2009;20:1993-1999. DOI: 10.1093/annonc/mdp238

[42] Ilić I, Randjelović P, Ilić R. Granular-cell tumor: a rare variant of mammary tumor. Vojnosanit Pregl. 2008;65(6):488-91.DOI: 10.2298/vsp0806488I

[43] Ryan G, Martinelli G, Kuper-Hommel M. Primary diffuse large B-cell lymphoma of the breast: prognostic factors and outcomes of a study by the International ExtranodalLymphoma Study Group. Ann Oncol. 2008;19:233-241.DOI:10.1093/annonc/mdm471

[44] Kell RM, Morrow M. Multifocal, multicentric and bilateral breast cancer. In: Winchester JD, Hudis AC, Norton L (Eds). Breast cancer. 2nd edition. PMPH-USA, 2006.

[45] Chen Y, Thompson W, Semenciw R. Epidemiology of contralateral breast cancer. Cancer Epidemiol Biomarkers Prev.1999;8(10):855-861PMID:10548312

[46] Mejdahl KM, Wohlfahrt J, Holm M. Synchronous bilateral breast cancer: a nationwide study on histopathology and etiology. Breast Cancer Res Treat. 2020;182(1):229-238.r4. DOI:10.1007/s10549-020-05689-0

[47] Ilic I, Djordjevic N, RandjelovicP. Seven-year survey of classical and pleomorphic invasive lobular breast carcinomas in women from southeastern Serbia: Differences in clinicopathological and immunohistochemical features. J BUON. 2016; 21(5):1113-1120.PMID: 27837612

[48] Pestalozzi BC, Zahrieh D, Mallon E. Distinct clinical and prognostic features of infiltrating lobular carcinoma of

the breast: combined results of 15 International Breast Cancer Study Group clinical trials. J Clin Oncol. 2008;26:3006-3014.DOI: 10.1200/JCO.2007.14.9336

[49] Silverstein MJ, Lewinsky BS, Waisman JR. Infiltrating lobular carcinoma. Is it different from infiltrating duct carcinoma? Cancer.1994;73:1673-1677.DOI: 10.1002/1097-0142(19940315)73:6

[50] McCrorie DA, Ashfield S, Begley A. Multifocal breast cancers are more prevalent in BRCA2 versus BRCA1 mutation carriers. J Pathol Clin Res. 2020;6(2):146-153.DOI: 10.1002/cjp2.155

[51] Karakas Y, Dizdar O, Aksoy S. The Effect of Total Size of Lesions in Multifocal/Multicentric Breast Cancer on Survival. Clin Breast Cancer.2018;18(4):320-327.DOI: 10.1016/j.clbc.2017.11.002

[52] Hooning MJ, Aleman BM, Hauptmann M. Roles of radiotherapy and chemotherapy in the development of contralateral breast cancer. J ClinOncol.2008;26:5561-5568.DOI: 10.1200/jco.2007.16.0192

[53] Berg WA, Gilbreath PL. Multicentric and multifocal cancer: Whole-breastUS in preoperative evaluation. Radiology. 2000;214:59-66.DOI:10.1148/radiology.214.1.r00ja2559

[54] Wang L, Di LJ. BRCA1 and estrogen/estrogen receptor in breast cancer: where they interact? Int J BiolSci. 2014;10:566-575.DOI: 10.7150/ijbs.8579

[55] Vera-Badillo FE, Napoleone M, Ocana A. Effect of multifocality and multicentricity on outcome in early stage breast cancer: a systematic review and meta-analysis. Breast Cancer Res Treat. 2014;146:235-244.DOI:10.1007/s10549-014-3018-3

[56] Kurian AW, McClure LA, John EM. Second primary breast cancer occurrence according to hormone receptor status. J Natl Cancer Inst. 2009;101:1058-65.DOI: 10.1093/jnci/djp181

[57] Dixon JM, Anderson TJ, Page DL. Infiltrating lobular carcinoma of the breast: an evaluation of the incidence and consequence of bilateral disease. Br J Surg. 1983;70:513-6.DOI: 10.1002/bjs.1800700902

[58] Malone KE, Begg CB, Haile RW. Population-based study of the risk of second primary contralateral breast cancer associated with carrying a mutation in BRCA1 or BRCA2. J Clin Oncol. 2010;28:2404-2410.DOI:10.1200/jco.2009.24.2495

[59] Concannon P, Haile RW, Borresen-Dale AL. Variants in the ATM gene associated with a reduced risk of contralateral breast cancer. Cancer Res.2008;68:6486-6491. DOI:10.1158/0008-5472.can-08-0134

[60] Senkus E, Kyriakides S, Penault-Llorca F. Primary breast cancer: ESMO Clinical Practice Guidelines for diagnosis, treatment and follow-up. Ann Oncol. 2013;24(Suppl. 6):7-23.DOI: 10.1093/annonc/mdv298

[61] Lopez JK, Bassett LW. Invasive lobular carcinoma of the breast: spectrum of mammographic, US, and MR imaging findings. Radiographics. 2009;29(1):165-176.DOI: 10.1148/rg.291085100

[62] Brem RF, Ioffe M, Rapelyea JA. Invasive lobular carcinoma: detection with mammography, sonography, MRI, and breast-specific gamma imaging. Am. J. Roentgenol. 2009;192(2):379-383. DOI: 10.2214/AJR.07.3827

[63] Ilić I, Stojanović N, Randjelović P. Evaluation of pathological parameters and morphometric data of desmoplastic

lobular breast carcinoma. Indian J Pathol Microbiol. 2016;59(4):463-8. DOI: 10.4103/0377-4929.191775

[64] Johnson K, Sarma D, Hwang ES. Lobular breast cancer series: imaging. Breast Cancer Res. 2015;17(1): 94.DOI: 10.1186/s13058-015-0605-0

[65] Dietzel M, Baltzer PA, Vag T. Magnetic resonance mammography of invasive lobular versus ductal carcinoma: systematic comparison of 811 patients reveals high diagnostic accuracy irrespective of typing. J Comput Assist Tomogr. 2010;34:587-595.DOI: 10.1097/rct.0b013e3181db9f0e

[66] Schelfout K, Van Goethem M, Kersschot E. Preoperative breast MRI in patients with invasive lobular breast cancer. EurRadiol. 2004;14:1209-1216. DOI:10.1007/s00330-004-2275-7

[67] Lebris A, Vildé A, Marret H. Role of imaging procedures in the diagnosis of synchronous bilateral breast cancer. GynecolObstetFertil. 2014;42:14-19. DOI: 10.1016/j.gyobfe.2013.08.004

[68] Petrovic A, Abramovic M, Mihailovic D. Multicolor counterstaining for immunohistochemistry - a modified Movat'spentachrome. Biotech Histochem. 2011;86(6):429-435.DOI: 10.3109/10520295.2010.528026

[69] Tot T. The role of large-format histopathology in assessing subgross morphological prognostic parameters: a single institution report of 1000 consecutive breast cancer cases. Int J Breast Cancer. 2012;2012:395-415. DOI:10.1155/2012/395415

[70] Mruthyunjayappa S, Zhang K, Zhang L. Synchronous and metachronous bilateral breast cancer: clinicopathologic characteristics and prognostic outcomes. Human Pathology. 2019;92:1-9.DOI: 10.1016/j.humpath.2019.07.008

[71] Wu YY, Yen MF, Yu CP. Risk assessment of multistate progression of breast tumor with state-dependent genetic and environmental covariates. Risk Anal. 2014;34(2):367-379. DOI: 10.1111/risa.12116

[72] East EG, Pang JC, Kidwell KM. Utility of estrogen receptor, progesterone receptor, and HER-2/neu analysis of multiple foci in multifocal ipsilateral invasive breast carcinoma. Am J ClinPathol. 2015;144(6):952-959. DOI: 10.1309/ajcpfwxp54olilmu

[73] Desmedt C, Fumagalli D, Pietri E. Uncovering the genomic heterogeneity of multifocal breast cancer. J Pathol. 2015;236(4):457-466. DOI: 10.1002/path.4540

[74] Brommesson S, Jonsson G, Strand C. Tiling array-CGH for the assessment of genomic similarities among synchronous unilateral and bilateral invasive breast cancer tumor pairs. BMC ClinPathol. 2008;8:6. DOI: 10.1186/1472-6890-8-6

[75] Kim H, Kim CY, Park KH. Clonality analysis of multifocal ipsilateral breast carcinomas using X-chromosome inactivation patterns. Hum Pathol. 2018;78:106-114. DOI: 10.1016/j.humpath.2018.04.016

[76] Kanumuri P, Hayse B, Killelea BK. Characteristics of multifocal and multicentric breast cancers. Ann. Surg. Oncol. 2015;22(8):2475-2482. DOI:10.1245/s10434-015-4430-6

[77] Cabioglu N, Ozmen V, Kaya H. Increased Lymph Node Positivity in Multifocal and Multicentric Breast Cancer. J Am CollSurg. 2009;208:67-74. DOI: 10.1016/j.jamcollsurg.2008.09.001

[78] Weissenbacher T, Hirte E, Kuhn C. Multicentric and multifocal versus unifocal breast cancer: differences in the expression of E-cadherin suggest differences in tumor biology.

BMC Cancer. 2013;13(1):361.DOI: 10.1186/1471-2407-13-361

[79] Volante M, Sapino A, Croce S. Heterogeneous versus homogeneous genetic nature of multiple foci of in situ carcinoma of the breast. HumPathol. 2003;34:1163-9.DOI: 10.1053/j.humpath.2003.07.011

[80] Yerushalmi R, Kennecke H, Woods R. Does multicentric/multifocal breast cancer differ from unifocal breast cancer? An analysis of survival and contralateral breast cancer incidence. Breast Cancer Res Treat. 2009;117:365-70.DOI: 10.1007/s10549-008-0265-1

[81] Andea AA, Bouwman D, Wallis T. Correlation of tumor volume and surface area with lymph node status in patients with multifocal/multicentric breast carcinoma. Cancer. 2004;100: 20-7.DOI: 10.1002/cncr.11880

[82] Teixeira MR, Ribeiro FR, Torres L. Assessment of clonal relationships in ipsilateral and bilateral multiple breast carcinomas by comparative genomic hybridisation and hierarchical clustering analysis. Br J Cancer. 2004;91(4):775-82.DOI: 10.1038/sj.bjc.6602021

[83] Eeles R, Knee G, Jhavar S. Multicentric breast cancer: clonality and prognostic studies. Breast Cancer Res Treat. 2011;129(3):703-16.DOI: 10.1007/s10549-010-1230-3

[84] Norton N, Advani PP, Serie DJ. Assessment of tumor heterogeneity, as evidenced by gene expression profles, pathway activation, and gene copy number, in patients with multifocal invasive lobular breast tumors. PLoS One. 2016;11(4):e0153411. DOI:10.1371/journal.pone.01534 11

[85] De la Haba-Rodríguez JR, Ruiz Borrego M, Gómez España A. Comparative study of the immunohistochemical phenotype in breast cancer and its lymph node metastatic location. Cancer Invest. 2004;22:219-24.DOI: 10.1081/cnv-120030210

[86] Imyanitov EN, Suspitsin EN, Grigoriev MY. Concordance of allelic imbalance profiles in synchronous and metachronous bilateral breast carcinomas. Int J Cancer. 2002;100:557-564.DOI: 10.1002/ijc.10530

[87] Regitnig P, Ploner F, Maderbacher M. Bilateral carcinomas of the breast with local recurrence: analysis of genetic relationship of the tumors. Mod Pathol. 2004;17:597-602.DOI: 10.1038/modpathol.3800089

[88] Paik S, Shak S, Tang G. A multigene assay to predict recurrence of tamoxifen-treated, node-negative breast cancer. N Engl J Med. 2004;351(27):2817-26.DOI: 10.1056/nejmoa041588

[89] Giuliano AE, Connolly JL, Edge SB. Breast cancer–Major changes in the American Joint Committee on Cancer eighth edition cancer staging manual. CA Cancer J Clin. 2017;67(4):290-303. DOI: 10.3322/caac.21393

[90] Grabenstetter A, Brogi E, Chou FJ. Multifocal/MulticentricIpsilateral Invasive Breast Carcinomas with Similar Histology: Is Multigene Testing of All Individual Foci Necessary?. Ann Surg Oncol. 2019;26(2):329-335.DOI: 10.1245/s10434-018-6866-y

[91] Tsuda H, Hirohashi S. Identification of multiple breast cancers of multicentric origin by histological observations and distribution of allele loss on chromosome 16q. Cancer Res 1995;55:3395-8.PMID: 7614478

[92] Hortobagyi GN, Connolly JL, D'Orsi CJ. AJCC Cancer Staging Manual. 8th ed. NY: USA; 2017.DOI: 10.3322/caac.21393

[93] Boyages J, Jayasinghe UW, Coombs N. Multifocal breast cancer and survival: each focus does matter particularly for larger tumours. Eur J Cancer. 2010;46:1990-1996.DOI: 10.1016/j.ejca.2010.03.003

[94] Lester SC, Bose S, Chen YY. Protocol for the examination of specimens from patients with invasive carcinoma of the breast. Arch Pathol Lab Med. 2009;133(10):1515-38.DOI: 10.1043/1543-2165-133.10.1515

[95] Lynch SP, Lei X, Hsu L. Breast cancer multifocality and multicentricity and locoregional recurrence. Oncologist. 2013;18:1167-73.DOI: 10.1634/theoncologist.2013-0167

[96] Gentilini O, Botteri E, Rotmensz N. Conservative surgery in patients with multifocal/ multicentric breast cancer. Breast Cancer Res Treat. 2009;113:577-583.DOI: 10.1007/s10549-008-9959-7

[97] Kaur N, Petit JY, Rietjens M. Comparative study of surgical margins in oncoplastic surgery and quadrantectomy in breast cancer. Ann. Surg. Oncol. 2005;12(7):539-545. DOI:10.1245/aso.2005.12.046

[98] Clarke M, Collins R, Darby S. Effects of radiotherapy and of differences in the extent of surgery for early breast cancer on local recurrence and 15-year survival: an overview of the randomised trials. Lancet.2005;366(9503):2087-2106.DOI: 10.1016/S0140-6736(05)67887-7

[99] Stovall M, Smith SA, Langholz BM. Dose to the contralateral breast from radiotherapy and risk of second primary breast cancer in the WECARE study. Int J Radiat Oncol Biol Phys. 2008;72:1021-1030.DOI:10.1016/j.ijrobp.2008.02.040

[100] Early Breast Cancer Trialists' Collaborative G. Effects of chemotherapy and hormonal therapy for early breast cancer on recurrence and 15-year survival: an overview of the randomised trials. Lancet. 2005;365:1687-717.DOI: 10.1016/S0140-6736(05)66544-0

[101] Bertelsen L, Bernstein L, Olsen JH. Effect of systemic adjuvant treatment on risk for contralateral breast cancer in the Women's environment, Cancer and radiation epidemiology study. J Natl Cancer Inst. 2008;100:32-40.DOI: 10.1093/jnci/djm267

[102] Ilić I, Stojanović N, Radulović N. The Quantitative ER Immunohistochemical Analysis in Breast Cancer: Detecting the 3+0, 4+0, and 5+0 Allred Score Cases. MEDICINA-LITHUANIA. 2019;55(8):461-.DOI: 10.3390/medicina55080461

[103] Sparano JA, Gray RJ, Makower DF. Adjuvant chemotherapy guided by a 21-gene expression assay in breast cancer. N Engl J Med. 2018;379(2):111-21.DOI: 10.1056/nejmoa1804710

[104] Weissenbacher TM, Zschage M, Janni W, et al. Multicentric and multifocal versus unifocal breast cancer: is the tumor-node-metastasis classification justified? Breast Cancer Res Treat. 2010;122:27-34.DOI: 10.1007/s10549-010-0917-9

[105] Katz A, Strom EA, Buchholz TA, Theriault R, Singletary SE, McNeese MD. The influence of pathologic tumor characteristics on locoregional recurrence rates following mastectomy. Int J RadiatOncolBiol Phys. 2001;50(3):735-42.DOI: 10.1016/s0360-3016(01)01500-0

[106] Rakha EA, Reis-Filho JS, Baehner F. Breast cancer prognostic classification in the molecular era: the role of histological grade. Breast Cancer Res. 2010;12:207.DOI: 10.1186/bcr2607

[107] Carter CL, Allen C, Henson DE. Relation of tumor size, lymph node

status, and survival in 24,740 breast cancer cases. Cancer. 1989; 63: 181-187. DOI: 10.1002/1097-0142(19890101)63:1

[108] Hilton JF, Bouganim N, Dong B. Do alternative methods of measuring tumor size, including consideration of multicentric/multifocal disease, enhance prognostic information beyond TNM staging in women with early stage breast cancer: an analysis of the NCIC CTG MA.5 and MA.12 clinical trials. Breast Cancer Res Treat. 2013;142:143-51.DOI: 10.1007/s10549-013-2714-8

[109] Pedersen L, Gunnarsdottir K, Rasmussen B. The prognostic influence of multifocality in breast cancer patients. Breast 2004;13(3):188-193. DOI: 10.1016/j.breast.2003.11.004

[110] Irvine T, Allen DS, Gillett C. Prognosis of synchronous bilateral breast cancer. Br J Surg.2009;96:376-380. DOI: 10.1002/bjs.6553

[111] Kheirelseid EAH, Jumustafa H, Miller N. Bilateral breast cancer: analysis of incidence, outcome, survival and disease characteristics. Breast Cancer Res. Treat. 2011;126(1):131-140.DOI: 10.1007/s10549-010-1057-y

[112] Verkooijen HM, Chatelain V, Fioretta G. Survival after bilateral breast cancer: results from a population-based study. Breast Cancer Res Treat. 2007;105:347-57. DOI: 10.1007/s10549-006-9455-x

[113] Takahashi H, Watanabe K, Takahashi M. The impact of bilateral breast cancer on the prognosis of breast cancer: a comparative study with unilateral breast cancer. Breast Cancer. 2005;12:196-202.DOI: 10.2325/jbcs.12.196

[114] Jobsen JJ, van der Palen J, Ong F, Riemersma S, Struikmans H. Bilateral breast cancer, synchronous and metachronous; differences and outcome. Breast Cancer Res Treat. 2015;153:277-83.DOI:10.1007/s10549-015-3538-5

[115] Houssami N, Ciatto S, Macaskill P. Accuracy and surgical impact of magnetic resonance imaging in breast cancer staging: systematic review and meta-analysis in detection of multifocal and multicentric cancer. J Clin Oncol. 2008;26:3248-3258.DOI:10.1200/jco.2007.15.2108

[116] Gradishar WJ, Anderson BO, Balassanian R. NCCN guidelines insights: breast cancer, version 1.2017. J Natl Compr Canc Netw. 2017;15(4):433-51.DOI: 10.6004/jnccn.2017.0044

[117] Harris LN, Ismaila N, McShane LM. Use of biomarkers to guide decisions on adjuvant systemic therapy for women with early-stage invasive breast cancer: American Society of Clinical Oncology Clinical Practice Guideline. J ClinOncol. 2016;34(10):1134-50. DOI: 10.1200/jco.2015.65.2289

[118] Goldhirsch A, Winer EP, Coates AS. Panel members. Personalizing the treatment of women with early breast cancer: highlights of the St Gallen International Expert Consensus on the Primary Therapy of Early Breast Cancer 2013. Ann Oncol. 2013;24:2206-2223. DOI: 10.1093/annonc/mdt303

[119] Carlson RW, Allred DC, Anderson BO. National Comprehensive Cancer Network. Invasive breast cancer: clinical practice guidelines in oncology. JNatlCompr Cancer Netw. 2011;9:136-222.DOI: 10.6004/jnccn.2009.0012

[120] Kadioğlu H, Özbaş S, Akcan A. Comparison of the histopathology and prognosis of bilateral versus unilateral multifocal multicentric breast cancers. World J Surg Oncol. 2014;12:266.DOI: 10.1186/1477-7819-12-266

[121] Fushimi A, Yoshida A, Yagata H. Prognostic impact of multifocal and multicentric breast cancer versus

unifocal breast cancer. Surg Today. 2019;49(3):224-230.DOI: 10.1007/s00595-018-1725-9

[122] Perry N, Broeders M, De Wolf C. European Guidelines for Quality Assurance in Breast Cancer Screening and Diagnosis. 4th ed. Office for Official Publications of the European Communities: Luxemburg; 2006. 219-313.DOI: 10.1093/annonc/mdm481

[123] Winters ZE, Bernaudo L. Evaluating the current evidence to support therapeutic mammoplasty or breast-conserving surgery as an alternative to mastectomy in the treatment of multifocal and multicentric breast cancers. Gland. Surg. 2018;7(6):525-535.DOI: 10.21037/gs.2018.07.01

Section 2

Breast Cancer Biomarkers

Chapter 2

Potential Biomarkers for Therapeutic Monitoring and Clinical Outcome in Breast Cancer

Yuki Yamamoto, Sabrina La Salvia, Sahoo Susmita and Hidetoshi Tahara

Abstract

Non-coding RNAs are a species of RNA that are not translated to proteins. These include transfer RNAs and ribosomal RNAs, microRNAs, transfer RNA-derived fragments, and long non-coding RNA. It is known that expression levels of some non-coding RNAs included microRNAs are altered in cancer cells or tumor tissues. Moreover, expression profiles of such non-coding RNAs correlate between tissues and body fluids. Therefore, several non-coding RNAs are being used as diagnostic/prognosis biomarkers or therapeutic targets in cancer. In this chapter, we review about representative non-coding RNAs and introduce especially microRNA as diagnosis/prognosis biomarkers and therapeutic targets.

Keywords: microRNA, isomiR, exosome, biomarker, therapeutics

1. Introduction

Non-coding RNAs (ncRNAs) are generic terms of RNA that are not translated to protein. For example, ribosomal RNA (rRNA) and transfer RNA (tRNA) are included in ncRNAs. In the body, ncRNA does not encode proteins but has important functions.

MicroRNAs (miRNA), one of the ncRNAs, are small non-coding RNAs with an average length of 22 nucleotides. miRNA is transcribed from genomic DNA, the transcribed miRNA is called "primary microRNA (pri-miRNA)," which is long transcripts having stem-loop structures. Pri-miRNA is processed by Drosha and DGCR8 (DiGeorge syndrome critical region 8), one of the microprocessors, to "precursor miRNA (pre-miRNA)." In the next step, there is pre-miRNA transition from nuclei to the cytoplasm through Exportin-5. Cytoplasmic pre-miRNA is processed by Dicer, one of RNaseIII, to double-strand miRNA. The double-strand miRNA binds to AGO (Argonaute) protein and forms RISC (RNA-induced silencing complex). RISC binds 3′ UTR (3′ untranslated region) of target mRNAs, and downregulate gene expression *via* mRNA cleavage, translational repression, or mRNA degradation (**Figure 1**) [1]. Recently, it is known that miRNA also binds to 5′ UTR (5′ untranslated region) and CDS (coding sequence) of target mRNAs [2, 3]. miRNAs may have over hundreds of target genes, regulating various biological phenomena. In cancer patients, many miRNAs are aberrantly expressed, caused by chromosomal aberration, epigenetic regulation, and genomic mutation [4–6]. Therefore, miRNAs

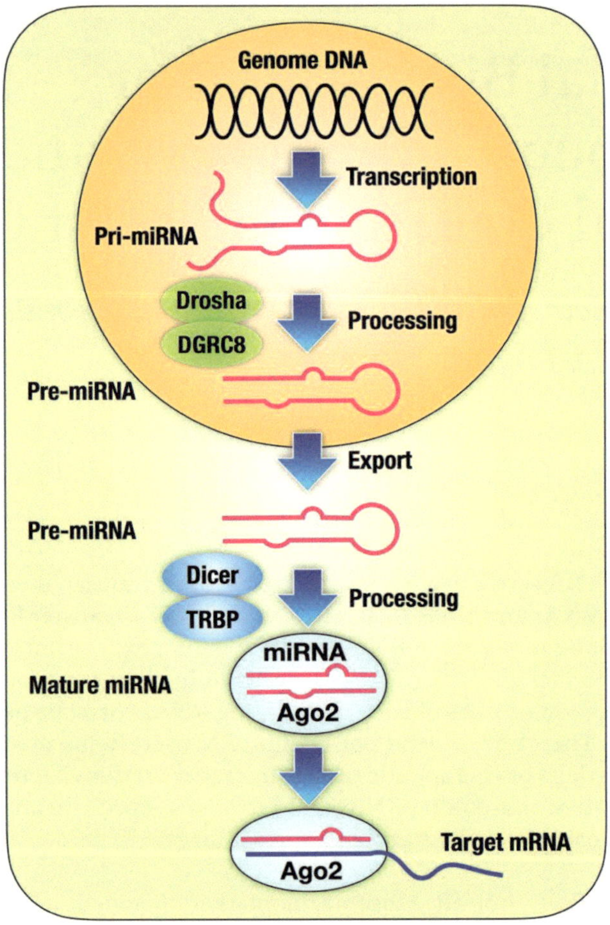

Figure 1.
The overview of miRNA biogenesis. miRNA is transcribed from genomic DNA to primary miRNA (pri-miRNA), which is long transcripts having stem-loop structures. Pri-miRNA is processed by Drosha and DGCR8 (DiGeorge syndrome critical region 8), one of the microprocessors, to precursor miRNA (pre-miRNA). After the transition of pre-miRNA from nuclei to the cytoplasm through Exportin-5, cytoplasmic pre-miRNA is processed by TRBP (transactivation response RNA-binding protein) and dicer, one of RNaseIII, to double-strand miRNA. The double-strand miRNA binds to AGO (Argonaute) protein and forms RISC (RNA-induced silencing complex). RISC binds 3′ UTR (3′ untranslated region) of target mRNAs.

with altered expression under pathological conditions are valuable for biomarkers and targets of therapeutics.

Interestingly, recent studies revealed that miRNA sequences have the variation compared with the reference sequences. As miRNAs are called isomiRs, isomiRs are the miRNA variants that have different sequences and/or lengths [7–10]. These isomiRs are classified as 5′ isomiR, 3′ isomiR, and polymorphic isomiR. isomiRs are generated through the slice site variation by Drosha or Dicer, the nucleotide addition, RNA editing, etc. [11]. Some isomiRs are abnormally expressed in cancer cells caused by chromosomal and/or miRNA processing aberration (**Figure 2**) [12, 13]. Thus, isomiR is also focused on as novel biomarker for cancer detection.

Long non-coding RNA (lncRNA) that is also one of ncRNAs consisting of over 200 nucleotides has multiple functions. LncRNA up- or downregulation has been shown to regulate several biological processes, such as transcription, translation, epigenetic modification, and miRNA expression [14]. It has been shown that lncRNA expressions are altered in various diseases. Therefore, similar to miRNAs, lncRNA has the potential of biomarkers and therapeutics. Moreover, recently it

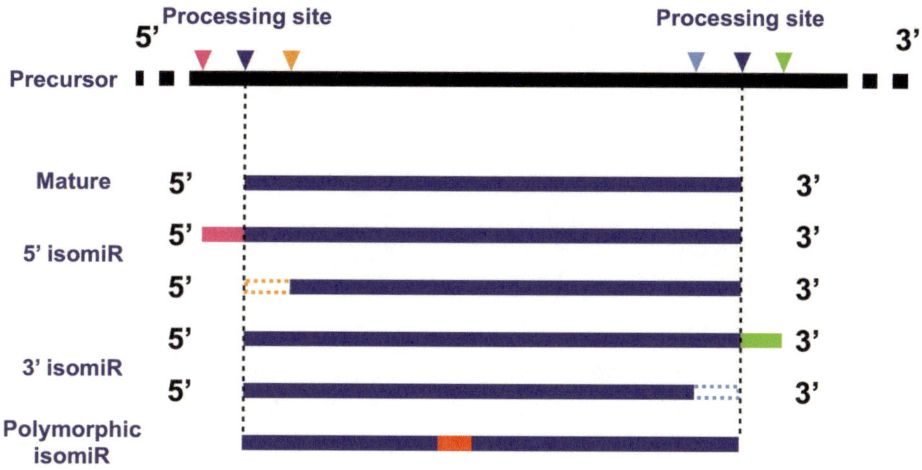

Figure 2.
The classification and generation of isomiRs. The isomiRs have a different length or sequence with mature miRNAs. These isomiRs are generated by a variation of Drosha or dicer variation. The aberrant processing in 5′ site generates 5′ isomiR. On the other hand, 3′ isomiR is generated by the aberrant processing in 3′ site. Polymorphic isomiR is generated by RNA editing. Navy arrow shows the correct processing site. Magenta and green arrows show the aberrant processing sites for isomiRs, which have a longer length. Orange and blue arrows show the aberrant processing sites for isomiRs, which have a shorter length. The red bar indicates the variati of sequence.

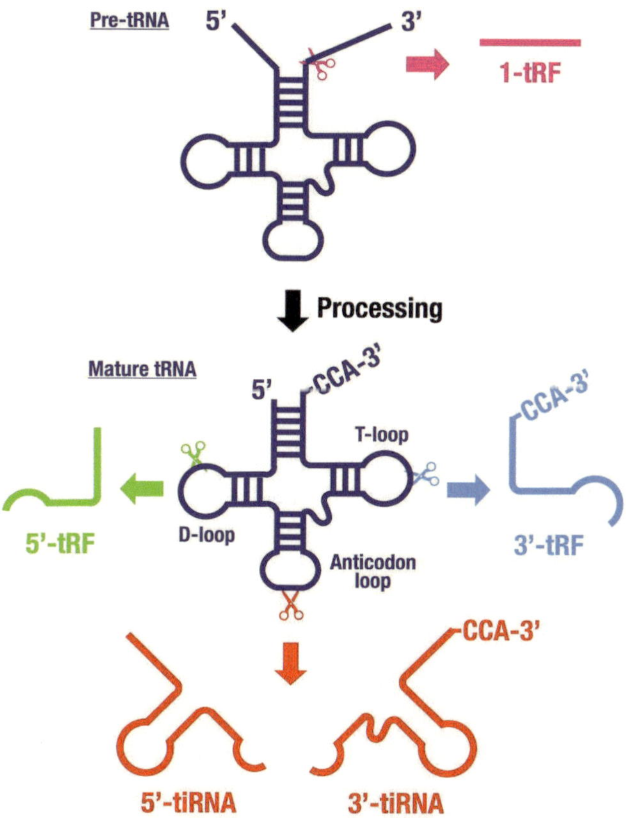

Figure 3.
The classification and various modes of generation of tRFs. tRNA-derived fragments (tRFs) are generated by cleavage of transfer RNA (tRNA). 1-tRFs are cleaved from pre-tRNA. The cleavage of the D-loop generates 5′-tRF. The cleavage of the T-loop generates 3′-tRF. 5′- and 3′-tRNA-derived stress-induced RNAs (tiRNAs) are generated by cleavage of the anticodon loop.

was uncovered that tRNA fragments are functional. Its non-coding RNA is called at tRNA-derived RNA fragment (tRF), and classified as 1-tRF, which is generated from the 3′-end of pre-tRNA, 5′-tRFs, which is generated by the cleavage of 5′ end in D-loop, 3′-tRFs, which is generated by the cleavage of 3′ end in T-loop, and tRNA-derived, stress-induced RNAs (tiRNAs), which is generated by specific cleavage in the anticodon loop. Some tRFs are identified as novel biomarkers for disease diagnosis (**Figure 3**) [15].

2. Liquid biopsy

A biopsy is a method for disease diagnosis using a part of tissues or cells of the lesion. The tissue specimens are sampled by surgery and the cells derived from the lesion are sampled by fine-needle aspiration. The biopsy is useful for diagnosing diseases and malignancies, because it is possible to observe tissues or cells directly.

Generally, to diagnose breast cancer, inspection, palpation, and mammography are performed at first. Then, if the patients are suspected of tumors, the biopsies using tissue or cells derived from the lesion are performed, resulting in diagnosing breast cancer. However, conventional biopsy, surgery, needle biopsy, fine-needle aspiration, etc., are high invasiveness and have the risk of needle tract seeding. As with other problems, it is also concerned that young women are diagnosed as false positive on mammography, caused by high breast density.

Recently, to solve a problem like this, some researchers focus on "liquid biopsy." Liquid biopsy is the method for disease diagnosis using body fluid. Body fluids using in the liquid biopsy are mainly blood, but also saliva, urine, and spinal fluid [16, 17]. Because using body fluid like blood, sampling the specimen is capable of low invasiveness and repetitive. These are one of the features and usefulness of liquid biopsy. In the field of cancer research, circulating tumor cells (CTCs) and circulating cell-free DNAs (cfDNAs) are detected and evaluated, resulting in the diagnosis of cancers. However, a recent study uncovered that circulating miRNA in body fluid is reflected in pathology. Many researchers show that specific miRNAs are aberrantly expressed in each disease. More interestingly, some miRNA expressions are altered from an early stage of cancer. Therefore, investigating the alteration of miRNA expression leads to the early diagnosis of cancer.

2.1 Circulating tumor cells (CTCs)

The cancer cells leak to the bloodstream from the primary tumor in the tumor metastasis phase. In the detection of CTCs, cancer cells that are derived from metastatic tumors are directly evaluated. However, detecting CTCs is not easy, because the number of CTCs is too low. To detect and gather CTCs, cell surface markers are recognized by the specific antibodies. Then, evaluating the shape and gene profile of cancer cells results in the diagnosis of malignancy and specific mutation of each tumor. However, the detection in the early stage of cancer is not useful, because the CTCs are detected in the late stage of cancer.

2.2 Cell-free DNAs (cfDNAs)

In the bloodstream, DNA derived from various dead cells containing hematopoietic cells or other cells derived from tissues are circulating. Additionally, it is known that DNA fragments derived from cancer cells are circulating in the bloodstream of cancer patients. These DNA fragments are generated by apoptosis or clearance by immune cells. In the detection of cfDNAs, the tumor-specific somatic mutation is detected, resulting in the diagnosis of cancer. However, the detection of cfDNA derived from cancer cells is not useful for the early diagnosis of cancer, because cfDNAs were derived from the dead cells.

2.3 Non-coding RNAs (ncRNAs)

Recent studies have uncovered that the ncRNAs included miRNAs, tRFs, and other ncRNAs circulate in different body fluids [15, 18]. Generally, circulating RNAs are easily degraded by RNase present in plasma. However, ncRNAs secreted to body fluids *via* extracellular vesicles like exosomes, or bound to proteins, are resistant to RNase and therefore can be stable in circulation. Exosomes are a type of extracellular vesicles, ranging in size from 50 to 150 nm. Exosomes that are secreted from donor cells circulate in the body fluids and are transferred to target recipient cells. The uptake of exosomes in recipient cells leads to various physiological functions. These functions are caused by ncRNAs and/or proteins contained in exosomes. In this regard, it is thought that exosomes are required for cell-to-cell communications. For example, it is reported that miRNA contained in exosomes secreted from cancer cells, contributing to the metastasis of cancer [19]. Recently, it is thought that exosomes derided from cancer cells educate metastasis site and help the cancer metastasis *via* the transfer of ncRNA and protein as like this report [20]. Moreover, recent studies uncovered that circulating ncRNA in body fluid is reflected in the pathology. Many researchers show that specific miRNAs are aberrantly expressed in each disease. More interestingly, some miRNA expressions are altered from an early stage of cancer. Therefore, investigating the alteration of miRNA expression leads to the early diagnosis of cancer. In this regard, many researchers focus on the ncRNAs circulating in the body fluids. In particular, miRNAs circulating in the blood are focused on.

3. The method of screening the ncRNAs in the liquid biopsy

In liquid biopsy, there are several methods of screening for the circulating ncRNAs in the body fluids. In the case of using blood, commonly, it is necessary to isolate plasma or serum from blood. Then, RNA purification is performed from plasma or serum. Using purified RNA, the expression profiles of ncRNAs are assessed by real-time PCR or microarray, resulting in the identification of a novel biomarker. Examples are shown below:

3.1 Real-time PCR

In the method using real-time PCR, the specific ncRNA is detected with its primer pair, and the alteration of the ncRNA expression is evaluated. The real-time PCR method is not suited for screening and identification of a novel biomarker, because of using the specific primer pair corresponding to each ncRNAs. On the other hand, this method is available for detecting the already identified ncRNA or the particular ncRNA, because the experimental procedure is easier and the detection sensitivity is more specific than other methods.

3.2 Microarray

In the method using microarray, the alteration of ncRNAs existing on microarray chips is capable of a comprehensive evaluation, because the multiple ncRNAs are detectable at the same time. In the microarray method, the ncRNA expression is detected by the binding between cDNAs synthesized from RNA and probes anchored to the microarray chip. Therefore, the microarray method is not available for unknown ncRNAs.

3.3 Next-generation sequencing (NGS)

In the NGS, the alteration of ncRNA expression is comprehensively evaluated by direct reading the RNA sequence of whole ncRNAs. In this regard, it is possible to identify and compare the expression pattern of ncRNAs like as microarray method. Additionally, it is also possible to identify unknown ncRNAs because of the directly determining ncRNA sequence. Moreover, isomiRs, that many researchers recently focused on, are also detectable. However, experimental procedures and data analyses are more difficult and complex than the other methods, and the experimental cost is also high.

4. microRNA for breast cancer diagnosis

Some miRNAs are altered in the tumor tissue compared with normal tissue. For example, the expression level of miR-21 is increased in various cancers included breast cancer and associated with tumorigenesis. Additionally, some miRNAs have a specific expression level in breast cancers. Recent studies also reported that the expression of some miRNAs is altered by the difference of subtype or stage and with/without the receptors. Furthermore, it is known that some of these miRNAs are circulating in body fluids. Therefore, such miRNAs are available for the biomarkers in liquid biopsy. Specific ncRNAs are described below, and recent reports are summarized in **Table 1**.

4.1 Circulating miRNAs

Francesca Maria Orlandella and colleagues focused on miR-622 that known to act as a tumor suppressor in several types of cancer. They reported that miR-622 was downregulated in the plasma and tissues of breast cancer patients. Moreover, it was revealed that the expression level of miR-622 correlated with the breast cancer subtypes and the advance of tumor stages. Additionally, miR-622 inhibited the migration of breast cancer cells *via* targeting NUAK family kinase 1 (NUAK1). In this regard, circulating miR-622 is useful for the biomarker of breast cancer [27].

To identify miRNAs that are useful for the early diagnosis of invasive breast cancers, Mio Yoshikawa and colleagues screened exosomal miRNAs of the plasma by microarray analysis. Using exosomal miRNAs of ductal carcinoma in situ (DCIS) and invasive ductal carcinoma (IDC), five miRNAs, miR-223-3p, miR-130-3p, miR-191-5p, miR-146a, and miR-221-3p, were upregulated in IDC compared with healthy control and DCIS. In this study, they revealed that the expression level of miR-223-3p was correlated between the tissue and plasma exosome. Furthermore, the expression level of miR-223-3p was upregulated according to the advance of tumor stages. In these findings, it is suggested that the expression level of exosomal miR-223-3p reflected the tissue pathogenesis, and the miR-223-3p has the potential as a biomarker for early diagnosing of invasive lesions from DCIS patients in liquid biopsy [37].

4.2 isomiR

Yumiko Koi and colleagues investigated the comprehensive expression profile of ncRNA using the NGS method and focused on the expression level of isomiR.

NcRNAs	Source	Alteration	Method	Characters	Reference
Let-7i	Urine	Down	qRT-PCR	Down in breast cancer	[21]
miR-15a	Serum	Down	qRT-PCR	Down in TNBC	[22]
miR-17	Serum	Down	qRT-PCR	Down in TNBC	[22]
miR-18a	Serum Urine	Down	qRT-PCR	Down in TNBC	[22]
miR-19b	Serum	Down	qRT-PCR	Down in TNBC	[22]
miR-30b	Serum Urine	Down	qRT-PCR	Down in TNBC	[22]
miR-92a	Serum	Down	qRT-PCR	Down during tumor progression	[23]
miR-145	Plasma	Down	Microarray	Down in breast cancer	[24]
miR-194-5p	Plasma	Down	NGS	Down in brain metastasis	[25]
miR-195	Plasma	Down	NGS	Down in metastatic breast cancer	[26]
miR-222	Urine	Down	qRT-PCR	Down in TNBC	[22]
miR-320c	Urine	Down	qRT-PCR	Down in TNBC	[22]
miR-423	Urine	Down	qRT-PCR	Down in breast cancer	[21]
miR-622	Plasma	Down	qRT-PCR	Down in breast cancer	[27]
miR-660	Urine	Down	qRT-PCR	Down in breast cancer	[21]
miR-802-5p	Plasma	Down	NGS	Down in brain metastasis	[25]
Let-7a	Serum	Up	qRT-PCR	Up in TNBC	[22]
Let-7e	Serum	Up	qRT-PCR	Up in TNBC	[22]
miR-16	Plasma	Up	Microarray	Up in breast cancer	[24]
miR-21	Serum Plasma	Up	qRT-PCR Microarray	Up during tumor progression Up in TNBC	[22–24, 28]
miR-21-5p (3′ isoRNA)	Serum	Up	NGS	Up in breast cancer	[29]
miR-23a-3p	Serum	Up	NGS	Up in breast cancer	[29]
miR-29c	Serum	Up	qRT-PCR	Up in early breast cancer	[30]
miR-99a-5p	Plasma	Up	qRT-PCR	Up in early breast cancer	[31]
miR-142-5p	Serum	Up	NGS	Up in luminal A breast cancer and TNBC	[32]
miR-150-5p	Plasma Serum	Up	NGS NGS	Prognostic biomarker (recurrence) Up in luminal A breast cancer and TNBC	[32, 33]
miR-155	Serum	Up	qRT-PCR Microarray	Up in breast cancer Prognostic biomarker (drug resistance)	[34, 35]
miR-199a	Serum	Up	qRT-PCR	Up in early breast cancer	[30]
miR-210	Plasma	Up	qRT-PCR	Up in breast cancer	[36]
miR-223-3p	Plasma	Up	Microarray	Up during tumor progression	[37]
miR-331	Plasma	Up	NGS	Up in metastatic breast cancer	[26]
miR-424	Serum Urine	Up Up	qRT-PCR	Up in early breast cancer	[21, 30]

NcRNAs	Source	Alteration	Method	Characters	Reference
miR-451	Plasma	Up	Microarray	Up in breast cancer	[24]
miR-488	Serum	Up	Microarray	Prognostic biomarker (recurrence)	[38]
miR-576-3p	Plasma	Up	NGS	Prognostic biomarker (recurrence)	[33]
miR-1246	Serum	Up	Microarray	Prognostic biomarker (drug resistance)	[35]
miR-1910-3p	Serum	Up	qRT-PCR	Up in breast cancer	[39]
miR-4433b-5p	Serum	Up	NGS	Up in luminal A breast cancer and TNBC	[32]
miR-4665-5p	Plasma	Up	NGS	Prognostic biomarker (recurrence)	[33]

"Up" indicates upregulation in breast cancer and "Down" indicates downregulation in breast cancer. qRT-PCR, quantitative reverse transcription-polymerase chain reaction; NGS, next-generation sequencing; TNBC, triple-negative breast cancer.

Table 1.
The alteration of circulating miRNAs in breast cancer.

They used the exosomal RNA of serum derived from breast cancer patients. At first, they revealed that 11 circulating small RNAs were upregulated in breast cancer serum compared with healthy controls. Then, 3′-isomiR of miR-21-5p was identified as one of the biomarkers for the diagnosis of breast cancer. Additionally, miR-23a-3p and tRF-Lys-TTT were also identified as biomarkers for the diagnosis of breast cancer. Interestingly, they proposed a discriminant model using the expression levels of these small ncRNAs, and this model was more significantly able to diagnose breast cancer than individual small ncRNA. It was revealed that this model was able to diagnose the stage 0 breast cancer. Moreover, the model also could diagnose the breast cancer irrespective of subtypes. In this regard, the model that included the alteration of isomiR is available for the early diagnosis of breast cancer [29].

4.3 tRFs

As mentioned above, it is clear that tRFs are generated in cancers. Yue Huang and colleagues investigated the expression profile of tRFs in normal breast epithelial cell lines and non-triple negative breast cancer (non-TNBC) cells using RNA sequencing. In further investigation, they revealed that the expression level of tDR-7816 (drives from $tRNA^{Gln-CTG-3-1}$), tDR-5334 (derived from $tRNA^{Gly-CCC-5-1}$), and tDR-4733 (derived from $tRNA^{Phe-GAA-2-1}$) is altered in the serum of non-TNBC patients compared with healthy controls. It is suggested that these tRFs are useful for the diagnosis of breast cancer [40].

In addition, Jingyi Wang and colleagues explored the expression profiles of tRFs in plasma derived from breast cancer patients. As the result, six tRFs, tRF-Glu-CTC-003, tRF-Gly-CCC-007, tRF-Gly-CCC-008, tRF-Leu-CAA-003, tRF-Ser-TGA-001, and tRF-Ser-TGA-002, were altered in the early stage of breast cancers compared with healthy controls. These six tRFs are also downregulated in the plasma derived from DCIS. Moreover, they also revealed that these tRFs which excluded tRF-Glu-CTC-003 in HER2+ type and tRF-Gly-CCC-008 in luminal type are downregulated in each subtype. In this regard, it is suggested that these tRFs are useful as a novel biomarker for the diagnosis of early-stage breast cancer [41].

4.4 Urinary miRNAs

In the liquid biopsy, urine as the specimens has the advantage of easy and non-invasive collection. Thalia Erbes and colleagues investigated whether miRNAs in serum/plasma that are already identified as the candidates of biomarkers for breast cancer are altered in also urine [42]. The expression level of miR-155 which is known to be upregulated in serum from the breast cancer patients, and useful for the diagnostic biomarker, was upregulated also in urine from the breast cancer patients [42, 43]. Moreover, they revealed that the expression levels of urinary miR-21, miR-125, and miR-451 were also downregulated in the breast cancer patients like serum miRNAs [24, 42, 44, 45]. In the recent study, it is revealed that the expression level of urinary miR-423, miR-424, miR-660, and let-7i was altered in the breast cancer patients compared with healthy controls. Moreover, this study reported that the combination of these miRNA's alterations more significantly diagnoses the breast cancer than the biomarker using individual miRNA's alteration [21]. In this regard, urinary miRNAs are useful for the diagnostic and prognosis biomarkers.

5. microRNA for breast cancer therapeutics

As mentioned above, the expression level of various miRNAs is dramatically altered in the development and progression of diseases including the tumors. In this regard, it is thought that the alteration of miRNA expression contributes to the development and progression of several diseases. Moreover, the expression profiles of miRNAs are different in each type of diseases. Then, such miRNAs are available for the therapeutic target of the disease. In cancer research, miRNAs that are over-expressed in tumors are called "oncogenic microRNA (OncomiR)", and are associated with tumor development and malignancy. On the other hand, miRNAs that are downregulated in tumors are called at "tumor suppressive microRNA (TS-miRNA)" and are contributed to the suppression of tumor progression *via* targeting genes that are associated with the cancer cell proliferation and survival. It is hoped that miRNA mimics and miRNA inhibitors targeting TS-miRNA or OncomiR are developed as therapeutic drugs. Specific ncRNAs are described below, and recent reports are summarized in **Table 2**.

5.1 miR-22

It is reported that a lot of miRNAs regulate tumor progression and malignancy. Previously, we revealed that miR-22, which induce cellular senescence, suppressed the proliferation of breast tumors. MiR-22 is upregulated during cellular senescence induction. Such miRNAs are called "senescence-associated microRNA (SA-miRNA)." We reported that miR-22 induces cellular senescence *via* targeting CDK6 and SIRT1. Moreover, it was suggested that miR-22 was the therapeutic target of breast cancer, because miR-22 was downregulated in the breast cancer cells. In an additional investigation, it is reported that the replacement of miR-22 expression repressed the breast tumors through the experiment using the xenograft model mouse model [56].

5.2 miR-155

Jiang and colleagues reported that the expression level of miR-155 was upregulated in breast cancer. Then, they suggested that miR-155 functions as OncomiR,

ncRNAs	Types	Targets	Functions	Reference
miR-429	Anti-sense oligonucleotide	VHL	Inhibit the proliferation of HER2+ breast cancer	[46]
miR-302b	inhibitor	RUNX2	Inhibit the proliferation	[47]
miR-532-5p	inhibitor	RERG	Inhibit the proliferation and migration	[48]
miR-1910-3p	inhibitor	MTMR3	Inhibit proliferation and migration	[39]
miR-99a	mimic	FGFR3	Inhibit the tumor proliferation and migration	[49]
miR-128-3p	mimic	NEK2	Inhibit tumorigenicity and tumor growth of breast cancer stem cells	[50]
miR-188-5p	mimic	RAP2C	Induce apoptosis and inhibit the proliferation	[51]
miR-299-5p	mimic	STK39	Inhibit the migration and invasion	[52]
miR-342	mimic	CFL1	Inhibit the migration and invasion	[53]
miR-424-5p	mimic	PD-L1	Induced apoptosis and cell cycle arrest	[54]
miR-590-3p	mimic	SLUG	Inhibit the metastasis in TNBCs	[55]

HER2, human epidermal growth factor receptor 2; TNBCs, triple-negative breast cancers.

Table 2.
The miRNAs as therapeutic targets in breast cancer.

because its target gene is a suppressor of cytokine signaling 1 (SOCS1) known as one of the tumor suppressor genes. This study revealed that the inhibition of the miR-155 expression and function by the antisense oligonucleotide against miR-155 repressed the tumor progression in the investigation using both the breast cancer cells and the xenograft mouse models. In this regard, the inhibition of OncomiR functions is available for the therapeutic targets [57].

5.3 miR-424/503 cluster

It is reported that the miR-424/503 cluster that was coded on X-chromosome was deficient in luminal B breast cancer. It is also clear that the deletion of this locus significantly correlated with the poor prognosis. Therefore, it is suggested that the miR-424/503 cluster functions as TS-miRNA. Moreover, the miR-424/503 cluster targets insulin-like growth factor 1 receptor (IGF1R) and B-cell lymphoma 2 (BCL-2) that contribute to anti-apoptosis. The deletion of this cluster leads to upregulating these gene expressions, resulting in the acquisition of drug resistance [58].

5.4 miR-539

A recent study reported that miR-539 was downregulated in tumor tissues, and it is suggested that miR-539 has the tumor suppressive effects. In the investigation using breast cancer cells, miR-539 mimics repressed the proliferation and migration of cancer cells *via* targeting epithelial growth factor receptor (EGFR). Additionally, miR-539 also repressed the tumor proliferation [59]. Moreover, it is uncovered that miR-539 was downregulated in TNBC, and miR-539 suppressed the proliferation, invasion, and migration *via* targeting Laminin subunit alpha 4 (LAMA4) [60].

5.5 miR-142

It is reported that miR-142 is also downregulated in breast tumor tissue compared with normal tissue and suggested that miR-142 functions as TS-miRNA. It is revealed that miR-142 inhibits the expression of the BTB domain and CNC homolog 1 (BACH1), which is associated with the metastasis of breast cancer, resulting in the suppression of the proliferation, invasion, and migration. Moreover, Mansoori and colleagues reported that miR-142 induced apoptosis *via* targeting estrogen receptor 1 (ESR1) that coded estrogen receptor in the estrogen receptor-positive breast cancer [61, 62].

5.6 miR-34a

miR-34a is the most famous TS-miRNAs that was reported to upregulate in the p53-dependent manner and downregulate in the colorectal cancer patients compared with healthy, and progressed in the development as the nucleic acid drug against cancer. MiR-34a suppressed colorectal cancer progression through the induction of cellular senescence *via* E2F pathway [63]. In further investigation, it is uncovered that miR-34a downregulates the gene expression *via* targeting sirtuin 1 (SIRT1), cyclin D1, cyclin-dependent kinase 4/6 (CDK4/6), and MYC [64–66]. In this regard, the clinical trial of MRX34, the liposomal miR-34a mimic, for various solid tumors included breast cancer was performed in miRNA Therapeutics Inc. Unfortunately, this clinical trial was dropped [67]. However, a recently study reported that miR-34a targets programmed death ligand 1 (PD-L1) in acute myeloid leukemia [68]. Moreover, it is reported that miR-34a expression level is downregulated in TNBC and inversely correlated with PD-L1 expression [69]. Therefore, a novel clinical trial of miR-34a is expected.

6. Conclusions

In this review, we summarized several ncRNAs that are available for the biomarkers diagnosing breast cancer or predicting poor prognosis and the targets of breast cancer therapeutics. The finding and studying of isomiRs or tRFs are leading to the development of highly specific biomarkers, which could lead to early diagnosis of breast cancer. Moreover, it is useful for comparing the alteration of several ncRNA expressions multidimensionally with the comprehensive analysis of the expression profiles of ncRNAs using microarray or NGS method. These approaches and results may lead to highly specific diagnostics of the disease and can correctly predict several different types of breast cancers. In regard to cancer therapeutics, the studies about isomiRs or tRFs may result in the development of novel therapeutic targets for breast cancers. Further research on the ncRNAs will aid to improve the diagnosis and therapeutics of breast cancers.

Conflict of interest

Professor Hidetoshi Tahara is the representative director of a university-originated venture, MiRTeL Co.

Author details

Yuki Yamamoto[1], Sabrina La Salvia[1,2], Sahoo Susmita[2] and Hidetoshi Tahara[1*]

1 Department of Cellular and Molecular Biology, Graduate School of Biomedical and Health Sciences, Hiroshima University, Hiroshima, Japan

2 Cardiovascular Research Institute, Icahn School of Medicine at Mount Sinai, New York, USA

*Address all correspondence to: toshi@hiroshima-u.ac.jp

References

[1] Winter J, Jung S, Keller S, Gregory RI, Diederichs S. Many roads to maturity: microRNA biogenesis pathways and their regulation. Nature Cell Biology. 2009;**11**(3):228-234

[2] Hausser J, Syed AP, Bilen B, Zavolan M. Analysis of CDS-located miRNA target sites suggests that they can effectively inhibit translation. Genome Research. 2013;**23**(4): 604-615

[3] Lee I, Ajay SS, Yook JI, Kim HS, Hong SH, Kim NH, et al. New class of microRNA targets containing simultaneous 5′-UTR and 3′-UTR interaction sites. Genome Research. 2009;**19**(7):1175-1183

[4] Aure M, Leivonen S-K, Fleischer T, Zhu Q, Overgaard J, Alsner J, et al. Individual and combined effects of DNA methylation and copy number alterations on miRNA expression in breast tumors. Genome Biology. 2013;**14**(11):R126

[5] Calin GA, Croce CM. MicroRNA signatures in human cancers. Nature Reviews. Cancer. 2006;**6**(11):857-866

[6] Lu J, Getz G, Miska EA, Alvarez-Saavedra E, Lamb J, Peck D, et al. MicroRNA expression profiles classify human cancers. Nature. 2005;**435**(7043):834-838

[7] Tan GC, Chan E, Molnar A, Sarkar R, Alexieva D, Isa IM, et al. 5′ isomiR variation is of functional and evolutionary importance. Nucleic Acids Research. 2014;**42**(14):9424-9435

[8] Morin RD, O'Connor MD, Griffith M, Kuchenbauer F, Delaney A, Prabhu A-L, et al. Application of massively parallel sequencing to microRNA profiling and discovery in human embryonic stem cells. Genome Research. 2008;**18**(4):610-621

[9] Landgraf P, Rusu M, Sheridan R, Sewer A, Iovino N, Aravin A, et al. A mammalian microRNA expression atlas based on small RNA library sequencing. Cell. 2007;**129**(7):1401-1414

[10] Kawahara Y, Zinshteyn B, Sethupathy P, Iizasa H, Hatzigeorgiou AG, Nishikura K. Redirection of silencing targets by adenosine-to-inosine editing of miRNAs. Science. 2007;**315**(5815):1137-1140

[11] Gebert LFR, Macrae IJ. Regulation of microRNA function in animals. Nature Reviews. Molecular Cell Biology. 2019;**20**(1):21-37

[12] Wang S, Zheng Z, Chen P, Wu M. Tumor classification and biomarker discovery based on the 5′isomiR expression level. BMC Cancer. 2019;**19**(1):127

[13] Telonis AG, Magee R, Loher P, Chervoneva I, Londin E, Rigoutsos I. Knowledge about the presence or absence of miRNA isoforms (isomiRs) can successfully discriminate amongst 32 TCGA cancer types. Nucleic Acids Research. 2017;**45**(6):2973-2985

[14] Yao R-W, Wang Y, Chen L-L. Cellular functions of long noncoding RNAs. Nature Cell Biology. 2019;**21**(5):542-551

[15] Yu M, Lu B, Zhang J, Ding J, Liu P, Lu Y. tRNA-derived RNA fragments in cancer: Current status and future perspectives. Journal of Hematology & Oncology. 2020;**13**(1):121

[16] Mattox AK, Yan H, Bettegowda C. The potential of cerebrospinal fluid–based liquid biopsy approaches in CNS tumors. Neuro-Oncology. 2019;**21**(12):1509-1518

[17] Rapado-González Ó, Majem B, Muinelo-Romay L, López-López R,

Suarez-Cunqueiro M. Cancer salivary biomarkers for tumours distant to the oral cavity. International Journal of Molecular Sciences. 2016;**17**(9):1531

[18] Kosaka N, Iguchi H, Ochiya T. Circulating microRNA in body fluid: A new potential biomarker for cancer diagnosis and prognosis. Cancer Science. 2010;**101**(10):2087-2092

[19] Fong MY, Zhou W, Liu L, Alontaga AY, Chandra M, Ashby J, et al. Breast-cancer-secreted miR-122 reprograms glucose metabolism in premetastatic niche to promote metastasis. Nature Cell Biology. 2015;**17**(2):183-194

[20] Xu R, Rai A, Chen M, Suwakulsiri W, Greening DW, Simpson RJ. Extracellular vesicles in cancer—Implications for future improvements in cancer care. Nature Reviews. Clinical Oncology. 2018;**15**(10):617-638

[21] Hirschfeld M, Rücker G, Weiß D, Berner K, Ritter A, Jäger M, et al. Urinary exosomal microRNAs as potential non-invasive biomarkers in breast cancer detection. Molecular Diagnosis & Therapy. 2020;**24**(2):215-232

[22] Ritter A, Hirschfeld M, Berner K, Rücker G, Jäger M, Weiss D, et al. Circulating non-coding RNA-biomarker potential in neoadjuvant chemotherapy of triple negative breast cancer? International Journal of Oncology. 2020;**56**(1):47-68

[23] Si H, Sun X, Chen Y, Cao Y, Chen S, Wang H, et al. Circulating microRNA-92a and microRNA-21 as novel minimally invasive biomarkers for primary breast cancer. Journal of Cancer Research and Clinical Oncology. 2013;**139**(2):223-229

[24] Ng EKO, Li R, Shin VY, Jin HC, Leung CPH, Ma ESK, et al. Circulating microRNAs as specific biomarkers for breast cancer detection. PLoS One. 2013;**8**(1):e53141

[25] Sereno M, Haskó J, Molnár K, Medina SJ, Reisz Z, Malhó R, et al. Downregulation of circulating miR 802-5p and miR 194-5p and upregulation of brain MEF2C along breast cancer brain metastasization. Molecular Oncology. 2020;**14**(3): 520-538

[26] Mcanena P, Tanriverdi K, Curran C, Gilligan K, Freedman JE, Brown JAL, et al. Circulating microRNAs miR-331 and miR-195 differentiate local luminal a from metastatic breast cancer. BMC Cancer. 2019;**19**(1):436

[27] Orlandella FM, Mariniello RM, Mirabelli P, De Stefano AE, Iervolino PLC, Lasorsa VA, et al. miR-622 is a novel potential biomarker of breast carcinoma and impairs motility of breast cancer cells through targeting NUAK1 kinase. British Journal of Cancer. 2020;**123**(3):426-437

[28] Anwar SL, Sari DNI, Kartika AI, Fitria MS, Tanjung DS, Rakhmina D, et al. Upregulation of circulating MiR-21 expression as a potential biomarker for therapeutic monitoring and clinical outcome in breast cancer. Asian Pacific Journal of Cancer Prevention. 2019;**20**(4):1223-1228

[29] Koi Y, Tsutani Y, Nishiyama Y, Ueda D, Ibuki Y, Sasada S, et al. Predicting the presence of breast cancer using circulating small RNAs, including those in the extracellular vesicles. Cancer Science. 2020;**111**(6):2104-2115

[30] Zhang L, Xu Y, Jin X, Wang Z, Wu Y, Zhao D, et al. A circulating miRNA signature as a diagnostic biomarker for non-invasive early detection of breast cancer. Breast Cancer Research and Treatment. 2015;**154**(2):423-434

[31] Garrido-Cano I, Constâncio V, Adam-Artigues A, Lameirinhas A, Simón S, Ortega B, et al. Circulating miR-99a-5p expression in plasma: A potential biomarker for early diagnosis of breast cancer. International Journal of Molecular Sciences. 2020; **21**(19):7427

[32] Ozawa PMM, Vieira E, Lemos DS, Souza ILM, Zanata SM, Pankievicz VC, et al. Identification of miRNAs enriched in extracellular vesicles derived from serum samples of breast cancer patients. Biomolecules. 2020;**10**(1):150

[33] Wu H, Wang Q, Zhong H, Li L, Zhang Q, Huang Q, et al. Differentially expressed microRNAs in exosomes of patients with breast cancer revealed by next-generation sequencing. Oncology Reports. 2020;**43**(1):240-250

[34] Sun Y, Wang M, Lin G, Sun S, Li X, Qi J, et al. Serum microRNA-155 as a potential biomarker to track disease in breast cancer. PLoS One. 2012;**7**(10):e47003

[35] Zhang Z, Zhang L, Yu G, Sun Z, Wang T, Tian X, et al. Exosomal miR-1246 and miR-155 as predictive and prognostic biomarkers for trastuzumab-based therapy resistance in HER2-positive breast cancer. Cancer Chemotherapy and Pharmacology. 2020;**86**(6):761-772

[36] Lopes BC, Braga CZ, Ventura FV, De Oliveira JG, Kato-Junior EM, Bordin-Junior NA, et al. miR-210 and miR-152 as biomarkers by liquid biopsy in invasive ductal carcinoma. Journal of Personalized Medicine. 2021;**11**(1):31

[37] Yoshikawa M, Iinuma H, Umemoto Y, Yanagisawa T, Matsumoto A, Jinno H. Exosome-encapsulated microRNA-223-3p as a minimally invasive biomarker for the early detection of invasive breast cancer. Oncology Letters. 2018;**15**(6):9584-9592

[38] Masuda T, Shinden Y, Noda M, Ueo H, Hu Q, Yoshikawa Y, et al. Circulating pre-microRNA-488 in peripheral blood is a potential biomarker for predicting recurrence in breast cancer. Anticancer Research. 2018;**38**(8):4515-4523

[39] Wang B, Mao J-H, Wang B-Y, Wang L-X, Wen H-Y, Xu L-J, et al. Exosomal miR-1910-3p promotes proliferation, metastasis, and autophagy of breast cancer cells by targeting MTMR3 and activating the NF-κB signaling pathway. Cancer Letters. 2020;**489**:87-99

[40] Huang Y, Ge H, Zheng M, Cui Y, Fu Z, Wu X, et al. Serum tRNA-derived fragments (tRFs) as potential candidates for diagnosis of nontriple negative breast cancer. Journal of Cellular Physiology. 2020;**235**(3):2809-2824

[41] Wang J, Ma G, Li M, Han X, Xu J, Liang M, et al. Plasma tRNA fragments derived from 5′ ends as novel diagnostic biomarkers for early-stage breast cancer. Molecular Therapy--Nucleic Acids. 2020;**21**:954-964

[42] Erbes T, Hirschfeld M, Rücker G, Jaeger M, Boas J, Iborra S, et al. Feasibility of urinary microRNA detection in breast cancer patients and its potential as an innovative non-invasive biomarker. BMC Cancer. 2015;**15**(1):193

[43] Sochor M, Basova P, Pesta M, Dusilkova N, Bartos J, Burda P, et al. Oncogenic MicroRNAs: miR-155, miR-19a, miR-181b, and miR-24 enable monitoring of early breast cancer in serum. BMC Cancer. 2014;**14**(1):448

[44] Mar-Aguilar F, Mendoza-Ramírez JA, Malagón-Santiago I, Espino-Silva PK, Santuario-Facio SK, Ruiz-Flores P, et al. Serum circulating microRNA profiling for identification of potential breast cancer biomarkers. Disease Markers. 2013;**34**:259454

[45] Asaga S, Kuo C, Nguyen T, Terpenning M, Giuliano AE, Hoon DS. Direct serum assay for microRNA-21 concentrations in early and advanced breast cancer. Clinical Chemistry. 2011;**57**(1):84-91

[46] Cava C, Novello C, Martelli C, Lodico A, Ottobrini L, Piccotti F, et al. Theranostic application of miR-429 in HER2+ breast cancer. Theranostics. 2020;**10**(1):50-61

[47] Ma J, Zhou Z. Downregulation of miR-302b is associated with poor prognosis and tumor progression of breast cancer. Breast Cancer. 2020;**27**(2):291-298

[48] Huang L, Tang X, Shi X, Su L. miR-532-5p promotes breast cancer proliferation and migration by targeting RERG. Experimental and Therapeutic Medicine. 2020;**19**(1):400-408

[49] Long X, Shi Y, Ye P, Guo J, Zhou Q, Tang Y. MicroRNA-99a suppresses breast cancer progression by targeting FGFR3. Frontiers in Oncology. 2020;**9**:1473

[50] Chen Y, Wu N, Liu L, Dong H, Liu X. microRNA-128-3p overexpression inhibits breast cancer stem cell characteristics through suppression of Wnt signalling pathway by down-regulating NEK2. Journal of Cellular and Molecular Medicine. 2020;**24**(13): 7353-7369

[51] Zhu X, Qiu J, Zhang T, Yang Y, Guo S, Li T, et al. MicroRNA-188-5p promotes apoptosis and inhibits cell proliferation of breast cancer cells via the MAPK signaling pathway by targeting Rap2c. Journal of Cellular Physiology. 2020;**235**(3):2389-2402

[52] Li C, Wang A, Chen Y, Liu Y, Zhang H, Zhou J. MicroRNA-299-5p inhibits cell metastasis in breast cancer by directly targeting serine/threonine kinase 39. Oncology Reports. 2020;**43**(4):1221-1233

[53] Liu C, Xing H, Luo X, Wang Y. MicroRNA-342 targets Cofilin 1 to suppress the growth, migration and invasion of human breast cancer cells. Archives of Biochemistry and Biophysics. 2020;**687**:108385

[54] Dastmalchi N, Hosseinpourfeizi MA, Khojasteh SMB, Baradaran B, Safaralizadeh R. Tumor suppressive activity of miR-424-5p in breast cancer cells through targeting PD-L1 and modulating PTEN/PI3K/AKT/mTOR signaling pathway. Life Sciences. 2020;**259**:118239

[55] Yan M, Ye L, Feng X, Shi R, Sun Z, Li Z, et al. MicroRNA-590-3p inhibits invasion and metastasis in triple-negative breast cancer by targeting Slug. American Journal of Cancer Research. 2020;**10**(3):965-974

[56] Xu D, Takeshita F, Hino Y, Fukunaga S, Kudo Y, Tamaki A, et al. miR-22 represses cancer progression by inducing cellular senescence. The Journal of Cell Biology. 2011;**193**(2): 409-424

[57] Jiang S, Zhang H-W, Lu M-H, He X-H, Li Y, Gu H, et al. MicroRNA-155 functions as an OncomiR in breast cancer by targeting the suppressor of cytokine signaling 1 gene. Cancer Research. 2010;**70**(8):3119-3127

[58] Rodriguez-Barrueco R, Nekritz EA, Bertucci F, Yu J, Sanchez-Garcia F, Zeleke TZ, et al. miR-424(322)/503 is a breast cancer tumor suppressor whose loss promotes resistance to chemotherapy. Genes and Development. 2017;**31**(6):553-566

[59] Guo J, Gong G, Zhang B. miR-539 acts as a tumor suppressor by targeting epidermal growth factor receptor in breast cancer. Scientific Reports. 2018;**8**(1):2073

[60] Yang Z-X, Zhang B, Wei J, Jiang G-Q, Wu Y-L, Leng B-J, et al. MiR-539

inhibits proliferation and migration of triple-negative breast cancer cells by down-regulating LAMA4 expression. Cancer Cell International. 2018;**18**(1):16

[61] Mansoori B, Mohammadi A, Ghasabi M, Shirjang S, Dehghan R, Montazeri V, et al. miR-142-3p as tumor suppressor miRNA in the regulation of tumorigenicity, invasion and migration of human breast cancer by targeting Bach-1 expression. Journal of Cellular Physiology. 2019;**234**(6):9816-9825

[62] Mansoori B, Mohammadi A, Gjerstorff MF, Shirjang S, Asadzadeh Z, Khaze V, et al. miR-142-3p is a tumor suppressor that inhibits estrogen receptor expression in ER-positive breast cancer. Journal of Cellular Physiology. 2019;**234**(9):16043-16053

[63] Tazawa H, Tsuchiya N, Izumiya M, Nakagama H. Tumor-suppressive miR-34a induces senescence-like growth arrest through modulation of the E2F pathway in human colon cancer cells. Proceedings of the National Academy of Sciences. 2007;**104**(39): 15472-15477

[64] Sun F, Fu H, Liu Q, Tie Y, Zhu J, Xing R, et al. Downregulation of CCND1 and CDK6 by miR-34a induces cell cycle arrest. FEBS Letters. 2008,**582**(10):1564-1568

[65] Wei JS, Song YK, Durinck S, Chen Q-R, Cheuk ATC, Tsang P, et al. The MYCN oncogene is a direct target of miR-34a. Oncogene. 2008;**27**(39): 5204-5213

[66] Yamakuchi M, Ferlito M, Lowenstein CJ. miR-34a repression of SIRT1 regulates apoptosis. Proceedings of the National Academy of Sciences. 2008;**105**(36):13421-13426

[67] Hong DS, Kang Y-K, Borad M, Sachdev J, Ejadi S, Lim HY, et al. Phase 1 study of MRX34, a liposomal miR-34a mimic, in patients with advanced solid tumours. British Journal of Cancer. 2020;**122**(11):1630-1637

[68] Wang X, Li J, Dong K, Lin F, Long M, Ouyang Y, et al. Tumor suppressor miR-34a targets PD-L1 and functions as a potential immunotherapeutic target in acute myeloid leukemia. Cellular Signalling. 2015;**27**(3):443-452

[69] Huang X, Xie X, Wang H, Xiao X, Yang L, Tian Z, et al. PDL1 And LDHA act as ceRNAs in triple negative breast cancer by regulating miR-34a. Journal of Experimental & Clinical Cancer Research. 2017;**36**(1):129

Chapter 3

Molecular Prognostic and Predictive Markers in Triple - Negative Breast Cancer

Marketa Koleckova, Katherine Vomackova and Zdenek Kolar

Abstract

Triple-negative breast cancer (TNBC) is defined as a molecular subtype of breast cancer that lacks expression of hormone receptors (oestrogen and progesterone receptor) and HER2/neu/ErbB2 protein. It accounts for 15–20% of all invasive breast cancers. The occurrence of TNBC is often associated with younger age at the time of diagnosis and pre-menopausal status, early onset of menarche, higher body mass index (BMI) in the pre-menopausal period, race and ethnicity (African, Hispanic) and the presence of germline mutation in the BRCA1/2 genes or somatic mutation in the TP53 or PTEN genes. TNBCs are specific in its aggressive biological behaviour, shorter interval to disease progression and more frequent relapse within five years (19 to 40 months). The most of TNBCs are represented by high-grade invasive carcinomas of no special type (NST) with high proliferation index measured by Ki-67 nuclear expression, followed by metaplastic carcinomas, secretory carcinomas, and adenoid cystic carcinomas. Genetical and morphological heterogeneity inside TNBC is responsible for the higher frequency of primary and secondary resistance to systemic therapy. The scope of this chapter is to summarise the potential therapeutic agents involved in regulation of cell proliferation, migration, angiogenesis, apoptosis, gene expression and DNA damage or immune response. The insight into this issue is essential for the setting of the optimal chemotherapy regimen and targeted therapeutic strategy.

Keywords: Triple-negative breast cancer, prognosis, prediction, molecular target

1. Introduction

Triple - negative breast cancer (TNBC) represents a morphologically and genetically heterogeneous molecular subtype of breast cancer lacking the expression of hormone receptors (oestrogen and progesterone receptor) and HER2/neu/ErbB2 protein. It accounts for 15–20% of all cases [1]. The occurrence of TNBC is often associated with younger age at the time of diagnosis and pre-menopausal status, early onset of menarche, higher body mass index (BMI) in the pre-menopausal period, race and ethnicity (African, Hispanic) and the presence of germline mutation in the *BRCA1/2* genes or somatic mutation in the *TP53* or *PTEN* genes [2, 3]. In addition, for BRCA1/2 mutant gene carriers, the risk of developing TNBC multiplies after therapeutic exposure to ionising radiation. Other genetic alterations include mutations in the *RB1*, *NF1*, *ERBB3*, *ERBB4*, *ALK* and *EGFR* genes, changes in the

NOTCH1/2, *MAST1/2* gene copy number or *MAGI3 - AKT3* gene fusion. The gain on chromosomes 1q, 8q, 10q and the loss on chromosomes 5q and 8p were also demonstrated.

From a clinical point of view, TNBC is specific in its aggressive biological behaviour, shorter interval to disease progression and more frequent relapse within five years (19 to 40 months vs. 35 to 65 months) [4]. The median overall survival (OS) for metastatic TNBC is reported to be 9 to 12 months [5]. Due to these tumour characteristics, chemotherapy is often indicated already during the initial phase of treatment. Heterogeneity inside TNBC is responsible for the higher frequency of primary and secondary resistance to treatment [6]. The current research trends therefore focus on finding the new potentially therapeutically manageable molecules, which could significantly help to decrease the risk of metastasis development and disease recurrence.

Compared to other molecular subtypes, TNBCs differ in their high degree of gene instability. Based on the gene expression profiling, TNBC can be subclassified into several distinct molecular subtypes. Lehmann et al. represent one of the first research groups using this approach in practical diagnostics [7, 8]. Since then, a couple of classification schemes have been introduced; see **Table 1** [9–13].

The essential clue for effective breast cancer management is comprehensive evaluation of number of prognostic and predictive molecular indicators. While prognostic factors correlate with patient survival, predictive factors provide

Authors	TNBC subtype	Basic molecular characteristics
Ma et al. [9]	BL	Increased CK5/6, EGFR expression
	LAR	Increased AR expression
	"Claudin - low"	CD44+/CD24- immunophenotype
		Decreased claudin 3, 4, 7 expression
Lehmann et al. [7]	BL1	Increased Ki-67 expression
	BL2	Increased CD10, p63 expression
	LAR	Increased AR expression
		Aberrant *FOXA1, KRT18, XBP1* gene activation
	M	Aberrant regulation of Wnt, ALK, TGF-β
	MSL	Aberrant regulation of Rho, ALK, TGF-β, Wnt/β-catenin, ERK1/2, EGFR, PDGF, PI3K
	IM	Aberrant regulation of NFKB, TNF, JAK/STAT
Burstein et al. [10]	LAR	Increased AR, MUC1 expression
		Aberrant *PIK3CA, AKT1, CDH1* gene activation
	M	Increased PDGF-A, c-Kit expression
	BLIA	Aberrant regulation of STAT
		Presence of B /T/NK immune cells
	BLIS	Aberrant regulation of VTCN1
Jézéquel et al. [11]	BL	Immune cells -, TAM – like cells +
	LAR	Increased AR expression Aberrant *FOXA1, KRT18, XBP1* gene activation
	"BL - enriched"	Immune cells +, TAM – like cells -

Authors	TNBC subtype	Basic molecular characteristics
Ahn et al. [12]	BL	Aberrant *ATR, BRCA1/2*, etc. gene activation
	M	*PIK3CA* gene mutation, *PTEN* gene inactivation
		Aberrant regulation of PI3K / AKT
	IM	Aberrant regulation of NFKB, TNF, JAK/STAT, VTCN1, presence of B/T/NK immune cells
	LAR	Increased AR expression Aberrant *FOXA1, KRT18, XBP1* gene activation
Zeng et al. [13]	BL	Increased CK5/6, EGFR expression
	NBL	Absence of CK5/6, EGFR expression

BL = basal – like; BL1/2 = basal – like 1/2; LAR = luminal androgen receptor; M = mesenchymal; MSL = mesenchymal stem – like; IM = immunomodulatory; BLIA = basal-like immune-activated; BLIS = basal-like immune-suppressed; NBL = normal breast - like.

Table 1.
History of proposed TNBC classification systems.

information on the response to a specific therapy. The all prognostic clinicopathological characteristics such as patient age at the time of diagnosis, clinical and pathological tumour stage, tumour type with detailed tumour morphology analysis including the intensity of tumour infiltrating lymphocytes (TILs), tumour grade, occurrence and extent of in situ carcinoma and family history of breast cancer should be taken into account.

The most of TNBCs are represented by high-grade invasive carcinomas of no special type (NST) with high proliferation index measured by Ki-67 nuclear expression, followed by metaplastic carcinomas, secretory carcinomas, and adenoid cystic carcinomas [14]. The morphological pattern of invasive carcinomas NST may involve medullary, lipid-rich, apocrine, pleomorphic or spindle cell areas. Carcinomas with spindle tumour cell transformation are usually related to "claudin-low" molecular subtype (CD44+/ D24−/low) and epithelial to mesenchymal transition (EMT) process [15–17]. Metaplastic breast cancers and secretory carcinomas account for 0.2 to 5%, respectively 0.02% of all breast cancers [14]. Adenoid-cystic carcinomas with typical fusion of the *MYB - NFIB* genes and mutations in the *EP300, NOTCH1, ER882* and *FGFR1* genes are described in 0.1 to 3.5% of breast tumours [14].

2. Molecular prognostic and predictive markers

Individual molecules involved in the process of TNBC carcinogenesis may be divided into several groups. The groups of proteins include proteins participating in mechanisms of repair of damaged DNA; proteins responsible for regulation of cell proliferation, migration, angiogenesis, programmed – cell death (apoptosis) and immune response (immune checkpoint proteins; and groups of proteins modifying gene expression (see **Table 2**).

2.1 Regulators in the DNA damage response

Genes and proteins involved in the repair of damaged DNA (poly (ADP-ribose) polymerase, genes with tumour suppressor function *PTEN, BRCA 1, BRCA2, TP53 a RB1)* are key factors in maintaining genome integrity, ensuring that the cell cycle

Regulators in the DNA damage response	BRCA1, BRCA2, PARP, PTEN, pRb, p53
Regulators of cell migration and proliferation	EGFR, VEGFR, FGFR
Regulators of apoptosis	Fas, TRAIL, p53, Bcl-2
Regulators of gene expression	microRNA, lncRNA, circRNA, siRNA
Steroid receptors	Androgen receptor
Immune checkpoint proteins	PD - 1, PD - L1

Table 2.
Classification of molecular prognostic and predictive markers.

proceeds correctly. Deoxyribonucleic acid (DNA) may be damaged due to physical, chemical, as well as biological processes. Repair of the damaged DNA is realised by several mechanisms, including repair of mismatched bases (mismatch repair - MMR), nucleotide and base excision repair (nucleotide excision repair"- NER; „base excision repair"- BER) or repair of double-strand DNA breaks by homologous recombination (HR) or by non-homologous end joining NHEJ).

The enzyme family **poly (ADP-ribose) polymerase** is responsible for the transfer of the subunit (ADP) – ribose from NAD+ to the acceptor protein creating long, branched and negatively charged polymers of poly - ADP ribose (**Figure 1**) [18–22]. PARP-1 is the most abundant, an evolutionally highly conserved enzyme involved in the repair of damaged DNA through BER. It is composed of an NH2-terminal domain with three „Zinc fingers", which binds to the damaged DNA, automodification domains and C-terminal catalytic domains. The conformation change arising from the binding of PARP to the site of damaged DNA enables catalysis of the transfer of ADP-ribose from NAD+ to its own molecule and histone H1.

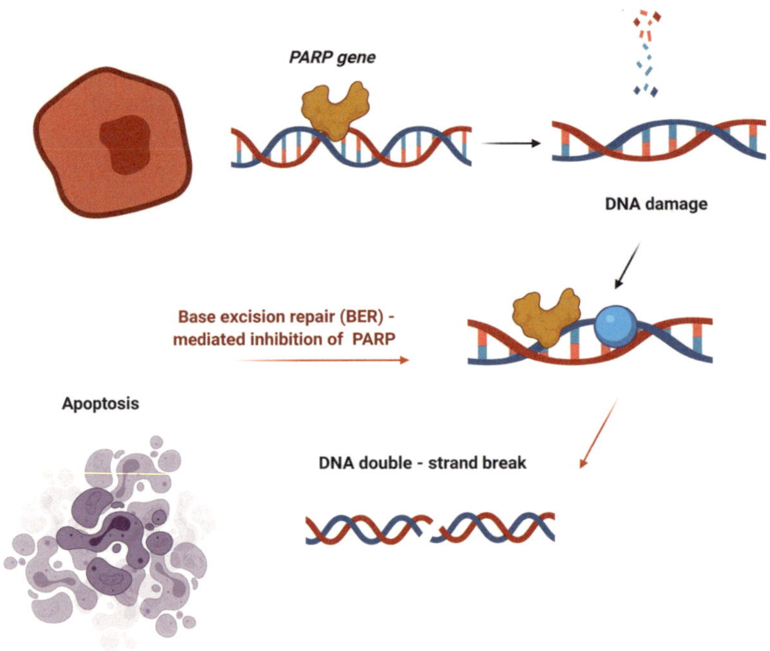

Figure 1.
Mechanism of action of PARP inhibitors (Koleckova M, www.biorender.com). Efficient single-strand breaks (SSB) repair provided by PARP is essential for the cell survival. The mechanism of action of PARP inhibitors include the suppression of this base excision repair (BER) – mediated pathway, resulting in the pathologic double-strand breaks (DSB) with homologous recombination (HR) – mediated repair and thus genome stability and the cell death.

Subsequently, degradation of the chromatin structure occurs and there is an influx of additional damaged DNA repair proteins (for example DNA ligase 3, DNA polymerase β and protein XRCC1). In patients with TNBC with a confirmed mutation in the gene *BRCA1* or *BRCA2*, PARP takes over a backup function, it inactivates the degradation of caspases and initiates apoptosis utilising so-called synthetic lethality. The direct inhibitory effect on the PI3K/AKT/mTOR and Wnt/β-catenin signalling pathways has also been established, with corresponding changes in miRNA and serine/threonine kinase ATM expression. *PARP inhibitors* may be administered in monotherapy as well as in combination. They amplify the effect of the administered chemotherapy and/or inhibitors of molecules of the signalling pathway PI3K/AKT/mTOR, inhibitors of deacetylation of histones, CDK1, EGFR, AR, ATM or MYC. In cases treated by *olaparib* versus the chemotherapy group (capecitabin, eribulin or vinorelbin based on selection of the examining physician), the progression-free survival (PFS) was prolonged from 4.2 months to 7 months. A higher rate of therapeutic response was also discovered (59.9%). A positive finding was also observed with *talazoparib* in monotherapy, where PFS was prolonged from 5.6 months to 8.6 months, while increasing the rate of therapeutic response to 62.6%. Finally, administration of *veliparib* in combination with paclitaxel and carboplatin seems to be effective. Mechanisms leading to the development of resistance to PARP inhibitors include secondary mutations in the *BRCA1* and *BRCA2* genes, in genes coding the P-glycoprotein pump or the loss of protein 1 binding protein p53 (53BP1).

Tumour suppressor gene *PTEN* participates in the regulation of cell proliferation, migration and apoptosis under physiological conditions [23–26]. Phosphatase and tensin homologue (PTEN) represent a protein belonging to the tyrosine-phosphatase family with phosphatidyl-inositol-phosphatase activity. After binding tensin, a focal adhesion complex is created, which affects cell integrity and the transfer of intercellular as well as intracellular signals. The catalytic domain C2 is responsible for PTEN binding to the cell's phospholipid membrane and ensures Ca2+ dependent membrane transport of signal proteins. The resulting action of protein PTEN is the inhibition of proteins of the signalling pathway PI3K/Akt/mTOR (**Figure 2**), whose aberrant activation via activation of genes *PI3CA*, *AKT1* and *MTOR* would lead to induction of the process of cancerogenesis. Indirect activation of protein PTEN is realised by the fully functional gene *TP53* (wild – type p53 protein). Alteration in the expression of gene *PTEN* is a result of its deletion or inactivating mutation. It occurs in up to 41% of cases of TNBC and correlates with a shorter PFS and overall survival (OS). Therapeutic inhibition of aberrantly activated PI3K/Akt/mTOR of the signalling pathway is possible by administering paclitaxel in combination with ATK inhibitor *ipatasertib*. Compared with placebo, ipatasertib led to a significant prolonging of PFS - from 4.9 months to 9 months, as well as OS – from 18.4 months to 23.1 months). Similarly, effective, but with a greater number of side effects, was the combination of paclitaxel with *capivasertib* (PFS – 5.9 months; OS – 19.1 months).

Tumour suppressor genes *BRCA1* **and** *BRCA2* are involved in the regulatory phases S and G2 of the cell cycle [27–29]. As transcription factors, they participate in the repair mechanism of DNA single-strand breaks via HR. In cases of DNA double-strand breaks, phosphorylation of protein BRCA1 by protein kinase ATM takes place, with subsequent interaction with protein RAD51, transported with the help of protein BRCA2, and leads to repair of the damaged DNA. In case there is a loss of function of genes *BRCA1* and *BRCA2*, the *PARP* genes take over their role, inactivates caspase degradation and initiates apoptosis through mechanism of synthetic lethality. Inactivating mutations in the *BRCA1* gene were determined in 40% of cases of familial breast cancer. Autosomal dominant inheritance was found in 5–10% of patients. Confirmation of a germline mutation in the *BRCA1* gene is

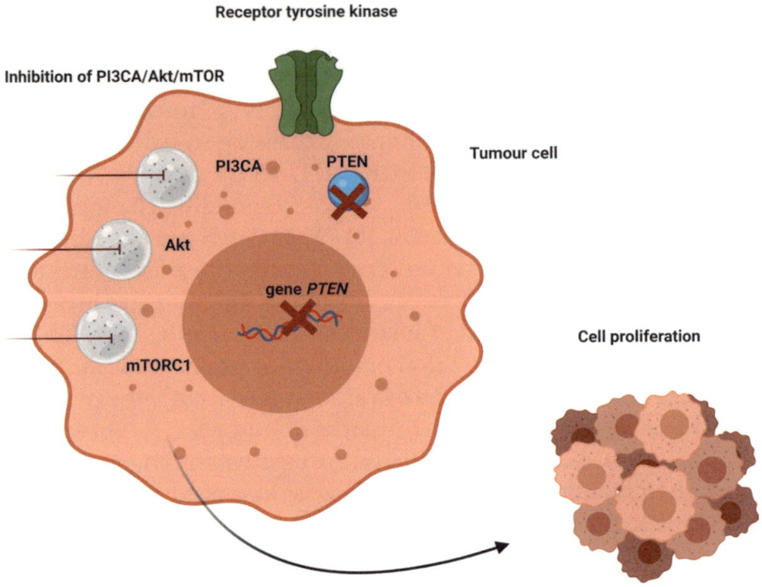

Figure 2.
Mechanism of action of PTEN protein (Koleckova M, www.biorender.com). PTEN protein (Phosphatase and tensin homologue) is essential for the regulation of intracellular levels of phosphorylation, cell migration, proliferation and survival. It plays a pivotal role in the phosphatidyl-inositol-3-kinase (PI3-K) pathway involved in the inhibition of proteins of the signalling pathway PI3K/Akt/mTOR. Inactivation of the PTEN tumour suppressor gene leads to the aberrant activation of PI3CA, Akt and mTORC1 genes associated with the initiation of the process of cancerogenesis.

considered to be an unfavourable prognostic marker. However, in NBC it predicts an increased therapeutic response to anthracyclines, taxanes, platinum derivatives, and in advanced disease stages, PARP inhibitors.

Protein Rb (pRb), a product of **tumour suppressor gene** *RB1,* inhibits the bound transcription factor E2F and thus is significant in regulating the cell cycle, chromatin structure, proliferation and differentiation of tumour cells and cell death [30, 31]. Lost expression of the gene *RB1* plays a role in the pathogenesis of tumour development. This is due to inactivation of deletion alleles, point mutation or hypermethylation of its promoter, increased expression and/or amplification of the gene for cyclin D1, decreased expression of inhibitor p16INK4A or binding protein pRb by oncoprotein E7 HPV. In addition, the concurrent presence of the mutation in genes *RB1* and *TP53* induces the process of epithelial-mesenchymal transition (EMT). In TNBC with confirmed inactivation of the *RB1* gene, this leads to induction of increased sensitivity to radiotherapy and cytotoxic drugs, such as doxorubicin, methotrexate or inhibitor of mitochondrial translation of proteins, tigecyclin. Inhibition of expression of glucose 1 transporter (GLUT1) by tumour cells with confirmed mutation of the *RB1* gene presents a new promising therapeutic goal.

2.2 Regulators of cell proliferation, migration and angiogenesis

The loss of effective mechanisms to repair damaged DNA during the cell cycle leads to uncontrolled cell division and their tumour transformation. Adequate nutrition for the tumour cells is provided by the process of angiogenesis. To initiate the metastatic cascade, there must be an increased expression of proteases by tumour cells with subsequent degradation of the basal membrane. Cells of the tumour stroma may amplify the aggressive potential of the tumour even further and thus participate in the EMT process.

Fibroblast growth factor receptor (FGFR) consists of an extracellular domain, transmembrane domain and an intracellular domain with tyrosine kinase activity [32–34]. The binding of fibroblast growth factor and its cofactor to the extracellular portion of one of four evolutionally conserved receptors leads to the dimerization of its polypeptide chain, autophosphorylation and subsequent activation of signalling molecules, which influence cell proliferation and differentiation (MAPK, PI3K-AKT), inflammatory reaction (MAPK – kinase p38, JNK), angiogenesis (MAPK - kinase p38; PI3K-AKT - FOXO1, TSC2), apoptosis (MAPK – JNK; PI3K-AKT - FOXO1, TSC2) and cell growth, metabolism and motility (PLCγ – IP3 – DAG, PKC). The therapeutic response to the administered FGFR inhibitors (for example dovitinib, lucitanib) differs greatly. While in cases of confirmed fusion of the genes *FGFR3-TACC3* or amplification of the gene for FGFR1, an excellent therapeutic response is observed, the mutation in specific genes is associated with a significantly reduced to zero therapeutic response. In breast cancer, the aberrant activation of receptors FGFR1 and FGFR4 is associated with resistance to chemotherapy (doxorubicin, cyclophosphamide), endocrine therapy (tamoxifen, fulvestrant) and VEGF inhibitors (bevacizumab).

Epidermal growth factor receptor (EGFR) consists of a glycoprotein with an extracellular domain for ligand binding (EGF and TNF-α), a transmembrane domain and cytoplasmic domain with tyrosine kinase activity [35–37]. The EGFR/ErbB1 receptor is significantly involved in the regulation of the cell cycle, cell migration, proliferation, differentiation and survival, by way of activating its secondary signalling pathways Ras/Raf/MEK/ERK, Ras/PI3K/AKT1/mTOR or Src/STAT3. After translocation to the nucleus, EGFR/ErbB1 regulates transcription and repair of damaged DNA. Aberrant activation and increased expression of EGFR/ErbB1 is caused by amplification or mutation of its gene. Increased expression of EGFR was proven in 13–76% of TNBC, whereas amplification of the gene in only 2–24% of cases and is more frequent in patients with mutation in the *BRCA1* gene. An increased number of copies of the *EGFR* gene was found in 8–27% TNBC. The use of EGFR inhibitors in monotherapy or in combination with chemotherapy is being considered especially in advanced and generalised forms of TNBC. The combination of docetaxel with cetuximab seems to be effective. In patients treated with a combination of cisplatin and cetuximab, a correlation between therapeutic response and intensity of CD8+ lymphocyte infiltration (tumour infiltrating lymphocytes – TILs) has been reported. Combination therapy with PARP inhibitors or immune checkpoint inhibitors (PD-1/PD-L1) has promising therapeutic potential. The synergistic effect of anti – EGFR therapy was also noted with radiation therapy. A possible mechanism of resistance development to EGFR inhibitors is methylation of the extracellular domain of the EGFR/ErB1 receptor by protein PRMT1 or increased expression of the Notch3 protein.

Vascular endothelial growth factor (VEGF) binds to its specific transmembrane receptors with tyrosine kinase activity (VEGFR-1 and VEGFR-2) by activating matrix metalloproteinases (MMP) and stimulates cell migration and endothelium proliferation with the creation of vascular lumen and fenestrations [38, 39]. Unregulated angiogenesis may be induced by genetic changes (mutations in tumour suppressor genes *TP53* or *VHL*, activation of oncogenes), as well as metabolic changes (hypoxia, effect of gonadal hormones, growth factors and cytokines). Increased VEGF expression is often observed in patients with advanced disease stages, resistant to therapy or with a mutation in the *BRCA1/2* genes. In TNBC, a synergic anti – angiogenic effect of the intravenously administered AAV2-VEGF-Trap and paclitaxel has been detected. Coenzyme Q0 has a similar effect, whereby its effect on signalling pathway PI3K/AKT/NFKB/MMP-9 and negative regulation of MMP-2/– 9, urokinase activator of plasminogen (uPA), receptors uPAR and VEGF lead to induction of apoptosis and inhibition of EMT. In advanced and metastasizing forms of TNBC, the benefits of combination therapy of bevacizumab and chemotherapy or mTOR inhibitors (temsirolimus, everolimus) or EGFR (erlotinib) are also being considered.

2.3 Proteins regulating apoptosis

Cell death receptors Fas and TRAIL of the tumour necrotizing factor (TNF) family are considered to be potential anti-tumour molecules. The **Fas receptor (CD95R)** is a transmembrane protein, composed of an extracellular, transmembrane and intracellular domain [40]. Binding the soluble membrane ligand of cytotoxic T-lymphocytes CD95 (CD95L, FasL) leads to the creation of complex DISC and activates the extrinsic apoptosis pathway. Soluble ligand CD95L, labelled cl-CD95L, is responsible for activating the immune response, EGFR and the oncogenic signalling pathway c-yes/Ca2+/PI3K. Increased expression of CD95R was found in almost 49% of TNBC. Decreased expression of the Fas receptor (CD95R) is a marker of poor prognosis. Expression of CD95L by tumour blood vessels and detection of serum levels of cl-CD95L predicts metastatic potential of the tumour in patients with TNBC. Excessive expression of protein Lifeguard by TNBC tumour cells inhibits the activity of CD95R receptor and thus presents a possible mechanism of resistance to systemic therapy with cisplatin. The **TRAIL receptor ligand (Apo2L)** activates the extrinsic apoptosis pathway in the mesenchymal subtype of TNBC [41]. Agonists of the TRAIL (TNF - related apoptosis -inducing ligand) receptor stimulate death receptors DR4 and/or DR5. In advanced and metastasizing forms of TNBC, molecule MEDI3039 has shown a positive therapeutic effect.

Gene *TP53* with tumour suppressor function plays the role of genome guardian. Its product, **protein p53**, acts as a transcription factor following translocation to the nucleus and has a fundamental influence on the regulation of checkpoints of the cell cycle, cellular response to damaged DNA and telomeres, aerobic cell metabolism, apoptosis, inhibition of angiogenesis and oncogene activation [42]. Protein p53 consists of an N – terminal domain activating transcription, DNA binding domain, oligomerization domain and protease-sensitive domain, which enables the binding of p53 to damaged DNA. Functional protein p53 exists in the form of a tetramer, where loss of function of one subunit causes nonfunction of the entire complex. Mutations in the *TP53* gene were discovered in 60–88% of TNBC. They are considered as a negative prognostic and predictive marker in terms of disease-free survival (DFS), overall survival (OS) and therapeutic response to chemotherapy. Manipulating genes involved in the regulation of protein p53 and its isoforms (Cyclin G2, Sharp-1, PI3K/AKT/mTOR, Chk1, CDK, Hsp90, Mdm2, histone deacetylase) may lead to new therapeutic strategies for TNBC.

Anti-apoptotic protein Bcl-2 is reported to be an independent negative prognostic marker of survival in patients with TNBC [43–45]. Expression of protein Bcl-2 in TNBC positively correlates with the size of the tumour and the development of metastases to regional axillary lymph nodes. It is also associated with a lower sensitivity to neoadjuvant and adjuvant chemotherapy with anthracyclines and resistance of the tumour to radiation therapy due to activation of the *STAT3* gene. The use of Bcl-2 inhibitors may have a protective effect against resistance development to chemotherapy and immunotherapy.

2.4 Regulation of gene expression

Detection of epigenetic changes taking place in breast cancer may aid in determining disease prognosis and in predicting the response to treatment. These primarily include changes in DNA methylation, modification of histones and altering miRNA expression [46–53]. Recently, the regulatory role of lncRNA, circRNA and siRNA has been described.

DNA methylation is among the most important modifications, ensured by the action of DNA methyltranferases, regulated by genes *DNMT1, DNMT3a* and especially *DNMT3b*. Also associated with the development and progression of breast cancer is hypermethylation of CpG promoters of tumour suppressor genes (*RASSF1A, CDKN2A, CDKN1B, CCND2a*), genes regulating repair of damaged DNA (*BRCA1, MLH1, MGMT*), cellular detoxification genes (*GSTP1*), adhesion, invasion (*TWIST1, CDH1, TIMP3*), hormone receptors (*ER, PR*) and apoptosis (*HOXA5, TMS1*).

Post-translational modification of histones includes their phosphorylation, ubiquitination, methylation and demythylation, acetylation and deacetylation. Methylation of histone H3K27 by protein EZH2 is described in aggressive and metastasizing forms of breast cancer. A therapeutic response may be reached using histone deacetylase inhibitors (vorinostat, entinostat and panobinostat) in monotherapy or in combination with cytotoxic, hormonal or targeted anti - HER2 and anti - VEGF therapy.

MiRNA represent endogenous short non-coding single strand RNA molecules with a length of 18 to 25 nucleotides. The miRNA sequence is phylogenetically conserved. They are partially or completely complementary to one or more mediator RNA (mRNA) and may also regulate other miRNAs. MiRNAs are significant regulators of gene expression and participate in the regulation of more than 50% of human genes. They are involved in angiogenesis, cell growth, proliferation, differentiation, effectiveness of mechanisms of damaged DNA repair and apoptosis. Changes in miRNA expression are therefore responsible for the development of many diseases, including dysfunctions of the immune system, tumours or resistance to pharmacological or radiation therapy. Depending on their role in the pathogenesis of tumour development, they can be divided into two types, miRNA with oncogenic or with tumour suppressor function. The positive influence on the EMT process also potentiates tumour metastasis. In the past years, miRNA has received much attention in connection with changes in its serum concentrations and its possible prognostic and predictive potential.

The miRNA biosynthesis is predominantly enabled by two major pathways - canonical and non-canonical pathway. The first pathway is initiated by the generation of the pri-miRNA transcript which is cleaved by microprocessor complex (Drosha and DGCR8) into precursor-miRNA (pre-miRNA). Pre-miRNA is transferred by the Exportin5/RanGTP to the cytoplasm and processed by the RNase III endonuclease Dicer to produce the mature miRNA duplex. The load of 5p or 3p strands of the mature miRNA duplex into the Argonaute (AGO) family of proteins to form a miRNA-induced silencing complex (miRISC). The second pathway begins by microprocessor complex – mediated cleavage of small hairpin RNA (shRNA) with following its export to the cytoplasm via Exportin5/RanGTP. Nevertheless, the further possible pathways were identified (e.g. Dicer-independent cleavage, miirtrons and 7-methylguanine capped (m7G)-pre-miRNA formation).

Long non-coding RNA (lncRNA) are, contrarily, molecules with a length of 200 and more nucleotides. Aberrantly increased lncRNA expression is able to stimulate the oncogenic signalling pathway PI3K/AKT, as well as changes in miRNA expression. They participate in the regulation of the biological behaviour of tumours and may induce a therapeutic response to administered systemic therapy. Newly described lncRNA includes DANCR (lncRNA - differentiation antagonising non-protein coding RNA), sONE, CCAT1 or GAS5. So-called **circular RNA (circRNA)** has a similar significance.

Short interfering RNA molecules of siRNA are due to their ability to reduce the expression of protein Bcl-2 and p-glycoprotein considered to be one of the possible mechanisms for developing resistance to chemotherapy in TNBC. Formation of conjugates with nanoparticles of silicon dioxide, or in combination with chemotherapy, may enhance therapeutic possibilities in the future.

2.5 Steroid androgen receptor

The androgen receptor (AR) is a nuclear steroid hormone receptor which is expressed in 70–90% of all breast cancers [54–56]. It contains a transactivation N-terminal domain, a DNA-binding domain and a C-terminal domain. The function of AR as a transcription factor is to modulate the activity of steroid-regulated genes, or to alter post-transcription processes, which leads to changes in levels of specific mRNA and proteins. Inactive form of AR is kept in the cytoplasm by a heterocomplex with heat-shock proteins and a chaperone complex (HSP-70, HSP-90). There exist two mechanisms of AR activation – genomic modality and non-genomic modality. Genomic modality is implemented by androgen binding to the C-terminal domain of AR, its conformational change, dimerization and translocation into the nucleus, leading to a promotion of a co-activator-mediated transcription of target genes. Non – genomic modality activates AR through ERK dependent (interaction with PI3K, Src proteins, Ras GTPase) or ERK independent signal transduction (mTOR phosphorylation, FOXO1 inactivation, PKA activation)

In TNBC, increased expression of AR was observed in 10–50% of cases. Although several studies concerning ER-related breast cancers confirm a positive correlation between its increased expression and disease-free survival (DFS) as well as overall survival (OS), others claim the opposite. Expression of AR in TNBC is associated with lower grade, lower proliferation activity and lower disease stage. The lack of AR expression is thus considered to be a factor associated with a higher risk of disease recurrence and development of distant tumour metastases. Taking into account the sensitivity of the tumour to systemic therapy, the use of AR antagonists in clinical practice seems more than promising.

2.6 Immune checkpoint proteins

Physiologically, healthy tissue is protected from damage by its own immunocompetent cells by inducing immune tolerance. It is mediated by cells of the immune system (especially T – lymphocytes, B - lymphocytes, macrophages, dendritic cells), which are able to effectively detect tumour antigens and activate a cellular and humoral antitumour response. A more intense antitumour immune response correlates with longer overall patient survival, period without development of metastases, period without disease relapse and symptom-free interval.

Understanding the mechanism of how tumour cells escape from immune supervision (theory of immunosurveillance) led to the identification of immune checkpoint proteins as potential aims of immunotherapy. The signalling pathway PD1/PD-L1 under normal conditions inhibits the PI3K/Akt and MAP-kinase pathway (Ras/MEK/Er) and leads to the induction of apoptosis and termination of the cell cycle. It also limits the effector function of CD8+ T-lymphocytes in favour of regulatory CD4+ T-lymphocytes. Receptor protein PD-1 is encoded by the gene *PDCD1* on chromosome 2. Its role in the immune system is played by two ligands with co-inhibitive function, protein PD-L1 (CD274) and PD-L2 (CD273). PD-L1 is expressed on the surface of T - and B - lymphocytes, dendritic cells, macrophages, mesenchymal stem cells and mastocytes; PD-L2 is only expressed on the surface of antigen-presenting cells and mastocytes.

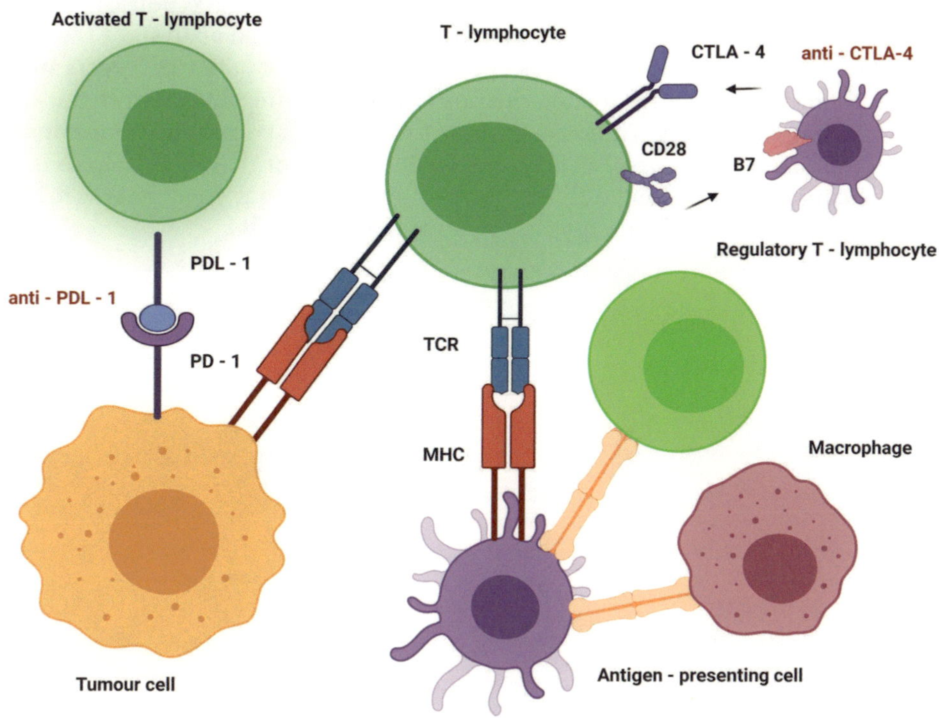

Figure 3.
Immune response to cancer - mechanism of action of PD-1/PD-L1 (Koleckova M, www.biorender.com). The mechanism of PD-1/PD-L1 axis action is based on the controlling of the anti-tumour immune response by the self-tolerance promotion. The activity of PD-1 and its ligand (PD-L1, PD-L2) is involved in the modulation of immune system accompanied by T cell activation, proliferation, cytotoxic secretion and apoptosis. Targeting the PD1 and PDL1 immune checkpoint proteins represents the new era of therapeutic strategy.

The testing of monoclonal antibodies with anti-PD-L1 inhibitory effect and their introduction into clinical practice signified a breakthrough in the treatment of a number of tumours [57–65]. Increased expression of PD-L1 in tumour cells is generally associated with poor disease prognosis. Contrarily, its increased expression by immune system cells (TILs) prolongs overall patient survival. Increased expression was observed in 20% of TNBC cases. Expression of PD – L1 in the tumour and its metastases in the lymph nodes is very heterogeneous and changes in time. Administration of immune checkpoint inhibitors (anti – PD1 - pembrolizumab, anti – PD-L1 - atezolizumab) with cytotoxic drugs is recommended in advanced forms of TNBC. Atezolizumab in combination with nab – paclitaxel has been shown to be effective; cases with increased expression of PD-L1 reported a prolongation of progression-free survival (PFS) from 5 months to 7.5 months and overall survival (OS) from 15.5 months to 25 months. Complete pathological response (pCR) was reached in 51.9% of cases receiving atezolizumab with nab – paclitaxel and carboplatin, and in 64.8% of cases receiving pembrolizumab with nab – paclitaxel and carboplatin (**Figure 3**).

3. Conclusions and future perspectives

The issue of TNBC is still a challenge for many investigators over the world. The current scientific interest is mainly focused on the development of promising therapeutic targets. Due to poor prognosis associated with tumour aggressive biological behaviour, high rates of metastases and unpredictable response to the primary systemic chemotherapy and radiotherapy, the detailed analysis of the mechanisms of TNBC genesis is asked. Identification of new potential targets and the development of specific targeted therapy is pivotal for improvement of the existing clinical outcomes. The knowledge of the crucial participation of immune system in carcinogenesis significantly extended the range of therapeutic options. Ongoing clinical trials testing different types of molecules may pave the way for effective pharmacological synergy and better treatment results.

Author details

Marketa Koleckova[1]*, Katherine Vomackova[2] and Zdenek Kolar[1]

1 Department of Clinical and Molecular Pathology, Faculty of Medicine and Dentistry, Palacky University and University Hospital, Olomouc, Czech Republic

2 Department of Surgery I, Faculty of Medicine and Dentistry, Palacky University and University Hospital, Olomouc, Czech Republic

*Address all correspondence to: m.koleckova@email.cz

References

[1] Yin L, Duan JJ, Bian XW, et al. Triple-negative breast cancer molecular subtyping and treatment progress. Breast Cancer Res. 2020; 22 (1): 61.

[2] Kumar P, Aggarwal R. An overview of triple-negative breast cancer. Arch Gynecol Obstet. 2016; 293 (2): 247-269.

[3] Morris GJ, Naidu S, Tophan AK, et al. Differences in breast carcinoma characteristics in newly diagnosed African-American and Caucasian patients: a single-institution compilation compared with the National Cancer Institute's Surveillance, Epidemiology, and End Results database. Cancer. 2007; 110 (4): 876-884.

[4] Lin NU, Claus E, Sohl J, et al. Sites of distant recurrence and clinical outcomes in patients with metastatic triple-negative breast cancer: high incidence of central nervous system metastases. Cancer. 2008; 113 (10): 2638-2645.

[5] Belli C, Duso BA, Ferraro E, et al. Homologous recombination deficiency in triple negative breast cancer. Breast. 2019; 45: 15-21.

[6] Gluz O, Liedtke C, Gottschalket N, al. Triple-negative breast cancer--current status and future directions. Ann Oncol. 2009; **20** (12): 1913-1927.

[7] Lehmann BD, Bauer JA, Chen X, et al. Identification of human triple-negative breast cancer subtypes and preclinical models for selection of targeted therapies. J Clin Invest. 2011; **121**(7): 2750-2767.

[8] Lehmann BD, Pietenpol JA. Identification and use of biomarkers in treatment strategies for triple-negative breast cancer subtypes. J Pathol. 2014; **232**(2): 142-150.

[9] Ma CX, Luo J, Ellis MJ. Molecular profiling of triple negative breast cancer. Breast Dis. 2010; 32 (1-2): 73-84.

[10] Burstein MD, Tsimelzon A, Poage GM, et al. Comprehensive genomic analysis identifies novel subtypes and targets of triple-negative b reast cancer. Clin Cancer Res. 2015; **21**(7): 1688-1698.

[11] Jézéquel P, Kerdraon O, Hondermarck H, et al. Identification of three subtypes of triple-negative breast cancer with potential therapeutic implications. Breast Cancer Res. 2019; 21(1): 65.

[12] Ahn SG, Kim SJ, Kim C, et al. Molecular Classification of Triple-Negative Breast Cancer. J Breast Cancer. 2016; 19(3): 223-230.

[13] Zeng Z, Hou CJ, Hu QH, et al. Mammography and ultrasound effective features in differentiating basal-like and normal-like subtypes of triple negative breast cancer. Oncotarget. 2017; 8 (45): 79670-79679.

[14] Lokuhetty D, White WA, Watanabe R, et al. Breast Tumours. WHO Classification of Tumours (5 th ed). Lyon: IARC, 2019. ISBN: 978-92-832-4500-1.

[15] Chiang SK, Chang WC, Chen SE, et al. DOCK1 Regulates Growth and Motility through the RRP1B-Claudin-1 Pathway in Claudin-Low Breast Cancer Cells. Cancers (Basel). 2019; 11(11): 1762.

[16] Sun L, Fang J. Epigenetic regulation of epithelial-mesenchymal transition. Cell Mol Life Sci. 2016; 73: 4493-4515.

[17] Zhang Y, Weinberg RA. Epithelial-to-mesenchymal transition in cancer: complexity and opportunities. Front Med. 2018;12(4): 361-373.

[18] Geenen JJJ, Linn SC, Beijnen JH, et al. PARP Inhibitors in the Treatment of Triple-Negative Breast Cancer. Clin Pharmacokinet. 2018; 57(4): 427-437.

[19] Lyons TG. Targeted Therapies for Triple-Negative Breast Cancer. Curr Treat Options Oncol. 2019; 20 (11): 82.

[20] Bergin ART, Loi S. Triple-negative breast cancer: recent treatment advances. F1000Res. 2019; 8: F1000

[21] Fasch Litton JK, Rugo HS, Ettl J, et al. Talazoparib in patients with advanced breast cancer with a germline BRCA mutation. N Engl J Med. 2018; 379(8): 753-763

[22] Loibl S, O'Shaughnessy J, Untch M, et al. Addition of the PARP inhibitor veliparib plus carboplatin or carboplatin alone to standard neoadjuvant chemotherapy in triple-negative breast cancer (BrighTNess): a randomised, phase 3 trial. Lancet Oncol. 2018; 19: 497-509.

[23] Barroso-Sousa R, Keenan TE, Pernas S, et al. Tumor Mutational Burden and PTEN Alterations as Molecular Correlates of Response to PD-1/L1 Blockade in Metastatic Triple-Negative Breast Cancer. Clin Cancer Res 2020; 26 (11): 2565-2572.

[24] Kim S-B, Dent R, Im S-A, et al. Ipatasertib plus paclitaxel versus placebo plus paclitaxel as first-line therapy for metastatic triple-negative breast cancer (LOTUS): a multicentre, randomised, double-blind, placebo-controlled, phase 2 trial. Lancet Oncol. 2017;18(10):1360-1372.

[25] Dent R, Im S-A, Espie M, et al. Overall survival (OS) update of the double-blind placebo (PBO)-controlled randomized phase 2 LOTUS trial of first-line ipatasertib (IPAT) + paclitaxel (PAC) for locally advanced/metastatic triple-negative breast cancer (mTNBC). J Clin Oncol. 2018; 36 (15_suppl,1008).

[26] Khan F, Esnakula A, Ricks-Santi LJ, et al. Loss of PTEN in high grade advanced stage triple negative breast ductal cancers in African American women. Pathol Res Pract. 2018; 214(5): 673-678.

[27] Fasching PA, Loibl S, Hu C, et al. BRCA1/2 Mutations and Bevacizumab in the Neoadjuvant Treatment of Breast Cancer: Response and Prognosis Results in Patients With Triple-Negative Breast Cancer From the Gepar Quinto Study. J Clin Oncol. 2018; 36(22): 2281-2287.

[28] Jacot W, Theillet C, Guiu S, et al. Targeting triple-negative breast cancer and high-grade ovarian carcinoma: refining BRCAness beyond BRCA1/2 mutations? Future Oncol. 2015; 11(4): 557-559.

[29] Jones RA, Robinson TJ, Liu JC, et al. RB1 deficiency in triple-negative breast cancer induces mitochondrial protein translation. J Clin Invest. 2016; 126(10): 3739-3757.

[30] Jones RA, Robinson TJ, Liu JC, et al. RB1 deficiency in triple-negative breast cancer induces mitochondrial protein translation. J Clin Invest. 2016; 126(10): 3739-3757.

[31] Wu Q, Ba-alawi W, Deblois G, et al. GLUT1 inhibition blocks growth of RB1-positive triple negative breast cancer. Nat Commun 2020; 11: 4205.

[32] Zhou Y, Wu C, Lu G, et al. FGF/FGFR signaling pathway involved resistance in various cancer types. J Cancer. 2020; 11(8): 2000-2007.

[33] Sharpe R, Pearson A, Herrera-Abreu MT, et al. FGFR signaling promotes the growth of triple-negative and basal-like breast cancer cell lines both in vitro and in vivo. Clin Cancer Res. 2011; 17 (16): 5275-5286.

[34] Sporikova Z, Koudelakova V, Trojanec R, et al. Genetic Markers in Triple-Negative Breast Cancer. Clin Breast Cancer. 2018; 18(5): e841-e850.

[35] Danzinger S, Tan YY, Rudas M, et al. Differential Claudin 3 and EGFR Expression Predicts BRCA1 Mutation in Triple-Negative Breast Cancer. Cancer Invest. 2018; 36(7): 378-388.

[36] Diluvio G, Del Gaudio F, Giuli MV, et al. NOTCH3 inactivation increases triple negative breast cancer sensitivity to gefitinib by promoting EGFR tyrosine dephosphorylation and its intracellular arrest. Oncogenesis. 2018; 7(5): 42.

[37] Nakai K, Hung MC, Yamaguchi H. A perspective on anti-EGFR therapies targeting triple-negative breast cancer. Am J Cancer Res. 2016; 6(8): 1609-1623.

[38] Nagini S. Breast Cancer: Current Molecular Therapeutic Targets and New Players. Anticancer Agents Med Chem. 2017;17(2):152-163.

[39] Ali AM, Ansari JAK, El-Aziz NMA, Abozeed WN, Warith AMA, Alsaleh K, Nabholtz JM. Triple Negative Breast Cancer: A Tale of Two Decades. Anticancer Agents Med Chem. 2017; 17(4): 491-499.

[40] Radin D, Lippa A, Patel P, Leonardi D. Lifeguard inhibition of Fas-mediated apoptosis: A possible mechanism for explaining the cisplatin resistance of triple-negative breast cancer cells. Biomed Pharmacother. 2016; 77: 161-166.

[41] Song C, Choi S, Oh KB, Sim T. Suppression of TRPM7 enhances TRAIL-induced apoptosis in triple-negative breast cancer cells. J Cell Physiol. 2020; 235(12): 10037-10050.

[42] Bykov VJN, Eriksson SE, Bianchi J, et al. Targeting mutant p53 for efficient cancer therapy. Nat Rev Cancer. 2018; 18(2): 89-102.

[43] Inao T, Iida Y, Moritani T, et al. Bcl-2 inhibition sensitizes triple-negative human breast cancer cells to doxorubicin. Oncotarget. 2018; 9(39): 25545-25556.

[44] Lu L, Dong J, Wang L, et al. Activation of STAT3 and Bcl-2 and reduction of reactive oxygen species (ROS) promote radioresistance in breast cancer and overcome of radioresistance with niclosamide. Oncogene. 2018; 37(39): 5292-5304.

[45] Bouchalova K, Svoboda M, Kharaishvili G, et al. BCL2 is an independent predictor of outcome in basal-like triple-negative breast cancers treated with adjuvant anthracycline-based chemotherapy. Tumour Biol. 2015; 36(6): 4243-4252.

[46] Mathe A, Scott RJ, Avery-Kiejda KA. MiRNAs and Other Epigenetic Changes as Biomarkers in Triple Negative Breast Cancer. Int J Mol Sci. 2015; 16(12): 28347-28376.

[47] Sempere LF. Celebrating 25 Years of MicroRNA Research: From Discovery to Clinical Application. Int J Mol Sci. 2019; 20(8): E1987.

[48] Adhikary J, Chakraborty S, Dalal S, et al. Circular PVT1: an oncogenic non-coding RNA with emerging clinical importace. J Clin Pathol 2019; 72: 513-519.

[49] Nabholtz J, Darvishi B, Farahmand L, et al. Stimuli-Responsive Mesoporous Silica NPs as Non-viral Dual siRNA/Chemotherapy Carriers for Triple Negative Breast Cancer. Mol Ther Nucleic Acids. 2017; 7: 164-180.

[50] Wang Y, Wu S, Zhu X, et al. LncRNA-encoded polypeptide ASRPS inhibits triple-negative breast cancer angiogenesis. J Exp Med. 2020; 217(3): jem.20190950.

[51] Koleckova M, Janikova M, Kolar Z. MicroRNAs in triple-negative breast cancer. Neoplasma. 2018; 65(1):1-13.

[52] Michlewski G, Cáceres JF. Post-transcriptional control of miRNA biogenesis. RNA. 2019; 25(1):1-16.

[53] Wu G, Zhou H, Li D, et al. LncRNA DANCR upregulation induced by TUFT1 promotes malignant progression in triple negative breast cancer via miR-874-3p-SOX2 axis. Exp Cell Res. 2020; 396(2): 112331.

[54] Rampurwala M, Wisinski KB, O'Regan R. Role of the androgen receptor in triple-negative breast cancer. Clin Adv Hematol Oncol. 2016;14(3):186-193.

[55] Lehmann BD, Bauer JA, Schafer JM, et al. PIK3CA mutations in androgen receptor-positive triple negative breast cancer confer sensitivity to the combination of PI3K and androgen receptor inhibitors. Breast Cancer Res. 2014; 16(4): 406.

[56] Gerratanaa L, Basilea D, Buonob G, et al. Androgen receptor in triple negative breast cancer: A potential target for the targetless subtype. Cancer Treatment Reviews 2018; 68: 102-110

[57] Adams S, Schmid P, Rugo HS, et al. Phase 2 study of pembrolizumab (pembro) monotherapy for previously treated metastatic triple-negative breast cancer (mTNBC): KEYNOTE-086 cohort a. J Clin Oncol. 2017;35(15_suppl):1008

[58] Pelekanou V, Carvajal-Hausdorf DE, Altan M, et al. Effect of neoadjuvant chemotherapy on tumor-infiltrating lymphocytes and PD-L1 expression in breast cancer and its clinical significance. Breast Cancer Res. 2017; 19(1): 91.

[59] Denkert C, Wienert S, Poterie A, et al. Standardized evaluation of tumor-infiltrating lymphocytes in breast cancer: results of the ring studies of the international immuno-oncology biomarker working group. Mod Pathol. 2016; 29(10): 1155-1164.

[60] Ganesan A, Ahmed M, Okoye I, et al. Comprehensive in vitro characterization of PD-L1 small molecule inhibitors. Sci Rep. 2019; 9(1): 12392.

[61] Wu Y, Chen W, Xu ZP, et al. PD-L1 Distribution and Perspective for Cancer Immunotherapy-Blockade, Knockdown, or Inhibition. Front Immunol. 2019; 10: 2022.

[62] García-Teijido P, Luque Cabal M, Peláez Ferandéz I, et al. Tumor-infiltrating lymhocytes in triple negative breast cancer: The future of immune targeting. Clinical Medicine Insights: Oncology 2016; 10: 31-39

[63] Huang W, Ran R, Shao B, et al. Prognostic and clinicopathological value of PD-L1 expression in primary breast cancer: a meta-analysis. Breast Cancer Res Treat. 2019; 178(1): 17-33.

[64] Mittendorf EA, Philips AV, Meric-Bernstam F, et al. PD-L1 expression intriple-negative breast cancer. Cancer Immunol Res. 2014; 2(4): 361-370.

[65] Li M, Li A, Zhou S, et al. Heterogeneity of PD-L1 expression in primary tumors and paired lymph node metastases of triple negative breast cancer. BMC Cancer. 2018; 18(1): 4.

Section 3

Breast Cancer *In vitro* Models

Chapter 4

In vitro Approaches to Model Breast Tumor Complexity

Heizel Rosado-Galindo, Lyanne Suarez and Maribella Domenech

Abstract

Cell culture technologies have provided biomedical researchers with fast and accessible tools to probe the breast tumor microenvironment. Exponential progress in fabrication methods combined with multiparametric approaches have enabled the development of cell culture model systems with enhanced biological complexity to identify key aspects that regulate breast cancer (BC) progression and therapeutic response. Yet, the culture parameters and conditions employed influence the behavior of tumor cells, thereby affecting its tissue biomimetic capabilities. In this chapter we review the wide range of culture platforms employed for the generation of breast tumor models and summarize their biomimetic capabilities, advantages, disadvantages and specific applications.

Keywords: culture platforms, microfluidics, organoids, 3D bioprinting, tumor microenvironment, co-culture

1. Introduction

Cell culture is an integral tool in biomedical research. It refers to the removal of cells from tissues or organs, into an artificial *in vitro* environment. The cells may be directly removed from the tissue before culturing, or they may be derived from a previously established cell line [1, 2]. Among their many applications, *in vitro* cell culture models allow for the evaluation of the physiology and biochemistry of cells; the study of mutagenesis and carcinogenesis; and drug research and development [1–3]. Furthermore, *in vitro* models provide a faster and more cost-effective alternative to *in vivo* animal models, while also allowing researchers to control and alter the cellular microenvironment.

Breast tumors are complex systems, composed of different cell subpopulations with distinct tumorigenic capabilities within the tumor. *In vitro* cell culture models have been one of the basic techniques utilized in BC research. Despite the many advances in the field, there is still a need for suitable tumor models that can accurately mimic the disease. Two-dimensional (2D) culture models have been commonly used in BC studies over the years. These have provided valuable insight about the molecular mechanisms involved in the pathology of the disease, yet 2D models are not able to properly model BC complexities [4]. Similarly, animal models require specialized animal facilities, are expensive, laborious, along with the consideration of pharmaco-and toxicokinetic differences between animal and humans which can make results unreliable [5]. Hence, the development of tumor models that can mimic to some extent the complexity present in the tumor microenvironment (TME) is imperative.

The TME is heterogeneous and plays a significant role in tumor development, progression and metastasis [6]. It is composed of multiple cell types such as fibroblasts, myoepithelial and endothelial cells, infiltrated immune cells (e.g., T cells, macrophages), adipocytes and mesenchymal stem cells (MSC), along with the extracellular matrix (ECM) and soluble factors [7, 8]. These cell types are important for modeling the disease as it has been shown that tumor prognosis is not solely based on the tumorigenic cells, but also on how those cells communicate with their environment [9]. For example, cancer associated fibroblasts (CAFs) have been demonstrated to promote cancer cell aggressiveness and survival by the secretion of growth factors and cytokines and the creation of a "protective niche" against drugs [8, 10, 11]. Similarly, immune cells promote angiogenesis [12], immunosuppression, invasion and metastasis [13, 14]. Furthermore, adipocytes and MSCs have been shown to be involved in the secretion of factors related to matrix remodeling, invasion and survival of the tumor [15, 16]. Thereby, models that include multiple cell types are likely to be more mimetic of the pathology and predictive of responses in tissues. As such, custom microscale platforms have been developed to accommodate multiple cell types in spatially defined patterns and locations to enable examination of multi-cell type interactions. Such models include those related to angiogenesis and metastatic processes [17–19], and due to the lack of spatial control it would have been difficult to recreate such interactions in traditional culture platforms highlighting the applicability of custom platforms for multi-cell type interactions.

The identification of relevant parameters from the tumor microenvironment is imperative for proper assessment and predictability of efficacy of experimental therapies. For this reason, 3D cell culture systems have become more popular due to its potential to better mimic the complexity of the TME and thereby increase the physiological relevance of the study [20, 21]. This modality incorporates scaffolds and 3D cell constructs that have been shown to impact cell proliferation, morphology, signaling and drug resistance in a more physiologically relevant manner [22–25].

Mimicking BC complexity is challenging, however, progress in microfabrication techniques, tissue engineering and cancer biology have paved the way to more sophisticated models with enhanced biomimetic capabilities that will help to elucidate the intricate nature of BC. In this chapter, we discuss the wide range of culture platforms employed for the generation of breast tumor models and summarize their biomimetic capabilities, advantages, disadvantages and specific applications.

2. Cell culture modalities

2.1 Two-dimensional and three-dimensional culture

The traditional cell culture methods for studying breast cancer employ two-dimensional monolayer cultures, where cells grow flat on a surface. Two-dimensional culture is still widely used, but with advances in microfabrication now surfaces can be modified with nanostructure topographies and different levels of stiffness to mimic to some extent the physical properties of the matrix surface. These topographies (e.g., roughness, surface geometry) have the capability of providing biomimetic surfaces that have been shown to modify the morphology, proliferation and signaling, among others, of cells [26]. Similarly, changes in the mechanical properties of the ECM (e.g., stiffness) are related to increasing malignant phenotype [27], cancer progression, signaling [28–30] and drug sensitivity [31]. Despite these technological advances in 2D cultures, multiple studies have shown that cell cultures in 2D felt short to mimic cell phenotypes associated with disease progress such as cell invasion, cell function and expression of pathological markers [4, 23, 32]. In some cases, utilizing 2D culture systems has resulted in the loss of essential cell signaling pathways, hence limiting the ability to fully evaluate cell–cell and cell-ECM interactions [33]. Evidence has also shown that there are inconsistencies when comparing cell morphology, receptor expression, and polarity between cells grown in 2D and the *in vivo* setting [34].

In order to bridge this gap in biological complexity, multiple methods employing 3D cell culture systems have emerged and continue to be steadily improving, aiming to produce the most *in vivo*-like structures. Essentially, 3D models can be divided into two groups: cell aggregates (spheroids) and biomaterial constructs [35]. The most basic 3D culture models use scaffolds of synthetic (e.g., polydimethylsiloxane-PDMS, polylactic acid-PLA) and natural (e.g., collagen, Matrigel®, hydrogels) biomaterials to investigate the effect of ECM properties on cancer behavior. Spheroids have been used mostly for drug screening applications since it has been demonstrated they more closely resemble the *in vivo* environment [36]. Growing BC cells in 3D has also revealed a more realistic drug response [21, 37], cell proliferation and morphology [38], and better representation of tumor heterotypic phenotype and TME [39, 40]. For example, single-cell RNA sequencing of breast cancer spheroids have uncovered cell clusters with specific functions (e.g., proliferation, invasion) that provide evidence of the heterotypic nature and complexity of breast tumors [41]. **Figure 1** below depicts the main *in vitro* 2D and 3D culture modalities along with the most predominant co-culture models (discussed in the next subsection) to study cell crosstalk.

2.2 Co-culture

Cancer is a heterogeneous disease and even though there have been various advances in cell culture modalities, thorough comprehension of the crosstalk between cancer and non-cancer cells is still not fully understood [42]. Co-culture and multi-culture models have been long established as appropriate tools for

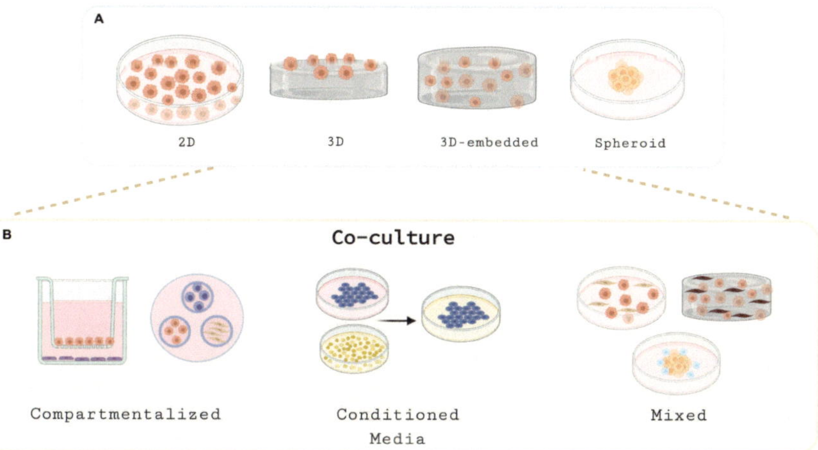

Figure 1.
In vitro *culture modalities. A) Cells can be cultured* in vitro *as 2D monolayers, over a 3D scaffold (synthetic or natural material), embedded into a scaffold material or as spheroid constructs. B) Yet, co-culture and multi-culture models are implemented in order to better understand tumor-stroma interactions and cross-talk. The three main co-culture modalities used are compartmentalized, conditioned media and mixed, which incorporate cells cultured in 2D monolayers, 3D scaffolds or spheroids. Created with BioRender.com*

evaluating breast cancer heterotypic interactions *in vitro* [6]. Co-culture refers to the culturing of two different cell lines, while multi-culture models involve three or more different cells. Historically, co-culture models have been the predominant approach in research. However, despite their ability to identify factors mediating cancer and stromal interactions, co-culture models are deficient in incorporating microenvironment structure, dimensionality, and functional response [42]. With the hopes of bridging the gap between *in vitro* and *in vivo* studies, new research has been moving away from the study of only two cell types, to studying multi-cell type systems. This type of model permits researchers to control and evaluate the influence of each cell culture component. It also allows the study of important cell–cell heterotypic signals, which would be impossible to study with a 2-cell type model [43].

There have been an increasing number of studies looking to compare tri-culture models with the more traditional mono-culture or co-culture methods. With the intention of better understanding the bone microenvironment, Pagani *et al.* compared a tri-culture model of osteoblasts, osteoclasts, and endothelial cells; to single and co-cultures. The results demonstrated that the behavior of the three cell types cultured together was very different from the single or the co-culture model, in terms of proliferation, activity, and viability. These results correlate with previously established data regarding their behavior *in vivo* [44]. Regier *et al.* evaluated how increased model complexity would affect gene expression. The results demonstrated that gene expression changes based on the type of model utilized; suggesting how tumor and stromal cells would respond to microenvironments of increased complexity *in vivo* [42]. Loy *et al.* investigated the effect a tri-culture model would have on angiogenesis and compared it to simpler models. The results showed that the tri-culture model promoted cell-matrix remodeling and early expression of elastic fiber-related proteins. It also reiterated the significance of multi-culture methods since culturing with fibroblasts, endothelial cells, and smooth muscle cells was required to obtain tissues with appropriate physiological-like properties [45]. All three of these studies highlight the increasing need and importance of more complex heterotypic cultures.

Co-culture models involve a cell growing arrangement, where two or more different cells are cultured with some amount of contact between them [46]. The communication between the cells may be bi-directional or multi-dimensional, and it can happen at the macro-scale or at the micro-scale [47]. The method of choice should be dependent on what is the focus of each individual study and can be grouped in: compartmentalized, conditioned media and mixed culture.

2.2.1 Compartmentalized

The segregated or compartmentalized model consists of two or more physically separated cells, cultured in a shared environment [6]. This type of culture is preferred when studying paracrine interactions of cells that are not located in close proximity in tissues. Also, this method is useful to identify target cells based on soluble factor signaling since the cells individual response can be examined, facilitating the identification of factors that may play a role in tumor growth and advancement. In compartmentalized co-cultures, one cell population is seeded in the bottom of the standard well, and the other is seeded on a top insert or in an adjacent compartment. By doing this, the cell types remain separated, while still being able to exchange soluble signals in their shared environment [48]. Indirect cell culture eliminates heterotypic interactions mediated by contact between the cell types, which can be seen in direct cell culture. It also allows for cell type specific readouts, which are unachievable in direct cell culture [6]. Such method has provided evidence on genes involved behind stromal invasiveness and metastasis, and the crucial role of fibroblasts in proliferation of estrogen-dependent human breast carcinomas [6, 49, 50]. Gonzalez *et al.* utilized a 2D indirect co-culture method with human BC cells and human umbilical vein endothelial cells to evaluate the process behind angiogenesis; concluding that melatonin may be an alternative for preventing tumor angiogenesis [51]. While Chiovaro *et al.* analyzed the role of ECM proteins in bone metastasis, showing that tenascin-W promotes cancer cell migration and proliferation [52].

If multiple cells need to be examined, co-culture platforms, such as transwells, are not useful since they are limited to only two compartments. Hence, the use of customizable culture systems such as microscale devices, is warranted [6]. Our group developed compartmentalized microwell culture platforms, in which we show the contribution of multiple cell types to the sensitivity to heat therapy in tumor cells [43]. The data shown indicates that the presence of macrophages and fibroblasts had a significant protective effect against heat stress in BC cells, thus, perturbing the effectiveness of heat therapy. Others have employed multi-cell type cultures to deconvolute cell communication of metastatic breast tumors. Regier *et al.* developed a compartmentalized multi-culture method, utilizing BC epithelial cells, bone marrow cells, and human monocytes. The platform allowed the creation of a substantial dataset made up of cell specific gene expression patterns. This was possible by collecting data from an individual cell type, while communicating through paracrine interactions in a heterotypic culture. The study also compared tri-culture to mono-culture and co-culture, which led to the demonstration of how stromal and tumor cells respond differently based on the complexity of the micro-environment [42]. This reiterates the importance of utilizing multi-cultures versus the more traditional co-cultures. A drawback with this method is that physical contact between cells cannot be completely prevented in the long term [47]. In addition, because cell-seeding sometimes requires more than one step, the process may be considered somewhat complicated and time-consuming [6].

2.2.2 Conditioned media

Conditioned media transfer utilizes two separately cultured cell populations, where one culture medium is utilized to nourish the other [48]. This type of method is simple and allows one-way signaling from effector to responder [6]. The advantage of utilizing this method is that conditioned media can be profiled for the identification of secreted soluble factor-related effects is possible [47]. Consequently, the role of signaling molecules could be tested in a specific response [6]. Also, this method is useful when the cells of interest cannot be cultured together such as studies involving tumor cells and microbes [53]. However, when employing multiple cell types, the method becomes a bit more complex since identification of the secretor and recipient cells can be complicated. Additionally, when this type of method is utilized, there is no cross-communication within the cells and it is not possible to study bi-directional signals [48]. For this reason, this type of method would not be ideal if the goal is to study multi-cell type interactions that naturally occur in the *in vivo* tumor environment.

2.2.3 Mixed co-culture

In mixed cell culture, different types of cells are cultured together. Just as with conditioned media transfer, this type of method is accessible and simple. It can be done in 2D or 3D using traditional well plates [6]. If the cells are cultured together in a standard plate, the method is referred to as direct or mixed cell culture.

However, if a transwell insert or adjacent compartments are utilized, the method is denoted as indirect or compartmentalized cell culture. Unlike the conditioned media method, mixed co-culture does allow for bi-directional paracrine and juxtacrine signaling, which is of great importance when studying multi-cell type interactions in breast cancer [6]. Because of the cellular arrangement, this method is also ideal for studying how cell–cell contact affects cell behavior [54]. When performing multi-cell type studies, the direct method simply requires the inclusion of the additional cell lines mixed.

Mixed co-culture experiments shed light on distinct microenvironment features based on cancer subtype; and potential mechanisms behind invasive phenotypes [55, 56]. Camp *et al.* compared the interaction of fibroblasts with the basal-like subtype versus the luminal subtype. The results were increased migration and expression of interleukins in the basal-like BC cell lines, which reiterates the important role of the TME in cancer progression [10]. Buess *et al.* also looked into evaluating the role of aspects of the TME by studying tumor-endothelial interactions and determining gene expression changes [56]. Multiple other studies have been done utilizing these culture modalities and have provided insight into further understanding the disease [6]. Yet, a disadvantage of this method is the lack of control of the spatial location of cells which can be important when examining and quantifying changes in some tumor cell behaviors such as cell migration and invasion. Also, single cell studies will require multiple cell separation steps that will make this method more time consuming and increase the number of cells needed for analysis due to cell loss during sample handling.

3. Culture platforms for enhanced biomimetic capabilities

Despite the development and application of the aforementioned cell culture methods, thorough understanding of cancer development and progression continues to be a challenge. As shown in **Figure 2**, *in vitro* cell models are mainly categorized in 2D and 3D (as discussed before) and thus, these models become more complex as research continues to be centered on creating experimental models that can mimic cell evolution on the bench with the goal of understanding the biology of the disease and identifying key therapeutic targets. Despite the advances that came with the implementation of 3D multi-culture systems, there still remains a scarcity of models that can recreate the biological complexity of the tumor microenvironment. Biomimetics can be defined as technology that utilizes or emulates tissue function with the intention of improving human lives [57]. Effective biomimetic models need to contribute a 3D environment permissive of cell phenotypic stages while enabling multi-cell type interactions [58]. As cell culture methods continue to evolve, innovative approaches are being created with the hopes of overcoming the limitations of the more traditional methods. **Table 1** summarizes the advantages, disadvantages and applications of advanced biomimetic *in vitro* 3D culture technologies.

3.1 Microfluidics

Microfluidic platforms can be utilized to scale down the traditional culture modalities, yet they enable to customize the culture environments to examine more complex interactions [64]. This technology employs microsystems that allow the manipulation of small fluid volumes and control over the spatial location of cell clusters [70]. Its application to improve 3D cell culture models has been increasing since 2012, particularly in BC research [71]. In comparison to macroscopic culture,

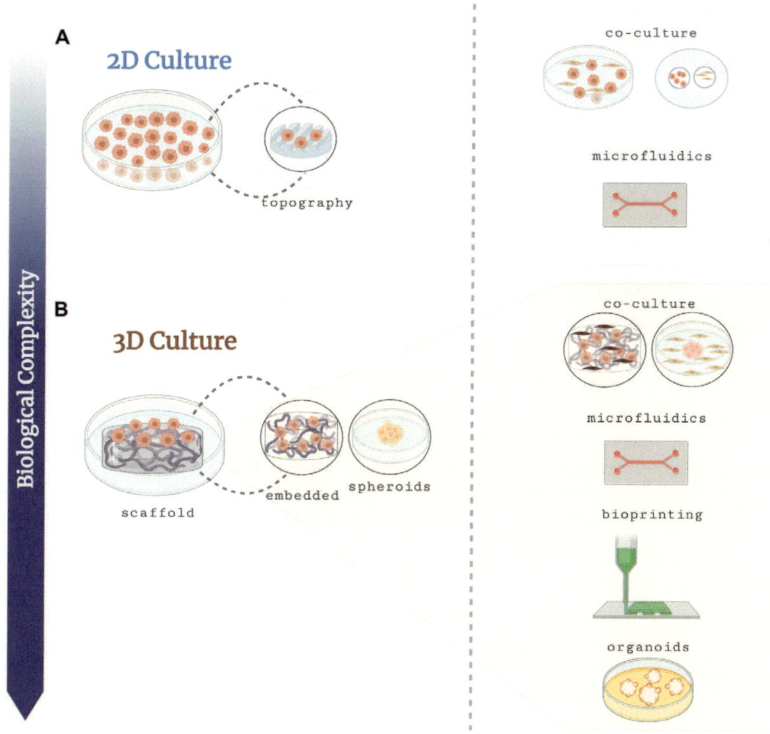

Figure 2.
Culture platforms employed in breast cancer models. A) Simple 2D platforms consist of cells cultured in flat, nano- or micro- structured substrates (left) that mimic to some extent tissue topography; or they can combine co-culture and microfluidic devices (right) to increase the complexity of the model and better resemble tumor-stroma interactions. B) In three-dimensional models, cells are culture in scaffolds and constructs that further imitate the architecture of the tumor (left). Co-culture and advanced 3D models such as microfluidics, bioprinting and organoids are capable of duplicating the TME and provide physiologically relevant insights about the disease (right). Created with BioRender.com

microfluidic cell culture models have several significant advantages that, when employed, lead towards better biomimetic models. Firstly, cells may be cultured in a spatially controlled environment by controlling fluid patterns and proximity across culture compartments [72–77]. This technology permits the combination of multiple cell types and to control cell patterning, to recapitulate to some extent tissue observations. For example, microfluidic devices permit the study of angiogenesis while also allowing the study of endothelial migration and evaluation of cell response in co-culture [71, 78]. Also, microfluidics can implement continuous perfusion conditions, and controlled gradients, which are both characteristics that also resemble the cancerous *in vivo* environment more closely. Gradients are found in angiogenesis, invasion, and migration whereas perfusion is crucial in vasculature and cell extravasation as well for nutrient replenishment. Finally, microfluidic systems enable high-throughput arrays and pose lower contamination risk and reagent consumption which make them very appealing for studies with limited cell samples such as those that employ patient-derived tissues [70, 71].

Recent studies in microfluidic systems have highlighted their capability to recreate and profile some of the biological complexity of the tumor microenvironment. Such studies have revealed important information regarding the processes involved in metastasis and how the tumor microenvironment contributes. For example, single cell RNA sequencing using microfluidic devices have revealed the diversity of the breast epithelium, which sheds light about early tumorigenesis and tumor progression [79, 80]. In addition, microfluidic devices pose as an advantage

Model	Advantages	Disadvantages	Application	Ref.
3D Microfluidics	Small size samples, spatial and temporal control, reduced reagent volumes, controlled gradients, high-throughput	Mechanical stress, complicated set-ups, material fabrication	Invasion, metastasis, vasculature, modeling TME	[20, 37, 59, 60]
Bioreactors	Long term culture, effective nutrient distribution, large scale	Contamination risk, expensive, specialized equipment, low throughput, limited spatial resolution, high cell numbers needed	Metastasis, drug discovery	[61–63]
3D bioprinting	Controlled spatial arrangement of cells and matrix, biomolecular gradients, high-throughput	Lower cell viability, material challenges, lack of standardized methods, high cell numbers needed	Migration, angiogenesis, drug discovery, modeling TME	[64–66]
Organoids	Small size samples, retain parental tumor phenotype, can be preserved as biobanks, mimetic of tissue function	Lack of standardized methods, heterogeneous cell samples, high variability across replicates	Drug discovery, invasion, metastasis	[67–69]

Table 1.
Comparison of in vitro *3D BC models.*

to personalized medicine by aiding in the selection of appropriate pharmacologic agents. In this regard, Lanz *et al.* developed a 3D microfluidic device, OrganoPlate®, to be utilized for therapy selection. They showed that MDA-MB-231 (cell line isolated at MD Anderson from a pleural effusion of a 51-year old Caucasian woman) cells embedded in Matrigel® became more sensitive to the drug, thus confirming along with previous studies that drug response is tuned by the ECM. The results were promising and even though further validation is warranted, it appears to be a fine tool for pharmacologic selection and response prediction [37]. Similarly, Yildiz-Ozturk *et al.* studied the cytotoxicity of carnosic acid and doxorubicin on MCF-7 and MDA-MB-231 BC cell lines and demonstrated the importance of biomimicry in *in vitro* platforms [20]. A breast metastatic microfluidic model was developed by Kong *et al.* to mimic the metastasis of circulating breast cancer cells (CBCCs) to the lung and other organs. Their microfluidic device allowed the flow of CBCCs over primary cell culture chambers, which would have been impossible with static conditions. They demonstrated that the metastatic potential of these cell lines was in concordance with animal models, providing a cost-effective and time-saving alternative [81]. Bersini *et al.* also developed a microfluidic co-culture model made up of metastatic BC cells, and collagen gel-embedded bone marrow-derived stem cells (hBM-MSC) lined with endothelial cells to create an osteo-conditioned microenvironment and access extravasation and micrometastases to bone tissue [59]. They found that BC receptors CXCR2 and bone-secreted chemokine CXCL5 play major roles in the extravasation process. However, due to the complexity of the design, their platform is not high throughput compatible, which adds many challenges, particularly to obtain multiple replicates in a short time. Also, in general it is important to notice that most of the organ on chip microfluidic platforms focus on the metastatic stage of the disease, leaving an evident need for research focusing on the early stages of breast cancer. Yet, some efforts are being done to overcome this gap. As an example, Choi *et al.* developed a compartmentalized microfluidic device that enabled co-culture of tumor spheroids and normal mammary epithelial cells in close proximity to fibroblasts, with the goal of providing a model that allows researchers to closely examine the mechanistic progression of early-stage breast ductal carcinoma *in situ* (DCIS) [82].

Even though microfluidic devices have given the opportunity to better replicate the tumor environment, there are still some caveats to its use. Silicone-based devices have been shown to sequester small hydrophobic molecules, which can compromise the results of some studies [70], yet researchers have been addressing this by modifying the material to make it more hydrophilic and reduce molecule sequestration [60]. Also, microfluidic devices in some cases can induce mechanical stress to the cells [83], which can modulate cell responses in an unpredictable manner, and are often limited by complicated set-ups [70], which limits their broad adoption by the scientific and clinical community. As such, simpler fabrication methods and commercial availability of customizable microscale platforms is desirable to overcome such limitations.

3.2 Bioreactors

Despite the numerous advantages of the aforementioned 3D culture methods, the duration of culture and nutrient availability can be a limitation in static cultures particularly to enable observations that occur in cells over periods of several weeks. In this case, perfusive systems, such as bioreactors, are more appropriate. A bioreactor is a canister that allows the 3D culture of cell clusters for extended periods of time. It is coupled to sensors and actuator components allowing for the controlled delivery of oxygen, nutrients and other parameters [84]. Goliwas *et al.* developed a perfused 3D BC surrogate model utilizing a bioreactor system that incorporated breast carcinoma epithelial cells and stromal fibroblasts into an extracellular matrix. The study demonstrated that using a bioreactor allowed for analysis of longer growth periods and a greater degree of growth when compared to solid models [85]. Bioreactors have also been utilized to study metastatic progression of breast cancer, and as potential drug development platforms for cancer treatment. Krishnan *et al.* utilized a compartmentalized bioreactor model, with osteoblasts and metastatic BC cells, to study the colonization of osteoblastic tissue. In their design, cultured osteoblasts were monitored over longer periods and exhibited more *in vivo*-like characteristics, compared to 2D cell cultures [86]. Marshall *et al.* developed a physiologically relevant bioreactor system that could be potentially used for pharmacologic development. Their construct was capable of supporting and perfusing larger volume, which poses as an advantage to lab-on-a-chip systems [62]. Other studies have also used bioreactors to assess drug response of BC tissue [63, 87]. Despite bioreactors being an ideal option for cultures that require long-term analysis, there are some factors that might damper their use. Membrane bioreactors may become contaminated and multilayer cell growth may cause transfer limitations [88]. Also, its complex composition and dimensionality limits their implementation in convectional labs and limits the number of experimental replicates [89].

3.3 Three-dimensional (3D) bioprinting

Another technology that has emerged in recent years and that is being applied to 3D culture technology is 3D bioprinting. Its development has been possible thanks to advances in 3D printing technology, biomaterials and tissue engineering methods. Three-dimensional (3D) bioprinting consists of printing cells together with ECM components, biomaterials and bioactive factors [90]. It has been shown that bioprinting techniques can be used to generate 3D tumor models that can better resemble the TME [90, 91]. This has been achieved as bioprinting provides the ability of controlling the spatial arrangement of cells, creating biomolecular gradients and well-organized vessel-like structures (vasculature) within a micron scale resolution [92, 93]. Therefore, bioprinted tumor models are used for angiogenesis, migration and drug development and screening studies as well as TME models [65, 94]. Although 3D bioprinting is widely used in tumor research, very few studies use bioprinted models for BC. Yet, most of these studies are focused on BC metastasis and drug resistance. A study performed by Zhou *et al.* evaluated the interaction between triple negative breast cancer cells (TNBC) and osteoblasts to assess metastatic progression in bone. They found that osteoblasts increased VEGF secretion and therefore, enhanced the proliferation of BC cells, while osteoblast proliferation was inhibited [58]. Bioprinted BC models have also been used for drug resistance studies. Swaminathan *et al.* bioprinted pre-formed MDA-MB-231 spheroids along with breast epithelial cells and vascular endothelial cells and evaluated plaxitacel chemoresistance in mono and co-culture. They demonstrated that bioprinted spheroids are more resistant to plaxitacel as it has been shown before in other studies. Yet, this resistance was decreased in co-culture with vascular endothelial cells highlighting the importance of replicating the TME complexities *in vitro* [95]. Another study by Duan *et al.* examined drug resistance using 3D bioprinted constructs of BC cells and adipose-derived mesenchymal stem cells (ADMSC). They found increased chemoresistance in BC cells cultured with ADMSC in comparison to monoculture and, thus provided a model to better understand the role of ADMSC in BC progression [66]. Likewise, Campbell et al. bioprinted MCF-7 cancer cells and showed higher resistance to Tamoxifen compared to monolayer culture, providing a more biological-like behavior [66, 96]. Despite the flexibility of 3D bioprinting systems, there are some challenges that need to be overcome to ease its application. Maintaining high viability and original phenotype is an issue in some bioprinting techniques due to exposure of cells to shear stress. Therefore, close control of bioink viscosities, extrusion rates, among other parameters, is imperative [97]. Also, lack of process standardization and guidelines pose another challenge for study comparison and reproducibility.

3.4 Organoids

The most recent 3D cell culture modality are organoids. These are 3D heterotypic *in vitro* tissue constructs, derived either from primary tissue or stem cells, that have the ability to mimic the *in vivo* organ [98, 99]. Historically, established cancer cell lines have been widely utilized as single cell models of the cancer disease. However, their use has several drawbacks in terms of their capability to mimic the pathology of the patient. Cell lines can undergo genetic changes, losing the genetic heterogeneity of the original tumor [100]. Organoids also possess substantial similarities to cancer cell lines 3D models (spheroids) such as cell–cell and cell-matrix interactions, gradients of nutrients, oxygen and metabolites, and can be replaced from frozen supplies with ease. They are also relatively easy to handle and can be grown in infinite quantities [101]. Yet, the main characteristic of organoids is their capability to closely resemble and retain the pathology of the parental tumor over several rounds of expansion *in vitro* [102, 103]. They also have shown therapeutic predictability for some drugs and can be preserved as biobanks and expanded, which allows extended incubation [98, 99]. Given the number of mutational processes involved in cancer development and progression, being able to study tumorigenesis in depth is crucial. Organoids allow for organ-specific mutations to be analyzed and their whole genomes to be sequenced. Intratumor heterogeneity can also be analyzed by growing organoids from separate sections of the same tumor [100]. Another area where organoids can play a major role is drug development. Organoids appear to be much better models for identifying and testing anticancer drugs yet in a patient specific manner. For instance, studies on single cell transcriptomics of organoids have detected differences in drug sensitivity, proving that organoids maintain tumor heterogeneity, which is considered a critical aspect of tumor models [104].

Studies with BC organoids are limited, since this modality has just started to be explored. However, they have gained more popularity in the last few years. Cheung *et al.* used breast carcinoma organoids to understand tumor invasiveness and metastasis. They found that the heterotypic interactions between epithelial subgroups are key to collective invasion [105]. Broutier *et al.* was able to demonstrate that liver cancer derived organoids could be utilized for drug screening testing and identification of potential pharmacologic targets [68]. Sachs *et al.* demonstrated the biomimetic nature of organoids by demonstrating the reflecting histopathology of *in vivo* tumors, as well as HER2 and hormone receptor status. Moreover, drug screening tests were consistent with patient response [69]. These promising findings suggest that organoids will be an ideal alternative model for cancer research. Nonetheless, successfully cultivating patient organoids from biopsy specimens is still a challenge mainly due to low cell recovery and heterogeneity of collected samples, and limited availability of standardized methods [103, 105].

4. Concluding remarks

Breast cancer is an evolutionary disease and cell culture modalities should continue to evolve concomitantly. Even though traditional 2D co-culture methods have provided valuable insights on disease development and progression, there is a need for more heterotypic biomimetic models that can replicate the tumor environment more closely. Some of the consequences of limited biomimetic models has been the large number of investigational drugs that never make it past clinical trials and the lack of clear understanding on the foundations of breast cancer malignant transformation. Aside from the need for more biomimetic models, most of the current research has been focused on the metastatic stage of the disease. Even though understanding tumor progression and the role of its microenvironment is of utmost importance, understanding the early and localized stages of breast cancer is also imperative. Not having an explicit grasp on the biological processes behind progression from early stage to invasive to metastasis has hindered the ability to make a predictive diagnosis in patients with early disease that have a greater probability of invasive cancer progression. Hence, designing new targeted pharmacologic agents becomes a challenge. Despite the continuous development of innovative cell culture modalities, there are still many unanswered questions. However, the hope is that with the emergence of the new methods (bioreactors, organoids, etc.), many of these questions can be interrogated in a controlled and user friendly cell culture environment.

Acknowledgements

This publication was supported by the National Institute of General Medical Sciences of the National Institutes of Health under award number SC1 GM131967 and partial support from the Puerto Rico Idea Network for Biomedical Research Excellence (PR-INBRE) under Grant No. P20-GM103475.

Conflict of interest

The authors declare no conflict of interest.

Author details

Heizel Rosado-Galindo[1], Lyanne Suarez[1] and Maribella Domenech[1,2*]

1 Bioengineering Graduate Program, University of Puerto Rico, Mayaguez, Puerto Rico, United States

2 Department of Chemical Engineering, University of Puerto Rico, Mayaguez, Puerto Rico, United States

*Address all correspondence to: maribella.domenech@upr.edu

References

[1] M. Arora, "Cell Culture Media: A Review," *Materials and Methods*, vol. 3. 2013, doi: 10.13070/mm.en.3.175.

[2] "Animal tissue culture principles and applications." https://paperpile.com/app/p/cdc4fc9e-d3fa-05a3-a615-4767c5f44774 (accessed Jan. 11, 2021).

[3] D. Antoni, H. Burckel, E. Josset, and G. Noel, "Three-dimensional cell culture: a breakthrough in vivo," *Int. J. Mol. Sci.*, vol. 16, no. 3, pp. 5517-5527, Mar. 2015.

[4] S. Breslin and L. O'Driscoll, "The relevance of using 3D cell cultures, in addition to 2D monolayer cultures, when evaluating breast cancer drug sensitivity and resistance," *Oncotarget*, vol. 7, no. 29, pp. 45745-45756, Jul. 2016.

[5] "Thoughts on limitations of animal models." https://paperpile.com/app/p/fa8e2678-e93f-006a-ab90-0534c3b2b38b (accessed Jan. 12, 2021).

[6] M. C. Regier, E. T. Alarid, and D. J. Beebe, "Progress towards understanding heterotypic interactions in multi-culture models of breast cancer," *Integr. Biol.* , vol. 8, no. 6, pp. 684-692, Jun. 2016.

[7] S. D. Soysal, A. Tzankov, and S. E. Muenst, "Role of the Tumor Microenvironment in Breast Cancer," *PAT*, vol. 82, no. 3-4, pp. 142-152, 2015, Accessed: Feb. 01, 2021. [Online].

[8] J. Plava, M. Cihova, M. Burikova, M. Matuskova, L. Kucerova, and S. Miklikova, "Recent advances in understanding tumor stroma-mediated chemoresistance in breast cancer," *Mol. Cancer*, vol. 18, no. 1, p. 67, Mar. 2019.

[9] N. A. Bhowmick and H. L. Moses, "Tumor-stroma interactions," *Curr. Opin. Genet. Dev.*, vol. 15, no. 1, pp. 97-101, Feb. 2005.

[10] J. T. Camp *et al.*, "Interactions with fibroblasts are distinct in Basal-like and luminal breast cancers," *Mol. Cancer Res.*, vol. 9, no. 1, pp. 3-13, Jan. 2011.

[11] R. Straussman *et al.*, "Tumour micro-environment elicits innate resistance to RAF inhibitors through HGF secretion," *Nature*, vol. 487, no. 7408, pp. 500-504, Jul. 2012.

[12] R. D. Leek, C. E. Lewis, R. Whitehouse, M. Greenall, J. Clarke, and A. L. Harris, "Association of macrophage infiltration with angiogenesis and prognosis in invasive breast carcinoma," *Cancer Res.*, vol. 56, no. 20, pp. 4625-4629, Oct. 1996.

[13] W. Tan *et al.*, "Tumour-infiltrating regulatory T cells stimulate mammary cancer metastasis through RANKL-RANK signalling," *Nature*, vol. 470, no. 7335, pp. 548-553, Feb. 2011.

[14] M. Yang *et al.*, "Microvesicles secreted by macrophages shuttle invasion-potentiating microRNAs into breast cancer cells," *Mol. Cancer*, vol. 10, p. 117, Sep. 2011.

[15] Y. Xiong *et al.*, "Hematopoietic stem cell-derived adipocytes and fibroblasts in the tumor microenvironment," *World J. Stem Cells*, vol. 7, no. 2, pp. 253-265, Mar. 2015.

[16] K. M. Bussard, L. Mutkus, K. Stumpf, C. Gomez-Manzano, and F. C. Marini, "Tumor-associated stromal cells as key contributors to the tumor microenvironment," *Breast Cancer Res.*, vol. 18, no. 1, p. 84, Aug. 2016.

[17] A. Amann *et al.*, "Development of a 3D angiogenesis model to study tumour – endothelial cell interactions and the effects of anti-angiogenic drugs," *Scientific Reports*, vol. 7, no. 1. 2017, doi: 10.1038/s41598-017-03010-6.

[18] C. A. Staton, S. M. Stribbling, S. Tazzyman, R. Hughes, N. J. Brown, and C. E. Lewis, "Current methods for assaying angiogenesis in vitro and in vivo," *Int. J. Exp. Pathol.*, vol. 85, no. 5, pp. 233-248, Oct. 2004.

[19] M. Montagner and E. Sahai, "Models of Breast Cancer Metastatic Dormancy," *Front Cell Dev Biol*, vol. 8, p. 37, Mar. 2020.

[20] E. Yildiz-Ozturk, S. Gulce-Iz, M. Anil, and O. Yesil-Celiktas, "Cytotoxic responses of carnosic acid and doxorubicin on breast cancer cells in butterfly-shaped microchips in comparison to 2D and 3D culture," *Cytotechnology*, vol. 69, no. 2, pp. 337-347, Apr. 2017.

[21] Y. Imamura *et al.*, "Comparison of 2D- and 3D-culture models as drug-testing platforms in breast cancer," *Oncol. Rep.*, vol. 33, no. 4, pp. 1837-1843, Apr. 2015.

[22] R. Edmondson, J. J. Broglie, A. F. Adcock, and L. Yang, "Three-dimensional cell culture systems and their applications in drug discovery and cell-based biosensors," *Assay Drug Dev. Technol.*, vol. 12, no. 4, pp. 207-218, May 2014.

[23] D. Lv, Z. Hu, L. Lu, H. Lu, and X. Xu, "Three-dimensional cell culture: A powerful tool in tumor research and drug discovery," *Oncol. Lett.*, vol. 14, no. 6, pp. 6999-7010, Dec. 2017.

[24] K. Duval *et al.*, "Modeling Physiological Events in 2D vs. 3D Cell Culture," *Physiology* , vol. 32, no. 4, pp. 266-277, Jul. 2017.

[25] A. K. Zuk, B. Burczynska, D. Li, L. Ghali, S. Dilworth, and X. Wen, "Modelling and Validating Three-Dimensional Human Breast and Cancerous Human Breast Tissues In Vitro," Science Repository OU, 2020.

[26] "Polystyrene Topography Sticker Array for Cell-Based Assays," *Recent Progress in Materials | Polystyrene Topography Sticker Array for Cell-Based Assays*, Accessed: Jan. 11, 2021. [Online]. Available: https://www.lidsen.com/journals/rpm/.

[27] I. Acerbi *et al.*, "Human breast cancer invasion and aggression correlates with ECM stiffening and immune cell infiltration," *Integr. Biol.* , vol. 7, no. 10, pp. 1120-1134, Oct. 2015.

[28] J. Piao, K. You, Y. Guo, Y. Zhang, Z. Li, and L. Geng, "Substrate stiffness affects epithelial-mesenchymal transition of cervical cancer cells through miR-106b and its target protein DAB2," *Int. J. Oncol.*, vol. 50, no. 6, pp. 2033-2042, Jun. 2017.

[29] J. K. Mouw *et al.*, "Tissue mechanics modulate microRNA-dependent PTEN expression to regulate malignant progression," *Nat. Med.*, vol. 20, no. 4, pp. 360-367, Apr. 2014.

[30] V. Gkretsi and T. Stylianopoulos, "Cell Adhesion and Matrix Stiffness: Coordinating Cancer Cell Invasion and Metastasis," *Front. Oncol.*, vol. 8, p. 145, May 2018.

[31] T. Ebata *et al.*, "Substrate Stiffness Influences Doxorubicin-Induced p53 Activation via ROCK2 Expression," *Biomed Res. Int.*, vol. 2017, p. 5158961, Jan. 2017.

[32] P.-A. Vidi, M. J. Bissell, and S. A. Lelièvre, "Three-dimensional culture of human breast epithelial cells: the how and the why," *Methods Mol. Biol.*, vol. 945, pp. 193-219, 2013.

[33] M. Cavo, M. Fato, L. Peñuela, F. Beltrame, R. Raiteri, and S. Scaglione, "Microenvironment complexity and matrix stiffness regulate breast cancer cell activity in a 3D in vitro model," *Scientific Reports*, vol. 6, no. 1. 2016, doi: 10.1038/srep35367.

[34] S. Breslin and L. O'Driscoll, "Three-dimensional cell culture: the missing link in drug discovery," *Drug Discov. Today*, vol. 18, no. 5-6, pp. 240-249, Mar. 2013.

[35] K. Guiro and T. L. Arinzeh, "Bioengineering Models for Breast Cancer Research," *Breast Cancer: Basic and Clinical Research*, vol. 9s2. p. BCBCR. S29424, 2015, doi: 10.4137/bcbcr.s29424.

[36] F. Hirschhaeuser, H. Menne, C. Dittfeld, J. West, W. Mueller-Klieser, and L. A. Kunz-Schughart, "Multicellular tumor spheroids: an underestimated tool is catching up again," *J. Biotechnol.*, vol. 148, no. 1, pp. 3-15, Jul. 2010.

[37] H. L. Lanz *et al.*, "Therapy response testing of breast cancer in a 3D high-throughput perfused microfluidic platform," *BMC Cancer*, vol. 17, no. 1. 2017, doi: 10.1186/s12885-017-3709-3.

[38] P. A. Kenny *et al.*, "The morphologies of breast cancer cell lines in three-dimensional assays correlate with their profiles of gene expression," *Mol. Oncol.*, vol. 1, no. 1, pp. 84-96, Jun. 2007.

[39] Y. Shin, S. Han, E. Chung, and S. Chung, "Intratumoral phenotypic heterogeneity as an encourager of cancer invasion," *Integr. Biol.* , vol. 6, no. 7, pp. 654-661, Jul. 2014

[40] J. He *et al.*, "3D modeling of cancer stem cell niche," *Oncotarget*, vol. 9, no. 1, pp. 1326-1345, Jan. 2018.

[41] E. A. Muciño-Olmos *et al.*, "Unveiling functional heterogeneity in breast cancer multicellular tumor spheroids through single-cell RNA-seq," *Sci. Rep.*, vol. 10, no. 1, p. 12728, Jul. 2020.

[42] M. C. Regier *et al.*, "Transitions from mono- to co- to tri-culture uniquely affect gene expression in breast cancer, stromal, and immune compartments," *Biomed. Microdevices*, vol. 18, no. 4, p. 70, Aug. 2016.

[43] Y. R. Álvarez-García *et al.*, "Open multi-culture platform for simple and flexible study of multi-cell type interactions," *Lab Chip*, vol. 18, no. 20, pp. 3184-3195, Oct. 2018.

[44] S. Pagani, P. Torricelli, F. Veronesi, F. Salamanna, S. Cepollaro, and M. Fini, "An advanced tri-culture model to evaluate the dynamic interplay among osteoblasts, osteoclasts, and endothelial cells," *J. Cell. Physiol.*, vol. 233, no. 1, pp. 291-301, Jan. 2018.

[45] C. Loy *et al.*, "A planar model of the vessel wall from cellularized-collagen scaffolds: focus on cell-matrix interactions in mono-, bi- and tri-culture models," *Biomater Sci*, vol. 5, no. 1, pp. 153-162, Dec. 2016.

[46] L. Goers, P. Freemont, and K. M. Polizzi, "Co-culture systems and technologies: taking synthetic biology to the next level," *J. R. Soc. Interface*, vol. 11, no. 96, Jul. 2014, doi: 10.1098/rsif.2014.0065.

[47] D. R. Bogdanowicz and H. H. Lu, "Studying cell-cell communication in co-culture," *Biotechnology journal*, vol. 8, no. 4. pp. 395-396, Apr. 2013.

[48] C. Arrigoni, S. Bersini, M. Gilardi, and M. Moretti, "In Vitro Co-Culture Models of Breast Cancer Metastatic Progression towards Bone," *Int. J. Mol. Sci.*, vol. 17, no. 9, Aug. 2016, doi: 10.3390/ijms17091405.

[49] Y. Miki *et al.*, "Aromatase localization in human breast cancer tissues: possible interactions between intratumoral stromal and parenchymal cells," *Cancer Res.*, vol. 67, no. 8, pp. 3945-3954, Apr. 2007.

[50] Z. S. Templeton *et al.*, "Breast Cancer Cell Colonization of the Human Bone Marrow Adipose Tissue Niche," *Neoplasia*, vol. 17, no. 12, pp. 849-861, Dec. 2015.

[51] A. González-González, A. González, C. Alonso-González, J. Menéndez-Menéndez, C. Martínez-Campa, and S. Cos, "Complementary actions of melatonin on angiogenic factors, the angiopoietin/Tie2 axis and VEGF, in co-cultures of human endothelial and breast cancer cells," *Oncol. Rep.*, vol. 39, no. 1, pp. 433-441, Jan. 2018.

[52] F. Chiovaro, E. Martina, A. Bottos, A. Scherberich, N. E. Hynes, and R. Chiquet-Ehrismann, "Transcriptional regulation of tenascin-W by TGF-beta signaling in the bone metastatic niche of breast cancer cells," *Int. J. Cancer*, vol. 137, no. 8, pp. 1842-1854, Oct. 2015.

[53] T. A. Sebrell *et al.*, "A Novel Gastric Spheroid Co-culture Model Reveals Chemokine-Dependent Recruitment of Human Dendritic Cells to the Gastric Epithelium," *Cell Mol Gastroenterol Hepatol*, vol. 8, no. 1, pp. 157-171.e3, Mar. 2019.

[54] D. R. Bogdanowicz and H. H. Lu, "Multifunction co-culture model for evaluating cell-cell interactions," *Methods Mol. Biol.*, vol. 1202, pp. 29-36, 2014.

[55] S. Goswami *et al.*, "Macrophages Promote the Invasion of Breast Carcinoma Cells via a Colony-Stimulating Factor-1/Epidermal Growth Factor Paracrine Loop," *Cancer Research*, vol. 65, no. 12. pp. 5278-5283, 2005, doi: 10.1158/0008-5472.can-04-1853.

[56] M. Buess, M. Rajski, B. M. L. Vogel-Durrer, R. Herrmann, and C. Rochlitz, "Tumor-Endothelial Interaction Links the CD44 /CD24- Phenotype with Poor Prognosis in Early-Stage Breast Cancer," *Neoplasia*, vol. 11, no. 10. pp. 987-1002, 2009, doi: 10.1593/neo.09670.

[57] J. Hwang, Y. Jeong, J. M. Park, K. H. Lee, J. W. Hong, and J. Choi, "Biomimetics: forecasting the future of science, engineering, and medicine," *Int. J. Nanomedicine*, vol. 10, pp. 5701-5713, Sep. 2015.

[58] X. Zhou *et al.*, "3D Bioprinting a Cell-Laden Bone Matrix for Breast Cancer Metastasis Study," *ACS Appl. Mater. Interfaces*, vol. 8, no. 44, pp. 30017-30026, Nov. 2016.

[59] S. Bersini *et al.*, "A microfluidic 3D in vitro model for specificity of breast cancer metastasis to bone," *Biomaterials*, vol. 35, no. 8, pp. 2454-2461, Mar. 2014.

[60] "Amphiphilic silicones to reduce the absorption of small hydrophobic molecules," *Acta Biomater.*, Nov. 2020, doi: 10.1016/j.actbio.2020.11.041.

[61] G. A. Thouas, J. Sheridan, and K. Hourigan, "A bioreactor model of mouse tumor progression," *J. Biomed. Biotechnol.*, vol. 2007, no. 9, p. 32754, 2007.

[62] L. E. Marshall, K. F. Goliwas, L. M. Miller, A. D. Penman, A. R. Frost, and J. L. Berry, "Flow-perfusion bioreactor system for engineered breast cancer surrogates to be used in preclinical testing," *J. Tissue Eng. Regen. Med.*, vol. 11, no. 4, pp. 1242-1250, Apr. 2017.

[63] O. Candini *et al.*, "A Novel 3D In Vitro Platform for Pre-Clinical Investigations in Drug Testing, Gene Therapy, and Immuno-oncology," *Sci. Rep.*, vol. 9, no. 1, p. 7154, May 2019.

[64] "Innovative in vitro models for breast cancer drug discovery," *Drug Discov. Today Dis. Models*, vol. 21, pp. 11-16, Sep. 2016, Accessed: Jan. 11, 2021. [Online].

[65] Y. Zhao *et al.*, "Three-dimensional printing of Hela cells for cervical tumor model in vitro," *Biofabrication*, vol. 6, no. 3, p. 035001, Sep. 2014.

[66] Y. Wang *et al.*, "3D Bioprinting of Breast Cancer Models for Drug Resistance Study," *ACS Biomater Sci Eng*, vol. 4, no. 12, pp. 4401-4411, Dec. 2018.

[67] V. Srivastava, T. R. Huycke, K. T. Phong, and Z. J. Gartner, "Organoid

models for mammary gland dynamics and breast cancer," *Curr. Opin. Cell Biol.*, vol. 66, pp. 51-58, Oct. 2020.

[68] L. Broutier *et al.*, "Human primary liver cancer–derived organoid cultures for disease modeling and drug screening," *Nature Medicine*, vol. 23, no. 12. pp. 1424-1435, 2017, doi: 10.1038/nm.4438.

[69] N. Sachs *et al.*, "A Living Biobank of Breast Cancer Organoids Captures Disease Heterogeneity," *Cell*, vol. 172, no. 1-2, pp. 373-386.e10, Jan. 2018.

[70] S. Halldorsson, E. Lucumi, R. Gómez-Sjöberg, and R. M. T. Fleming, "Advantages and challenges of microfluidic cell culture in polydimethylsiloxane devices," *Biosens. Bioelectron.*, vol. 63, pp. 218-231, Jan. 2015.

[71] V. van Duinen, S. J. Trietsch, J. Joore, P. Vulto, and T. Hankemeier, "Microfluidic 3D cell culture: from tools to tissue models," *Curr. Opin. Biotechnol.*, vol. 35, pp. 118-126, Dec. 2015.

[72] L. E. Stallcop *et al.*, "Razor-printed sticker microdevices for cell-based applications," *Lab Chip*, vol. 18, no. 3, pp. 451-462, Jan. 2018.

[73] M. Domenech *et al.*, "Cellular observations enabled by microculture: paracrine signaling and population demographics," *Integr. Biol.* , vol. 1, no. 3, pp. 267-274, Mar. 2009.

[74] A. L. Paguirigan and D. J. Beebe, "Microfluidics meet cell biology: bridging the gap by validation and application of microscale techniques for cell biological assays," *Bioessays*, vol. 30, no. 9, pp. 811-821, Sep. 2008.

[75] J. M. Ayuso *et al.*, "Microfluidic Tumor-on-a-Chip Model to Study Tumor Metabolic Vulnerability," *Int. J. Mol. Sci.*, vol. 21, no. 23, Nov. 2020, doi: 10.3390/ijms21239075.

[76] S. K. Sia and G. M. Whitesides, "Microfluidic devices fabricated in poly(dimethylsiloxane) for biological studies," *Electrophoresis*, vol. 24, no. 21, pp. 3563-3576, Nov. 2003.

[77] S. N. Bhatia and D. E. Ingber, "Microfluidic organs-on-chips," *Nat. Biotechnol.*, vol. 32, no. 8, pp. 760-772, Aug. 2014.

[78] S. Chung, R. Sudo, P. J. Mack, C.-R. Wan, V. Vickerman, and R. D. Kamm, "Cell migration into scaffolds under co-culture conditions in a microfluidic platform," *Lab Chip*, vol. 9, no. 2, pp. 269-275, Jan. 2009.

[79] Q. H. Nguyen *et al.*, "Profiling human breast epithelial cells using single cell RNA sequencing identifies cell diversity," *Nat. Commun.*, vol. 9, no. 1, p. 2028, May 2018.

[80] Y.-C. Chen *et al.*, "Single-cell RNA-sequencing of migratory breast cancer cells: discovering genes associated with cancer metastasis," *Analyst*, vol. 144, no. 24, pp. 7296-7309, Dec. 2019.

[81] J. Kong *et al.*, "A novel microfluidic model can mimic organ-specific metastasis of circulating tumor cells," *Oncotarget*, vol. 7, no. 48, pp. 78421-78432, Nov. 2016.

[82] Y. Choi *et al.*, "A microengineered pathophysiological model of early-stage breast cancer," *Lab Chip*, vol. 15, no. 16, pp. 3350-3357, Aug. 2015.

[83] J. Shemesh, I. Jalilian, A. Shi, G. H. Yeoh, M. L. Knothe Tate, and M. E. Warkiani, "Flow-induced stress on adherent cells in microfluidic devices," *Lab Chip*, vol. 15, no. 21, pp. 4114-4127, Oct. 2015, Accessed: Jan. 12, 2021. [Online].

[84] D. Huh, G. A. Hamilton, and D. E. Ingber, "From 3D cell culture to organs-on-chips," *Trends Cell Biol.*, vol. 21, no. 12, pp. 745-754, Dec. 2011.

[85] K. F. Goliwas, L. M. Miller, L. E. Marshall, J. L. Berry, and A. R. Frost, "Preparation and Analysis of In Vitro Three Dimensional Breast Carcinoma Surrogates," *J. Vis. Exp.*, no. 111, May 2016, doi: 10.3791/54004.

[86] V. Krishnan, L. A. Shuman, D. M. Sosnoski, R. Dhurjati, E. A. Vogler, and A. M. Mastro, "Dynamic interaction between breast cancer cells and osteoblastic tissue: comparison of two- and three-dimensional cultures," *J. Cell. Physiol.*, vol. 226, no. 8, pp. 2150-2158, Aug. 2011.

[87] M. G. Muraro *et al.*, "assessment of drug response on breast cancer primary tissue with preserved microenvironments," *Oncoimmunology*, vol. 6, no. 7, p. e1331798, May 2017.

[88] A. A. Narkhede, L. A. Shevde, and S. S. Rao, "Biomimetic strategies to recapitulate organ specific microenvironments for studying breast cancer metastasis," *Int. J. Cancer*, vol. 141, no. 6, pp. 1091-1109, Sep. 2017.

[89] P. Kaur *et al.*, "Human Breast Cancer Histoid," *Journal of Histochemistry & Cytochemistry*, vol. 59, no. 12. pp. 1087-1100, 2011, doi: 10.1369/0022155411423680.

[90] J. Bae, S. Han, and S. Park, "Recent Advances in 3D Bioprinted Tumor Microenvironment," *BioChip Journal*, vol. 14, no. 2. pp. 137-147, 2020, doi: 10.1007/s13206-020-4201-8.

[91] S. Mao *et al.*, "Bioprinting of in vitro tumor models for personalized cancer treatment: a review," *Biofabrication*, vol. 12, no. 4, p. 042001, Jul. 2020.

[92] D. M. Kingsley *et al.*, "Laser-based 3D bioprinting for spatial and size control of tumor spheroids and embryoid bodies," *Acta Biomater.*, vol. 95, pp. 357-370, Sep. 2019.

[93] W. F. Hynes *et al.*, "Examining metastatic behavior within 3D bioprinted vasculature for the validation of a 3D computational flow model," *Sci Adv*, vol. 6, no. 35, p. eabb3308, Aug. 2020.

[94] S. Knowlton, S. Onal, C. H. Yu, J. J. Zhao, and S. Tasoglu, "Bioprinting for cancer research," *Trends Biotechnol.*, vol. 33, no. 9, pp. 504-513, Sep. 2015.

[95] S. Swaminathan, Q. Hamid, W. Sun, and A. M. Clyne, "Bioprinting of 3D breast epithelial spheroids for human cancer models," *Biofabrication*, vol. 11, no. 2, p. 025003, Jan. 2019.

[96] "[No title]." https://doi.org/10.1200/JCO.2019.37.15_suppl.2605 (accessed Jan. 11, 2021).

[97] Y. S. Zhang, M. Duchamp, R. Oklu, L. W. Ellisen, R. Langer, and A. Khademhosseini, "Bioprinting the Cancer Microenvironment," *ACS Biomater Sci Eng*, vol. 2, no. 10, pp. 1710-1721, Oct. 2016.

[98] M. Simian and M. J. Bissell, "Organoids: A historical perspective of thinking in three dimensions," *J. Cell Biol.*, vol. 216, no. 1, pp. 31-40, Jan. 2017.

[99] F. Weeber, S. N. Ooft, K. K. Dijkstra, and E. E. Voest, "Tumor Organoids as a Pre-clinical Cancer Model for Drug Discovery," *Cell Chem Biol*, vol. 24, no. 9, pp. 1092-1100, Sep. 2017.

[100] J. Drost and H. Clevers, "Organoids in cancer research," *Nature Reviews Cancer*, vol. 18, no. 7. pp. 407-418, 2018, doi: 10.1038/s41568-018-0007-6.

[101] S. E. Burdall, A. M. Hanby, M. R. J. Lansdown, and V. Speirs, "Breast cancer cell lines: friend or foe?," *Breast Cancer Res.*, vol. 5, no. 2, pp. 89-95, Feb. 2003.

[102] L. Grassi *et al.*, "Organoids as a new model for improving regenerative medicine and cancer personalized therapy in renal diseases," *Cell Death Dis.*, vol. 10, no. 3, p. 201, Feb. 2019.

[103] L. Yang *et al.*, "Progress in the application of organoids to breast cancer research," *J. Cell. Mol. Med.*, vol. 24, no. 10, pp. 5420-5427, May 2020.

[104] K.-Y. Chen *et al.*, "Single-Cell Transcriptomics Reveals Heterogeneity and Drug Response of Human Colorectal Cancer Organoids," *Conf. Proc. IEEE Eng. Med. Biol. Soc.*, vol. 2018, pp. 2378-2381, Jul. 2018.

[105] K. J. Cheung, E. Gabrielson, Z. Werb, and A. J. Ewald, "Collective invasion in breast cancer requires a conserved basal epithelial program," *Cell*, vol. 155, no. 7, pp. 1639-1651, Dec. 2013.

Section 4

Breast Cancer Pharmacotherapy

Chapter 5

The Use of Plants' Natural Products in Breast Cancer: Have We Already Found the New Anticancer Drug?

Isadora de Fátima Braga Magalhães, Kátia da Silva Calabrese, Ana Letícia Marinho Figueirêdo, Ana Lucia Abreu-Silva and Fernando Almeida-Souza

Abstract

The importance of a new anticancer drug for breast cancer is well established. Natural compounds that can prevent this disease or be used as an adjuvant treatment associated with conventional drugs could be the solution for this. This chapter is an overview of agents extracted from plants with outstand results in the last six years. Green tea, berberine, thymoquinone and cannabidiol are compounds isolated from medicinal plants. These agents showed action through induction of apoptosis, down regulation of inflammation, epigenetics, hormonal modulation, among other. In vitro effect against cancer cells, in vivo experiments mainly with murine model and clinical trials reassured their efficacy against breast cancer. A protective effect against recurrence cases and chemosensitization to standard drugs was also successful. The use of nanotechnology provided a optimize delivery of these therapeutical molecules. Taken together this information led us to acknowledgement that we do probably have the natural agents for a future adjuvant treatment against breast cancer.

Keywords: plants, phytotherapy, breast cancer, green tea, berberine, thymoquinone, cannabidiol, anticancer

1. Introduction

Breast cancer (BC) remains one of the leading causes of death [1] and one of the most common types of malignancies among women worldwide [2]. The conventional treatment includes chemotherapy, hormone therapy, radiotherapy and surgery. Problems such as high recurrence and toxicity to medication are frequent [1]. Due to this, the combination of the conventional treatment with a new approach is the key to a higher degree of success in the therapeutic of this disease.

Complementary therapies are already used among many women who have BC to help dealing with adverse effects or against recurrence. Phytotherapy is one of the most popular adjuvant therapies and a common target for a new BC drug [1]. Plant-derived anticancer therapeutics aim to reduce side effects and increase the sensitivity to chemotherapy and the overall effectiveness of the treatment [3].

IntechOpen

Although there is a false believe in the harmlessness of plants, they can cause negative effects and even reduce the therapeutic effects of standard drugs. Therefore, is crucial to understand their correct dosage and potential effects [1].

Over the past decades, many bioactive phytochemicals from medicinal plants have being studied and some of them have remarkable results. Among all these natural compounds, it is natural to ask ourselves: have we found the answer yet? What is the role of plant derived compounds in reducing breast cancer cells and promoting survival and less recurrence among breast cancer patients? This chapter is an overview of agents extracted from plants with outstand results in the last six years. Therefore, can be helpful in trying to answer these questions.

2. Green tea

Tea has become one of the most popular beverages all over the world. The consumption of green tea gained popularity in the last years and is now associated with a different lifestyle. Green tea, *Camellia sinensis* [4], has shown anticancer effect on different types of cancer [5] and apparently possess many chemopreventive qualities in primary breast cancer and recurrence [6].

In the search for different forms that green tea can act as an anticancer agent in BC, hormonal modulation has been considered. Supplementation with decaffeinated green tea extract significantly increases circulating of estradiol in healthy postmenopausal women. The consumption of green tea extract also reduces circulation of cholesterol and LDL-cholesterol [7], and the regular consume seems to facilitate lipid metabolisms in breast cancer survivors [8]. In a study among Chinese women in Hong Kong, drinking green tea was not associated with overall breast cancer risk, which may be masked by the differential effect in pre- and post-menopausal women, due to modified hormone receptor expression [9].

A great potential as a chemo-preventive agent against breast cancer can be attributed to green tea, especially for recurrence [6]. Drinking at least five cups of green tea per week may be associated with decreased breast cancer risk [10].

Tamoxifen is an adjuvant treatment for hormone receptor-positive breast cancer, but drug resistance related to genetic and epigenetic mechanisms is rising to dangerously levels [11]. Tamoxifen has no pharmacokinetic interaction with green tea [12] which can encourage this association.

Green tea high inhibited the proliferation of cell line derived from breast cancer in mouse, named 4TI cells, with upregulation of Casp8, Casp9, Casp3, Casp6, Casp8AP2, Aifm1, Aifm2 and Apopt1 genes [13]. When associated with silicon nanomaterials, this compound has action against breast cancer in vitro and in vivo with inhibition of tumor growth [14].

Catechin, epicatechin, epigallocatechin and epigallocatechin-3-gallate (EGCG) are the four major constituents of green tea [15]. EGCG has demonstrated potential anticancer effects on several preclinical and clinical researches [16].

Epigenetics are non-mutational events that alter the expression of genes [17]. Catechins from green tea, especially EGCG, are be able to modulate epigenetic processes by increasing transcription of tumor suppressor genes through attenuating the effect of DNA methyltransferase 1 (DNMT1) and consequently reversing DNA methylation [18].

The most active anticancer component in green tea is EGCG [19]. EGCC might act on breast cancer cells progression through inhibition of focal adhesion kinase (FAK) signaling pathway [20], by interfering in proteins involved in cell death and survival, DNA replication, recombination and repair [21]. It can also interfere on the expression of genes such as PTEN, CASP3, CASP9 [22] and through inhibition of protein tyrosine phosphatase 1B (PTP1B) activity [23], a protein that plays a crucial role in the development of breast cancer, with higher levels associated with tumor size and lymph node metastasis in patients [24]. EGCG also decreases BC cells with similar results as tamoxifen [22].

A protective effect of EGCG on BC was reaffirmed on several experimental models and different conditions with promising clinical implications for breast cancer prevention and therapy [25].

A lecithin formulation of a caffeine-free green tea catechin extract named green select phytosome (GSP) increased the bioavailability of EGCG on early breast cancer patients who received GSP in 300 mg dose, daily, for 4 weeks prior to surgery [26].

Capsules of green tea with a high dose (843 mg) of EGCG provided during 12 months reduced the percent of mammographic density in younger women similar to tamoxifen. This indicates a possible chemo preventive effect on breast cancer risk, although no effect was detected on older women [27]. The treatment with EGCG can also act through epigenetic by reduction of the expression and activity of DNA methyltransferase and decreasing of methylation of the domain-containing epidermal growth factor-like 2 (2SCUBE2), a tumor suppressor that inhibits BC cells migration and invasion [28].

EGCG and quercetin isolated from green tea and green tea alone had anticarcinogenic effect on estrogen receptor-positive and -negative breast cancer cells [29]. It also showed in vitro and in vivo effect, by inhibiting the growth of 4 T1 tumor and increasing the proportions of CD4+ and CD8+ T cells at tumor sites in mice. EGCG regulated the canonical and non-canonical pathways in myeloid-derived suppressor cells (MDSCs) [30].

The action of polyphenols from green tea on BC cells was mediated by apoptosis thought mitochondrial pathway with induction of DNA fragmentation and activation of caspase-3 and caspase-9 [31].

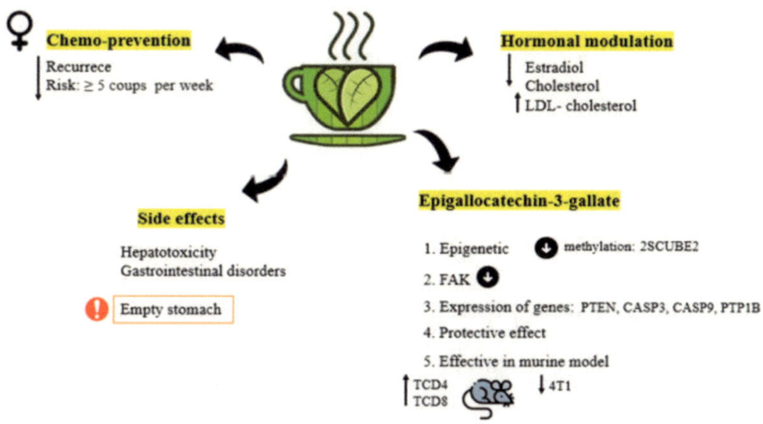

Figure 1.
Green tea and breast cancer. Hormonal modulation. The consumption of green tea causes hormonal modulation through depression of estradiol and cholesterol levels and increase of LDL-cholesterol levels. ***Epigallocatechin-3-gallate****. Epigallocatechin-3-gallate isolated from green tea causes effects in epigenetic by decreasing methylation of tumor suppressors such as epidermal growth factor-like 2 (2SCUBE2); inhibits focal adhesion kinase (FAK) signaling pathway; interferes in the expression of genes such as phosphatase and tensin homolog (PTEN), caspase-3 (CASP3), caspase-9 (CASP9) and protein-tyrosine phosphatase 1B (PTP1B); has protective effect against breast cancer and is effective in murine model by decreasing breast cancer cells 4 T1 and increasing the proportions of CD4+ and CD8+ T cells at tumor sites.* ***Side effects.*** *Hepatotoxicity and gastrointestinal disorders are reported mainly when tea is consumed with an empty stomach.* ***Chemo-prevention.*** *Green tea is a chemo-preventive in women causing less recurrence cases and also lower risk of breast cancer when at least 5 cups of tea are consumed per week.*

Matcha green tea (MGT), a special type of green tea with higher concentrations of catechins due to a different preparation [32] inhibits mTOR, stimulates an antioxidant response and interferes in interleukin signaling in BC cells [33].

Some side effects have been associated with green tea such as hepatotoxicity and gastrointestinal disorders, especially if consumed on an empty stomach (**Figure 1**). Although green tea and its main components are not major teratogen, mutagen or carcinogen substances and have a selective cytotoxicity against cancer cells, some caution needs to be taken in pregnant and breast-feeding women due to the lack of information [4]. Between Japanese women, green tea was the most commonly consumed non-alcoholic beverage, and it had no significant associations with breast cancer risk [34].

3. Berberine

Berberine(5,6-dihydro-9,10-dimethoxybenzo[g]-1,3-benzodioxolo[5,6-a] quinolizinium) is an alkaloid with several properties, such as hepatoprotective, immunomodulatory, cardioprotective and antioxidative. Plants containing this compound have been traditionally used in different parts of the world for the treatment of affections in the eyes, inflammatory diseases, dermatitis, wound healing, digestive and respiratory diseases and treatment of neoplasia [35].

A wide variety of different plant species contains berberine (BBR), such as *Coptis chinensis* [36], *Rhizoma coptidis* [37], *Berberis vulgaris* [38], *Arcangelisia flava*, *Berberis aquifolium* and *Berberis aristate*. The genus Berberis contains nearly 550 species [39].

Due to the ability to seize the cell cycle and induce apoptosis of cancer cells, berberine has received considerable research attention [40]. BBR can inhibit tumor growth and metastasis of triple negative breast cancer cells (TNBC) by suppression of transforming growth factor beta 1 (TGF-β1) expression, a multifunctional factor associated with poor prognosis on BC. It also decreased lung metastasis and tumor growth in MDA-MB-231, a cell line originated from an invasive ductal carcinoma, and 4 T1 breast cancer xenograft models [41]. Same effect was detected in tumor growth in MDA-MB-231 nude mouse xenografts, with binding of vasodilator-stimulated phosphoprotein (VASP), related to cell migration and overexpressed in high-motility BC cells [42] and throught caspase-9 pathway [43]. At a 50 mg/kg dose, BBR demonstrated a preventive role in rats with mammary ductal and invasive carcinoma [40].

BBR suppresses breast cancer cells through inhibition of transforming growth factor beta 1 (TGF-β1) expression [41], targeting ephrin-B2 [44], AMPK signaling pathway [45], inhibition of specific activator protein-1 (AP-1) activity [46], triggering to a caspase9-dependent apoptosis [43], affecting mRNA levels of chemokine receptors genes such as C-X-C motif chemokine receptor 1 (CXCR1) and C-X-C motif chemokine receptor 4 (CXCR4) [47] and by inducing nucleolar stress and upregulation of p53, a tumor suppressor gene [48].

The anti-cancer ability of BBR against BC may be partially dependent on the regulation of metadherin [49] and attenuation of inflammation through inhibition of nuclear factor kappa-light-chain-enhancer of activated B cells (NF-κB) activation [50] and reduction of secretion of proinflammatory cytokines such as interleukin-1α (IL-1α), interleukin-1β (IL-1β), interleukin-6 (IL-6) and tumor necrosis factor-α (TNF-α) [51]. BBR also reduces interleukin-8 (IL-8) secretion, which is associated with poor outcomes involving metastasis-free survival and relapse-free [52].

In animals, the inhibition of canine mammary gland carcinoma cells, highlights its potential against the most frequent cause of cancer in female dogs [53].

Salt-inducible kinases 3 (SIK3) belong to the AMPK-related family of kinases, and when highly expressed is associated with poor survival among BC patients. This kinase was significantly inhibited by the combination of emodin and BBR [54].

Another successful combination happened between lapatinib and BBR, and reversed the resistance to lapatinib through downregulating of c-Myc, a gene often expressed in cancer [55]. The association between BBR and doxorubicin increased chemosensitivity to this agent [45] and reverted the resistance by inhibiting autophagy [56].

The combination of theophylline and berberine showed a synergistic anti-proliferation effect on MDA-MB-231 cells, with a less necrotic effect and increased apoptotic cell death [57]. A sensibilization of BC cells to the chemotherapeutic drugs cisplatin, camptothecin and methyl methanesulfonate was provide by the association with BBR by a deoxyribonucleic acid (DNA) repair pathway involving XRCC1, a protein involved in the efficient repair of DNA [58].

Berberine and tamoxifen together induced cell growth inhibition more effectively than tamoxifen alone [59] and BBR with evodiamine synergistically induced cell cycle arrest and apoptosis of MCF-7 cells [60], an established breast cancer cell line originated from a pleural effusion of a patient with invasive breast ductal carcinoma.

Synergetic effect between poly (lactic-co-glycolic acid) nanoparticles with doxorubicin conjugate for encapsulation and BBR increased rat half-life and anti-proliferative action against BC cells [61]. The encapsulation with citrate-capped silver nanoparticles was also efficient [62].

The association of BBR and exercise, consider an immunotherapy treatment, against BC showed a synergistic effect in vitro and in mice, throught the improvement of the immune system, regulation of intestinal microbial metabolite and activation of apoptosis [36].

Although there are many positive outcomes on the therapy with BBR, a low dose of berberine caused attenuation on chemotherapeutic drugs fluorouracil (5-FU) and camptothecin activities [37] (**Figure 2**). Therefore, some caution needs to be taken in regards to its use.

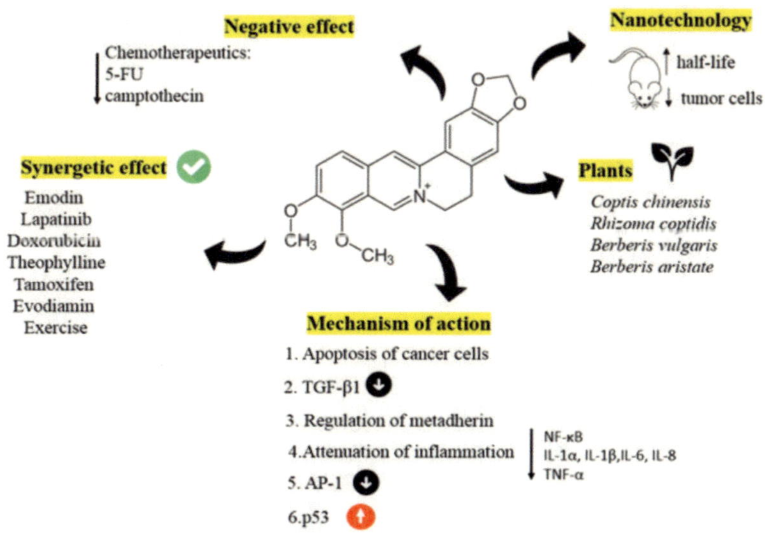

Figure 2.
Berberine and breast cancer. Plants. Many plants can contain berberine, such as Coptis chinensis, Rhizoma coptidis, Berberis vulgaris and Berberis aristate. ***Mechanism of action.*** *Berberine induces apoptosis of cancer cells; reduces transforming growth factor beta 1 (TGF-β1) expression; regulates metadherin; attenuates inflammation by inhibition of nuclear factor kappa B (NF-κB) activation and reduction of interleukins IL-1α, IL-1β, IL-6, IL-8 and tumor necrosis factor-α secretions.* ***Synergetic effect.*** *Between berberine and emodin, lapatinib, doxorubicin, theophylline, tamoxifen, evodiamin, and also with physical exercise.* ***Negative effect.*** *Berberine causes attenuation on chemotherapeutic drugs fluorouracil (5-FU) and camptothecin activities.* ***Nanotechnology.*** *Nanotechnology provides an increased half-life and reduced tumor cells in rats with induced breast cancer.*

4. Thymoquinone

Black cumin seed from *Nigella sativa*, also known as cumin, is used for centuries and it has unsurpassed traditional medicinal value and versatility to treat a wide range of diseases [63]. *N. sativa* is the source of the monoterpene thymoquinone, a compound that can cause anticancer effect in proliferation, migration and invasion in different human cancers including breast cancer lineages [64].

Thymoquinone (TQ) induces apoptosis through death receptors, inhibits TNBC cell line and also can cause in vivo effects on mouse tumor model [65]. TQ inhibits autophagic activity and expression of Beclin-1 and LC3 in TNBC cells and suppresses pathways related to cell invasion and angiogenesis, including integrin-β1, vascular endothelial growth fator (VEGF), matrix metalloproteinase-2 (MMP-2) and MMP-9, suggesting that TQ may be used to control autophagic activity and oncogenic signaling in TNBC [66]. In silico docking studies confirm the action against TNBC, with thymoquinone down-regulating poly (ADP-ribose) polymerase (PARP) gene expression, docking metastatic, apoptotic and cell proliferation targets [67].

TQ-induced ceramide accumulation and endoplasmic reticulum stress, decreased S1P, C1P and NF-κB, triggered apoptosis in BC cells [68] and also changed the cell cycle progression [69].

The combination between different anticancer drugs can be helpful to reduce dose causing less side effects and reducing multidrug resistance. Synergic effect was detected with a combination of TQ with paclitaxel [65] and also with resveratrol, causing a decrease in tumor size, enhanced apoptosis, decreased VEGF expression, elevated levels of interferon-gama (IFN-γ), angiogenesis inhibition with no toxic effect on liver or kidney [70].

TQ and piperine, another bioactive compound of *N. sativa*, together caused an anticancer action in vitro and in vivo in murine model by angiogenesis inhibition, induction of high degrees of apoptosis and shifting the immune response towards a T helper1 response [71], a similar result to the combination with melatonin [72]. When associated with gemcitabine, TQ caused a better anti-cancer activity via modulation of apoptotic and autophagic action [73].

A combined doxorubicin thymoquinone-loaded with aragonite calcium carbonate nanoparticle showed higher efficacy against BC cells at lower dose of doxorubicin and TQ [74]. In a clinical trial, combination between tamoxifen and TQ had a better effect than each of these drugs alone on patients with BC [2].

TQ and black cumin seed oil anticancer effect in BC in female rats induced by 7,12-dimethylbenz[a]anthracene (DMBA), caused alteration on rates of tumor markers such as malondialdehyde (MDA), lactate dehydrogenase (LDH), alkaline phosphatase (ALP) and aspartate aminotransferase (AST) and decrease of the expression of Brca1, Brca2, Id-1 and P53 mutations which highlights a protective effective against BC [63]. In xenograft tumors in mice, TQ inhibited metastasis through enhanced promotion of DNA methylation of the TWIST1 gene [75]. A reduced in drug resistance, anti-migratory potency and tumor size in ex-ovo xenograft was possible with TQ associated with Emodin [76].

Using a metastasis breast cancer mouse model, TQ treatment suppressed multiple metastases in bone, brain, lungs. This effect was attributed to down-regulation of NF-κB and chemokine receptor type 4 (CXCR4) expression, an indicator of poor prognosis in patients (**Figure 3**) [77].

Agents than can make a compound more available and deliver a more efficient effect are being searched. The encapsulation of TQ in nanoparticles improved the bioavailability of this compound [78], and a nanostructured lipid carrier enhanced the therapeutic qualities of TQ by increasing the survival rate of mice [79]. Same

DOI: http://dx.doi.org/10.5772/intechopen.96404

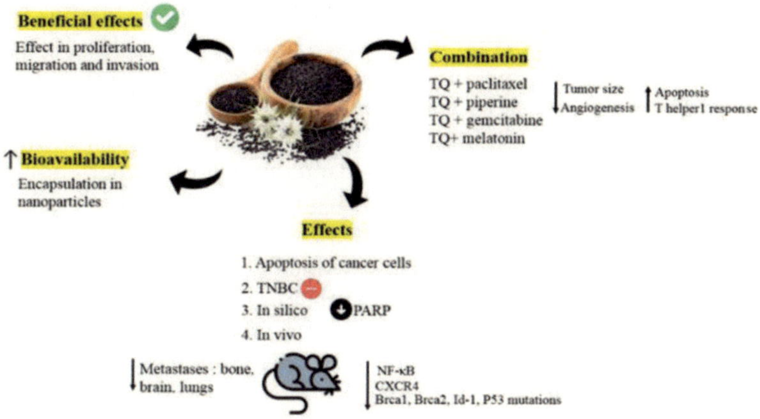

Figure 3.
Thymoquinone and breast cancer. Combination. The combination of thymoquinone (TQ) and paclitaxel, piperine, gemcitabine and melatonin have synergic effects including reduction of tumor size and angiogenesis, increasing of cancer cells apoptosis and shifting of the immune response towards a T helper1 response. ***Effects.*** *The effects in breast cancer includes induction of apoptosis; antiproliferative effect in triple negative breast cancer (TNBC) cells; anticancer effects in silico experiments by downregulation of poly (ADP-ribose) polymerase (PARP) gene expression; suppression of metastases in bone, brain and lungs, down-regulation of nuclear factor kappa B (NF-κB), chemokine receptor type 4 (CXCR4) and Brca1, Brca2, id-1 and P53 mutations expression.* ***Bioavailability.*** *The use of nanothenology increased the bioavailability of thymoquinone.* ***Beneficial effects.*** *Overall action against proliferation, migration and invasion of breast cancer cells was confirmed.*

effects were obtained with low-molecular-weight chitosan-grafted lipid nanocapsules to co-delivery docetaxel and TQ [80], cubosomal nanoparticles used to encapsulate TQ [81] and cabazitaxel and TQ co-loaded lipospheres [82].

5. Cannabidiol

Cannabidiol (CBD) is the main non-psychoactive component of *Cannabis sativa* [83]. Although researches related to cannabis derivates need to face a lot of misunderstanding due to association with psychoactive effects and recreation [84], cannabidiol has proven to stimulate apoptosis pathways and inhibit metastasis, angiogenesis and proliferation of different cancer cells [85].

Cannabidiol can act in cancer cells in a receptor-independent way but also thought CB-receptors such as CB1-R, with moderated expression in BC, and CB2-R with high expression related to tumor aggressiveness. Breast cancer positive for the protein human epidermal growth factor receptor 2 (HER2+), a protein that promotes cancer cells growth, when associated with expression of a cannabinoid receptor (CB2) is associated to poor patient prognosis, therefore can be used as a biomarker with prognostic value [86].

Cannabidiol has an antiproliferative effect against aggressive subtype of BC cells, and also inhibits tumor growth in murine model by interfering in the recruitment of macrophages [83]. The anti-cancer effects of CBD on BC cells are related to regulatory effects on the biogenesis of exosomes and microvesicles released by cells and involved in intercellular communication [87] and by inducing apoptosis with down-regulation of mammalian target of rapamycin (mTOR) and cyclin D1 and up-regulation of peroxisome proliferator-activated receptor gamma (PPARγ) protein expression [88]. CBD also blocks and reverts the effect of IL-1β involved in the change to a malignant phenotype through epithelial-mesenchymal transition [89].

Mice treated with a combination of CBD and doxorubicin had reduced tumor weight and increased apoptosis than the animals treated with CBD or doxorubicin alone [90]. The co-administration of CBD in solution and paclitaxel or doxorubicin showed a synergistic effect, and cannabidiol-loaded microparticles extended release of this compound, causing an optimized action [91]. The cannabinoid combination of tetrahydrocannabinol, cannabigerol, cannabinol and cannabidiol induced apoptosis in BC cell line in a reduced dose with good selectivity, killing BC cells with minimized harmful effects to normal cells [92].

In low dose of 40 mg/day, the treatment with CBD inhibited cytochrome P450 3A4 and P450 2D6, enzymes with important role in cancer treatment, and increased endoxifen levels in a woman with a history of bilateral breast carcinoma in remission [93]. Typical cannabinoids and abnormal cannabidiol had antiproliferative effects on paclitaxel-resistant BC cells and they both reduced tumor growth in zebrafish xenograft model [94].

A botanical drug preparation was more potent than delta-9-tetrahydrocannabinol, a pure compound, as an anticancer agent in cell culture and animal model, which highlights the potential of standardized cannabis drug preparations to manage BC [95]. Synthetic cannabidiol was analyzed in 119 cancer patients over a four-year period and it led to a reduced circulation of tumor cells or reduced tumor size with no side-effects [96].

A precursor of cannabidiol, cannabidiol acid, downregulates the proto-oncogene c-fos and the cyclooxygenase-2 (COX-2) signaling, an anti-inflammatory response that can be linked to the anticancer activity [97].

An effective result in reducing symptoms associated with tumors such as anorexia, nausea and neuropathic pain, and also to decelerate tumor progression in earlier breast cancer cases was attributed to cannabidiol (**Figure 4**) [98].

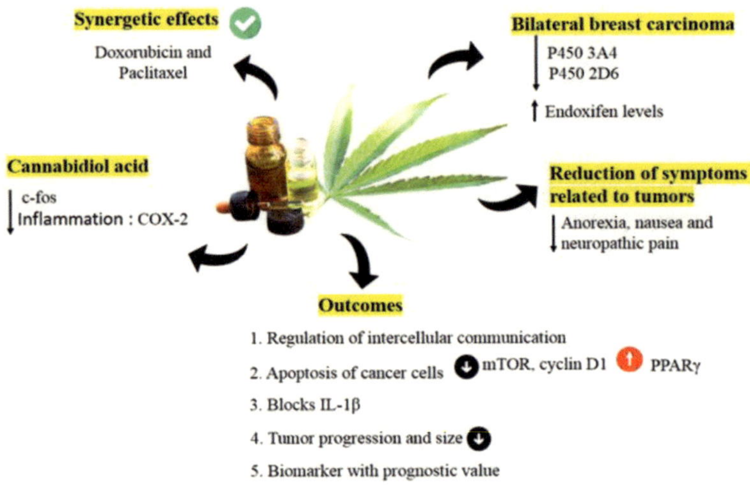

Figure 4.
Cannabidiol and breast cancer. Bilateral breast carcinoma. Treatment with cannabidiol inhibited cytochrome P450 3A4 and P450 2D6 and increased endoxifen levels in a woman with a history of bilateral breast carcinoma. ***Reduction of symptoms related to tumors.*** *Cannabidiol reduces symptoms associated with tumors such as anorexia, nausea and neuropathic pain.* ***Outcomes.*** *Cannabidiol regulates intercellular communication; induces apoptosis of breast cancer cells through down-regulation of mammalian target of rapamycin (mTOR) and cyclin D1 and up-regulation of peroxisome proliferator-activated receptor gamma (PPARγ) protein expression; blocks the effect of IL-1β; reduces tumor size and tumor progression; cannabinoid receptor can be used as biomarker with prognostic value.* ***Cannabidiol acid.*** *Demonstrated anti-inflammatory response by proto-oncogene c-fos and cyclooxygenase-2 (COX-2) signaling downregulation.* ***Synergetic effects.*** *The combination between cannabidiol with doxorubicin or paclitaxel increased the anticancer action.*

6. Conclusions

The need for a more efficient therapeutic to treat breast cancer is imminent, due to side effects and chemoresistance associated with the current treatment. In these chapter we demonstrated the potential of natural compounds to be used as a new anticancer drug against breast cancer.

A natural compound that can protect against one of the most lethal cancers can save thousands of women's lives, and green tea, berberine, thymoquinone and cannabidiol all showed this capability at different experiments.

In vitro action through multiple pathways involving apoptosis and epigenetics, and in vivo experiments, mainly with mouse model, showed decrease of tumor size and angiogenesis. A stimulation of an anti-inflammatory response with cannabidiol, thymoquinone or berberine treatment reveled another link to an anticancer response.

These agents promoted chemo sensitization, making breast cancer cells more sensible to the effect of drugs used in conventional treatment. A synergistic effect with other natural products or standard drugs such as tamoxifen, paclitaxel, doxorubicin and cisplatin were able to reaffirm the possibility of these combination to reduce dose and side effects.

Antiproliferative action against triple-negative breast cancer cells emphasizes the potential of these therapeutic molecules to treat aggressive and difficult cases of breast cancer. Several clinical trials including a large period of time demonstrated a protective and preventive role of these phytocompounds, with almost no side-effects.

Nanotechnology was often used to increase the bioavailability, create a target-oriented delivery and also to provide an effective lower dose of phytomedicine against breast cancer.

Taken together this information led us to acknowledgement that we do probably have the natural agents for a future adjuvant treatment against breast cancer.

Acknowledgements

This research was funded by the Coordination for the Improvement of Higher Education Personnel (Coordenação de Aper feiçoamento de Pessoal de Nível Superior do Brazil—CAPES) [grant number Finance Code 001]. Fernando Almeida-Souza is postdoctoral researcher fellow of CAPES [grant number 88887.363006/2019-2100]. Dra. Ana Lucia Abreu-Silva is research productivity fellow of National Scientific and Technological Development Council (Conselho Nacional de Desenvolvimento Científico e Tecnológico—CNPq) [grant number 309885/2017-5].

Conflict of interest

The authors declare no conflict of interest.

Author details

Isadora de Fátima Braga Magalhães[1,2*], Kátia da Silva Calabrese[3], Ana Letícia Marinho Figueirêdo[2], Ana Lucia Abreu-Silva[2] and Fernando Almeida-Souza[2,3]

1 Federal Fluminense University, Niterói, Brazil

2 State University of Maranhão, São Luís, Brazil

3 Oswaldo Cruz Institute, Rio de Janeiro, Brazil

*Address all correspondence to: isadoradefatimamagalhaes@gmail.com

References

[1] Lopes CM, Dourado A, Oliveira R. Phytotherapy and nutritional supplements on breast cancer. BioMed Research International. 2017;7207983. DOI: 10.1155/2017/7207983

[2] Elrashedy M, Kabel A, Omar M. Ameliorative potential of tamoxifen/thymoquinone combination in patients with breast cancer: a biochemical and immunohistochemical study. Journal of Cancer Science and Research.2016;1: 102.DOI: 10.4172/2576-1447.1000102

[3] GospodinovaZI, Zupkó I, Bózsity N, Manova VI, Georgieva MS, Todinova SJ, Taneva SG, Ocsovszki I, Krasteva ME. *Cotinus coggygria* Scop. induces cell cycle arrest, apoptosis, genotoxic effects, thermodynamic and epigenetic events in MCF7 breast cancer cells. Zeitschrift für Naturforschung C: A Journal of Biosciences. 2020.DOI: 10.1515/znc-2020-0087

[4] Bedrood Z, Rameshrad M, Hosseinzadeh H. Toxicological effects of Camellia sinensis (green tea): A review. Phytotherapy Research. 2018;32: 1163-1180.DOI: 10.1002/ptr.6063

[5] Saeed M, Naveed M, Arif M, Kakar MU, Manzoor R, Abd El-Hack ME, Alagawany M, Tiwari R, KhandiaR,MunjalA,KarthikK,DhamaK, Iqbal HMN, Dadar M, Sun C. Green tea (*Camellia sinensis*) and l-theanine: Medicinal values and beneficial applicationsinhumans-A comprehensive review. Biomedicine & Pharmacotherapy. 2017; 95:1260-1275. DOI: 10.1016/j.biopha.2017.09.024

[6] Gianfredi V, Nucci D, Abalsamo A, Acito M, Villarini M, Moretti M, Realdon, S. Green tea consumption and risk of breast cancer and recurrence-a systematic review and meta-analysis of observational studies. Nutrients.2018; 10:1886. DOI:10.3390/nu10121886

[7] Samavat H, Newman AR, Wang R, Yuan JM, Wu AH, Kurzer MS. Effects of green tea catechin extract on serum lipids in postmenopausal women: a randomized, placebo-controlled clinical trial. The American Journal of Clinical Nutrition. 2016; 104:1671-1682. DOI: 10.3945/ajcn.116.137075

[8] Zhang JY, Liao YH, Lin Y, Liu Q, Xie XM, Tang LY, Ren ZF. Effects of tea consumption and the interactions with lipids on breast cancer survival. Breast Cancer Research and Treatment.2019; 176:679-686. DOI: 10.1007/s10549-019-05253-5

[9] Mengjie Li, Lap Ah Tse, Wing-cheong Chan, Chi-hei Kwok, Siu-lan Leung, Cherry Wu, Wai-cho Yu, Ignatius Tak-sun Yu, Chloe Hui-Tung Yu, Feng Wang, Hyuna Sung, Xiaohong R. Yang. Evaluation of breast cancer risk associated with tea consumption by menopausal and estrogen receptor status among Chinese women in Hong Kong, Cancer Epidemiology. 2016; 40:73-78. DOI: 10.1016/j.canep.2015.11.013.

[10] Zhang D, Nichols HB, Troester M, Cai J, Bensen JT, Sandler DP. Tea consumption and breast cancer risk in a cohort of women with family history of breast cancer. International Journal of Cancer. 2020;147:876-886. DOI: 10.1002/ijc.32824

[11] Bezerra LS, Santos-Veloso MAO, Bezerra Junior NDS, Fonseca LCD, Sales WLA. Impacts of cytochrome P450 2D6 (CYP2D6) genetic polymorphism in tamoxifen therapy for breast cancer. Revista Brasileira de Ginecologia e Obstetrícia. 2018;40:794-799. DOI: 10.1055/s-0038-1676303

[12] Braal CL, Hussaarts KGAM, Seuren L, Oomen-de Hoop E, de Bruijn P, Buck SAJ, Bos MEMM, Thijs-Visser MF, Zuetenhorst HJM,

Mathijssen-van Stein D, Vastbinder MB, van Leeuwen RWF, van Gelder T, Koolen SLW, Jager A, Mathijssen RHJ. Influence of green tea consumption on endoxifen steady-state concentration in breast cancer patients treated with tamoxifen. Breast Cancer Research and Treatment. 2020;184:107-113. DOI: 10.1007/s10549-020-05829-6

[13] Mbuthia KS, Mireji PO, Ngure RM, Stomeo F, Kyallo M, Muoki C, Wachira FN. Tea (*Camellia sinensis*) infusions ameliorate cancer in 4TI metastatic breast cancer model. BMC Complementary and Alternative Medicine. 2017; 17:202. DOI: 10.1186/s12906-017-1683-6

[14] Chu B, Wu S, Ji X, Chen R, Song B, Tang J, Wang H, Su Y, He Y. Controllable silicon nanostructures featuring stable fluorescence and intrinsic in vitro and in vivo anti-cancer activity. Journal of Materials Chemistry B. 2019; 7:6247-6256. DOI: 10.1039/c9tb01191a.

[15] Farhan M, Khan HY, Oves M, Al-Harrasi A, Rehmani N, Arif H, Hadi SM, Ahmad A. Cancer therapy by catechins involves redox cycling of copper ions and generation of reactive oxygen species. Toxins.2016;8:37. DOI: 10.3390/toxins8020037.

[16] Sur S, Panda CK. Molecular aspects of cancer chemopreventive and therapeutic efficacies of tea and tea polyphenols. Nutrition. 2017;43-44:8-15. DOI: 10.1016/j.nut.2017.06.006

[17] Romagnolo DF, Daniels KD, Grunwald JT, Ramos SA, Propper CR, Selmin OI. Epigenetics of breast cancer: Modifying role of environmental and bioactive food compounds. Molecular Nutrition & Food Research. 2016; 60:1310-1329. DOI: 10.1002/mnfr.201501063

[18] Yiannakopoulou EC. Targeting DNA methylation with green tea catechins. Pharmacology. 2015; 95:111-116. DOI: 10.1159/000375503

[19] Chen H, Yao K, Chang X, Shim J-H, Kim HG, Malakhova M, et al. Computational and Biochemical Discovery of RSK2 as a novel target for Epigallocatechin Gallate (EGCG). PLoS ONE.2015;10: e0130049. DOI:10.1371/journal.pone.0130049

[20] Luo X, Guo L, Zhang L, Hu Y, Shang D, Ji D. Bioinformatics analysis of microarray profiling identifies the mechanism of focal adhesion kinase signalling pathway in proliferation and apoptosis of breast cancer cells modulated by green tea polyphenol epigallocatechin 3-gallate. Journal of Pharmacy and Pharmacology. 2018; 70:1606-1618. DOI: 10.1111/jphp.13010

[21] Song X, Zhang M, Chen L, Lin Q. Bioinformatic prediction of possible targets and mechanisms of action of the green tea compound epigallocatechin-3-gallate against breast cancer. Frontiers in Molecular Biosciences. 2017; 4:43. DOI: 10.3389/fmolb.2017.00043

[22] Moradzadeh M, Hosseini A, Erfanian S, Rezaei H. Epigallocatechin-3-gallate promotes apoptosis in human breast cancer T47D cells through down-regulation of PI3K/AKT and Telomerase. Pharmacological Reports. 2017; 69:924-928. DOI: 10.1016/j.pharep.2017.04.008.

[23] Kuban-Jankowska A, Kostrzewa T, Musial C, Barone G, Lo-Bosco G, Lo-Celso F, Gorska-Ponikowska M. Green Tea Catechins Induce Inhibition of PTP1B Phosphatase in Breast Cancer Cells with Potent Anti-Cancer Properties: In Vitro Assay, Molecular Docking, and Dynamics Studies. Antioxidants. 2020; 9:1208. DOI:10.3390/antiox9121208

[24] Liao SC, Li JX, Yu L, Sun SR. Protein tyrosine phosphatase 1B expression contributes to the development of breast cancer. Journal of Zheijang University SCIENCE B. 2017; 18:334-342. DOI: 10.1631/jzus. B1600184.

[25] Romano A, Martelb F. The Role of EGCG in Breast Cancer Prevention and Therapy. Mini-Reviews in Medicinal Chemistry. 2020. DOI:10.2174/1389557520999201211194445

[26] LazzeroniM, Guerrieri-Gonzaga A, Gandini S, Johansson H, Serrano D, Cazzaniga M, Aristarco V, Macis D, Mora S, Caldarella P, Pagani G, Pruneri G, Riva A, Petrangolini G, Morazzoni P, DeCensi A, Bonanni B. A presurgical study of lecithin formulation of green tea extract in women with early breast cancer. Cancer prevention research.2017;10:363-370. DOI: 10.1158/1940-6207.CAPR-16-0298

[27] Samavat H, Ursin G, Emory TH, Lee E, Wang R, Torkelson CJ, Dostal AM, Swenson K, Le CT, Yang CS, Yu MC, Yee D, Wu AH, Yuan JM, Kurzer MS. A randomized controlled trial of green tea extract supplementation and mammographic density in postmenopausal women at increased risk of breast cancer. Cancer Prevention Research. 2017; 10:710-718. DOI: 10.1158/1940-6207.CAPR-17-0187

[28] Sheng J, Shi W, Guo H, Long W, Wang Y, Qi J, Liu J, Xu Y. The Inhibitory Effect of (−)-Epigallocatechin-3-Gallate on Breast Cancer Progression via Reducing SCUBE2 Methylation and DNMT Activity. Molecules. 2019; 24:2899. DOI: 10.3390/molecules24162899

[29] Schröder L, Marahrens P, Koch JG, Heidegger H, Vilsmeier T, Phan-Brehm T, Hofmann S, Mahner S, Jeschke U, Richter DU. Effects of green tea, matcha tea and their components epigallocatechin gallate and quercetin on MCF 7 and MDA-MB-231 breast carcinoma cells. Oncology Reports. 2019;41:387-396. DOI: 10.3892/or.2018.6789

[30] Xu P, Yan F, Zhao Y, Chen X, Sun S, Wang Y, Ying L. Green tea polyphenol EGCG attenuates MDSCs-mediated immunosuppression through canonical and non-canonical pathways in a 4T1 murine breast cancer model. Nutrients. 2020;12:1042. DOI: 10.3390/nu12041042

[31] Liu SM, Ou SY, Huang HH. Green tea polyphenols induce cell death in breast cancer MCF-7 cells through induction of cell cycle arrest and mitochondrial-mediated apoptosis. Journal of Zheijang University SCIENCE B. 2017; 18:89-98. DOI: 10.1631/jzus.B1600022.

[32] Fujioka K, Iwamoto T, Shima H, Tomaru K, Saito H, Ohtsuka M, Yoshidome A, Kawamura Y, Manome Y. The powdering process with a set of ceramic mills for green tea promoted catechin extraction and the ROS inhibition effect. Molecules. 2016; 21:474. DOI: 10.3390/molecules21040474.

[33] Bonuccelli G, Sotgia F, Lisanti MP. Matcha green tea (MGT) inhibits the propagation of cancer stem cells (CSCs), by targeting mitochondrial metabolism, glycolysis and multiple cell signalling pathways. Aging (Albany NY). 2018; 10:1867-1883. DOI: 10.18632/aging.101483

[34] Sinnadurai S, Okabayashi S, Kawamura T, Mori M, Bhoo-Pathy N, Aishah Taib N, Ukawa S, Tamakoshi A, The Jacc Study Group -. Intake of Common Alcoholic and Non-Alcoholic Beverages and Breast Cancer Risk among Japanese Women: Findings from the Japan Collaborative Cohort Study. Asian Pacific Journal of Cancer Prevention. 2020; 21:1701-1707. DOI: 10.31557/APJCP.2020.21.6.1701

[35] Neag MA, Mocan A, Echeverría J, Pop RM, Bocsan CI, Crişan G, Buzoianu AD. Berberine: Botanical Occurrence, Traditional Uses, Extraction Methods, and Relevance in Cardiovascular, Metabolic, Hepatic, and Renal Disorders. Frontiers in Pharmacology. 2018; 9:557. DOI: 10.3389/fphar.2018.00557

[36] Ma W, Zhang Y, Yu M, Wang B, Xu S, Zhang J, Li X, Ye X. In-vitro and in-vivo anti-breast cancer activity of synergistic effect of berberine and exercise through promoting the apoptosis and immunomodulatory effects. International Immunopharmacology. 2020; 87:106787. DOI: 10.1016/j.intimp.2020.106787

[37] Han B, Wang K, Tu Y, Tan L, He C. Low-dose berberine attenuates the anti-breast cancer activity of chemotherapeutic agents via induction of autophagy and antioxidation. Dose Response. 2020; 18:1559325820939751. DOI: 10.1177/1559325820939751

[38] El Khalki L, Tilaoui M, Jaafari A, Ait Mouse H, Zyad A. Studies on the Dual Cytotoxicity and Antioxidant Properties of *Berberis vulgaris* Extracts and Its Main Constituent Berberine. Advances in Pharmacological Sciences. 2018; 2018:3018498. DOI: 10.1155/2018/3018498.

[39] Belwal T, Bisht A, Devkota HP, Ullah H, Khan H, Pandey A, Bhatt ID, Echeverría J. Phytopharmacology and Clinical Updates of Berberis Species Against Diabetes and Other Metabolic Diseases.Frontiers in Pharmacology. 2020;11:41. DOI: 10.3389/fphar.2020.00041

[40] Karnam KC, Ellutla M, Bodduluru LN, Kasala ER, Uppulapu SK, Kalyankumarraju M, Lahkar M. Preventive effect of berberine against DMBA-induced breast cancer in female Sprague Dawley rats. Biomedicine & Pharmacotherapy. 2017; 92:207-214. DOI: 10.1016/j.biopha.2017.05.069

[41] Kim S, Lee J, You D, Jeong Y, Jeon M, Yu J, Kim SW, Nam SJ, Lee JE. Berberine Suppresses Cell Motility Through Downregulation of TGF-β1 in Triple Negative Breast Cancer Cells. Cellular Physiology and Biochemistry. 2018; 45: 795-807. DOI: 10.1159/000487171

[42] Su K, Hu P, Wang X, Kuang C, Xiang Q, Yang F, Xiang J, Zhu S, Wei L, Zhang J. Tumor suppressor berberine binds VASP to inhibit cell migration in basal-like breast cancer. Oncotarget. 2016; 7:45849-45862. DOI: 10.18632/oncotarget.9968

[43] Zhao Y, Jing Z, Lv J, Zhang Z, Lin J, Cao X, Zhao Z, Liu P, Mao W. Berberine activates caspase-9/cytochrome c-mediated apoptosis to suppress triple-negative breast cancer cells in vitro and in vivo. Biomedicine and Pharmacotherapy. 2017; 95:18-24. DOI: 10.1016/j.biopha.2017.08.045

[44] Ma W, Zhu M, Zhang D, Yang L, Yang T, Li X, Zhang Y. Berberine inhibits the proliferation and migration of breast cancer ZR-75-30 cells by targeting Ephrin-B2. Phytomedicine. 2017; 25:45-51. DOI: 10.1016/j.phymed.2016.12.013

[45] Pan Y, Zhang F, Zhao Y, Shao D, Zheng X, Chen Y, He K, Li J, Chen L. Berberine enhances chemosensitivity and induces apoptosis through dose-orchestrated AMPK signaling in breast cancer. Journal of Cancer. 2017; 8:1679-1689. DOI: 10.7150/jca.19106

[46] Jeong Y, You D, Kang HG, Yu J, Kim SW, Nam SJ, Lee JE, Kim S. Berberine suppresses fibronectin expression through inhibition of c-Jun phosphorylation in breast cancer cells. Journal of Breast Cancer. 2018; 21:21-27. DOI: 10.4048/jbc.2018.21.1.21

[47] Ahmadiankia N, Moghaddam HK, Mishan MA, Bahrami AR, Naderi-Meshkin H, Bidkhori HR, Moghaddam M, Mirfeyzi SJ. Berberine suppresses migration of MCF-7 breast cancer cells through down-regulation of chemokine receptors. Iranian Journal of Basic Medical Sciences. 2016; 19:125-131. DOI:10.22038/IJBMS.2016.6531

[48] Sakaguchi M, Kitaguchi D, Morinami S, Kurashiki Y, Hashida H, Miyata S, Yamaguchi M, Sakai M,

Murata N, Tanaka S. Berberine-induced nucleolar stress response in a human breast cancer cell line. Biochemical and Biophysical Research Communications.2020 ;528:227-233. DOI: 10.1016/j.bbrc.2020.05.020

[49] Sun Y, Wang W, Tong Y. Berberine inhibits proliferative ability of breast cancer cells by reducing metadherin. Medical Science Monitor. 2019; 25:9058-9066. DOI: 10.12659/MSM.914486.

[50] Zhao L, Zhang C. Berberine Inhibits MDA-MB-231 Cells by attenuating their inflammatory responses. BioMed Research International. 2020; 16:3617514. DOI: 10.1155/2020/3617514

[51] Yao M, Fan X, Yuan B, Takagi N, Liu S, Han X, Ren J, Liu J. Berberine inhibits NLRP3 Inflammasome pathway in human triple-negative breast cancer MDA-MB-231 cell. BMC Complementary and Alternative Medicine. 2019;19:216. DOI: 10.1186/s12906-019-2615-4

[52] Kim S, You D, Jeong Y, Yu J, Kim SW, Nam SJ, Lee JE. Berberine down-regulates IL-8 expression through inhibition of the EGFR/MEK/ERK pathway in triple-negative breast cancer cells. Phytomedicine. 2018; 50:43-49. DOI: 10.1016/j.phymed.2018.08.004

[53] Sefidabi R, Mortazavi P, Hosseini S. Antiproliferative effect of berberine on canine mammary gland cancer cell culture. Biomedical Reports. 2017; 6:95-98. DOI: 10.3892/br.2016.809

[54] PonnusamyL, Kothandan G, Manoharan R. Berberine and Emodin abrogates breast cancer growth and facilitates apoptosis through inactivation of SIK3-induced mTOR and Akt signaling pathway. Biochimica et Biophysica Acta (BBA) - Molecular Basis of Disease. 2020; 1866:165897. DOI: 10.1016/j.bbadis.2020.165897

[55] Zhang R, Qiao H, Chen S, Chen X, Dou K, Wei L, Zhang J. Berberine reverses lapatinib resistance of HER2-positive breast cancer cells by increasing the level of ROS. Cancer Biology & Therapy. 2016; 17:925-934. DOI: 10.1080/15384047.2016.1210728

[56] Wang Y, Liu Y, Du X, Ma H, Yao J. Berberine reverses doxorubicin resistance by inhibiting autophagy through the PTEN/Akt/mTOR signaling pathway in breast cancer. OncoTargets and Therapy. 2020; 13:1909-1919. DOI: 10.2147/OTT.S241632

[57] Hashemi-Niasari F, Rabbani-Chadegani A, Razmi M, Fallah S. Synergy of theophylline reduces necrotic effect of berberine, induces cell cycle arrest and PARP, HMGB1, Bcl-2 family mediated apoptosis in MDA-MB-231 breast cancer cells. Biomedicine & Pharmacotherapy. 2018; 106:858-867. DOI: 10.1016/j.biopha.2018.07.019.

[58] Gao X, Wang J, Li M, Wang J, Lv J, Zhang L, Sun C, Ji J, Yang W, Zhao Z, Mao W. Berberine attenuates XRCC1-mediated base excision repair and sensitizes breast cancer cells to the chemotherapeutic drugs. Journal of Cellular and Molecular Medicine. 2019; 23:6797-6804. DOI: 10.1111/jcmm.14560

[59] Wen C, Wu L, Fu L, Zhang X, Zhou H. Berberine enhances the anti-tumor activity of tamoxifen in drug-sensitive MCF-7 and drug-resistant MCF-7/TAM cells. Molecular Medicine Reports.2016; 14:2250-2256. DOI: 10.3892/mmr.2016.5490

[60] Du J, Sun Y, Lu YY, Lau E, Zhao M, Zhou QM, Su SB. Berberine and Evodiamine act synergistically against human breast cancer MCF-7 Cells by inducing cell cycle arrest and apoptosis. Anticancer Research. 2017; 37:6141-6151. DOI: 10.21873/anticanres.12063

[61] Khan I, Joshi G, Nakhate KT, Ajazuddin, Kumar R, Gupta U. Nano-Co-Delivery of Berberine and

Anticancer Drug Using PLGA Nanoparticles: exploration of better anticancer activity and in vivo kinetics. Pharmaceutical Research. 2019; 36:149. DOI: 10.1007/s11095-019-2677-5.

[62] Bhanumathi R, Manivannan M, Thangaraj R, Kannan S. Drug-carrying capacity and anticancer effect of the folic acid- and berberine-loaded silver nanomaterial to regulate the AKT-ERK pathway in breast cancer. ACS Omega. 2018; 3:8317-8328. DOI: 10.1021/acsomega.7b01347

[63] Linjawi S A A, Khalil W K B, M. Hassanane M, Ahmed E S. Evaluation of the protective effect of *Nigella sativa* extract and its primary active component thymoquinone against DMBA-induced breast cancer in female rats. Archives of Medical Science. 2015; 11:220-229. DOI:10.5114/aoms.2013.33329.

[64] Imran M, Rauf A, Khan IA, Shahbaz M, Qaisrani TB, Fatmawati S, Abu-Izneid T, Imran A, Rahman KU, Gondal TA. Thymoquinone: A novel strategy to combat cancer: A review. Biomedicine & Pharmacotherapy. 2018; 106:390-402. DOI: 10.1016/j.biopha.2018.06.159

[65] Şakalar Ç, İzgi K, İskender B, Sezen S, Aksu H, Çakır M, Kurt B, Turan A, Canatan H. The combination of thymoquinone and paclitaxel shows anti-tumor activity through the interplay with apoptosis network in triple-negative breast cancer. Tumour Biology. 2016; 37:4467-77. DOI: 10.1007/s13277-015-4307-0

[66] Ünal TD, Hamurcu Z, Delibaşı N, Çınar V, Güler A, Gökçe S, Nurdinov N, Ozpolat B. Thymoquinone inhibits proliferation and migration of mda-mb-231 triple negative breast cancer cells by suppressing autophagy and beclin-1 and lc3. Anti-Cancer Agents in Medicinal Chemistry. 2020; 21: 355-364. DOI:10.2174/1871520620666200807221047

[67] Sundaravadivelu S, Raj SK, Kumar BS, Arumugamand P, Ragunathan PP. Reverse screening bioinformatics approach to identify potential anti breast cancer targets using thymoquinone from neutraceuticals Black Cumin Oil. Anti-Cancer Agents in Medicinal Chemistry.2019;19:599-609. DOI: 10.2174/1871520619666190124155359

[68] Aslan M, Afşar E, Kırımlıoglu E, Çeker T, Yılmaz Ç. Antiproliferative Effects of Thymoquinone in MCF-7 Breast and HepG2 Liver Cancer Cells: Possible Role of Ceramide and ER Stress. Nutrition and Cancer. 2020; 14:1-13. DOI: 10.1080/01635581.2020.1751216

[69] KhanA, AldebasiYH, AlsuhaibaniSA, Khan MA. Thymoquinone augments cyclophosphamide-mediated inhibition of cell proliferation in breast cancer cells. Asian Pacific Journal of Cancer Prevention. 2019; 20:1153-1160. DOI: 10.31557/APJCP.2019.20.4.1153.

[70] Alobaedi, O.H. W.H. Talib, I.A. Basheti.Antitumor effect of thymoquinone combined with resveratrol on mice transplanted with breast cancer. Asian Pacific Journal of Tropical Medicine.2017; 10:400-408. DOI: 10.1016/j.apjtm.2017.03.026

[71] Talib WH. Regressions of breast carcinoma syngraft following treatment with piperine in combination with thymoquinone. Scientia Pharmaceutica. 2017; 85:27. DOI: 10.3390/scipharm85030027.

[72] Odeh LH, Talib WH, Basheti IA. Synergistic effect of thymoquinone and melatonin against breast cancer implanted in mice. Journal of Cancer Research and Therapeutics. 2018 ;14: S324-S330. DOI: 10.4103/0973-1482.235349

[73] Bashmail HA, Alamoudi AA, Noorwali A, Hegazy GA, AJabnoor G, Choudhry H, Al-Abd AM. Thymoquinone synergizes gemcitabine anti-breast cancer activity via modulating its apoptotic and autophagic activities. Scientific Reports. 2018; 8:11674. DOI: 10.1038/s41598-018-30046-z

[74] Ibiyeye KM, Nordin N, Ajat M, Zuki ABZ. Ultrastructural changes and antitumor effects of doxorubicin/thymoquinone-loaded CaCO3 nanoparticles on breast cancer cell line. Frontiers in Oncology. 2019; 9:599. DOI: 10.3389/fonc.2019.00599.

[75] Khan M, Tania M, Wei C, Mei Z, Fu S, Cheng J, Xu J, Fu J. Thymoquinone inhibits cancer metastasis by downregulating TWIST1 expression to reduce epithelial to mesenchymal transition. Oncotarget. 2015; 6: 19580-19591.

[76] Bhattacharjee M, Upadhyay P, Sarker S, Basu A, Das S, Ghosh A, Ghosh S, Adhikary A. Combinatorial therapy of Thymoquinone and Emodin synergistically enhances apoptosis, attenuates cell migration and reduces stemness efficiently in breast cancer. Biochimica et Biophysica Acta General Subjects. 2020; 1864:129695. DOI: 10.1016/j.bbagen.2020.129695

[77] Shanmugam MK, Ahn KS, Hsu A, Woo CC, Yuan Y, Tan KHB, Chinnathambi A, Alahmadi TA, Alharbi SA, Koh APF, Arfuso F, Huang RY, Lim LHK, Sethi G, Kumar AP. Thymoquinone inhibits bone metastasis of breast cancer cells through abrogation of the cxcr4 signaling axis. Frontiers in Pharmacology. 2018; 9:1294. DOI: 10.3389/fphar.2018.01294

[78] Bhattacharya S, Ahir M, Patra P, Mukherjee S, Ghosh S, Mazumdar M, Chattopadhyay S, Das T, Chattopadhyay D, Adhikary A. PEGylated-thymoquinone-nanoparticle mediated retardation of breast cancer cell migration by deregulation of cytoskeletal actin polymerization through miR-34a. Biomaterials. 2015;51:91-107. DOI: 10.1016/j.biomaterials.2015.01.007

[79] Ong YS, Saiful Yazan L, Ng WK, Abdullah R, Mustapha NM, Sapuan S, Foo JB, Tor YS, How CW, Abd Rahman N, Zakarial Ansar FH. Thymoquinone loaded in nano-structured lipid carrier showed enhanced anticancer activity in 4T1 tumor-bearing mice. Nanomedicine. 2018; 13:1567-1582. DOI: 10.2217/nnm-2017-0322.

[80] Zafar S, Akhter S, Ahmad I, Hafeez Z, Alam Rizvi MM, Jain GK, Ahmad FJ. Improved chemotherapeutic efficacy against resistant human breast cancer cells with co-delivery of docetaxel and thymoquinone by chitosan grafted lipid nanocapsules: formulation optimization, in vitro and in vivo studies. Colloids and Surfaces B Biointerfaces. 2020;186:110603. DOI: 10.1016/j.colsurfb.2019.110603

[81] Mehanna MM, Sarieddine R, Alwattar JK, Chouaib R, Gali-Muhtasib H. Anticancer Activity of Thymoquinone Cubic Phase Nanoparticles Against Human Breast Cancer: Formulation, Cytotoxicity and Subcellular Localization. International Journal of Nanomedicine. 2020;15:9557-9570. DOI: 10.2147/IJN.S263797

[82] Kommineni N, Saka R, Bulbake U, Khan W. Cabazitaxel and thymoquinone co-loaded lipospheres as a synergistic combination for breast cancer. Chemistry and Physics of Lipids. 2019; 224:104707. DOI: 10.1016/j.chemphyslip.2018.11.009.

[83] Elbaz M, Nasser MW, Ravi J, Wani NA, Ahirwar DK, Zhao H, Oghumu S, Satoskar AR, Shilo K, Carson WE 3rd, Ganju RK. Modulation of the tumor microenvironment and inhibition of EGF/EGFR pathway: novel

anti-tumor mechanisms of Cannabidiol in breast cancer. Molecular Oncology. 2015; 9:906-919. DOI: 10.1016/j.molonc.2014.12.010

[84] Mokoena D, George B, Abrahamse H. Enhancing Breast Cancer Treatment Using a Combination of Cannabidiol and Gold Nanoparticles for Photodynamic Therapy. International Journal of Molecular Sciences.2019; 20:4771. DOI: 10.3390/ijms20194771

[85] Śledziński P, Zeyland J, Słomski R, Nowak A. The current state and future perspectives of cannabinoids in cancer biology. Cancer Medicine. 2018;7: 765-775.DOI: 10.1002/cam4.1312.

[86] Pérez-Gómez E, Andradas C, Blasco-Benito S, Caffarel MM, García-Taboada E, Villa-Morales M, Moreno E, Hamann S, Martín-Villar E, Flores JM, Wenners A, Alkatout I, Klapper W, Röcken C, Bronsert P, Stickeler E, Staebler A, Bauer M, Arnold N, Soriano J, Pérez-Martínez M, Megías D, Moreno-Bueno G, Ortega-Gutiérrez S, Artola M, Vázquez-Villa H, Quintanilla M, Fernández-Piqueras J, Canela EI, McCormick PJ, Guzmán M, Sánchez C. Role of cannabinoid receptor CB2 in HER2 pro-oncogenic signaling in breast cancer. Journal of the National Cancer Institute. 2015;107: djv077. DOI: 10.1093/jnci/djv077

[87] Kosgodage US, Mould R, Henley AB, Nunn AV, Guy GW, Thomas EL, Inal JM, Bell JD, Lange S. Cannabidiol (CBD) is a novel inhibitor for exosome and microvesicle (EMV) release in cancer. Frontiers in Pharmacology. 2018; 9:889. DOI: 10.3389/fphar.2018.00889

[88] Sultan AS, Marie MA, Sheweita SA. Novel mechanism of cannabidiol-induced apoptosis in breast cancer cell lines. Breast. 2018; 41:34-41. DOI: 10.1016/j.breast.2018.06.009

[89] García-Morales L, Castillo AM, Tapia Ramírez J, Zamudio-Meza H, Domínguez-Robles MDC, Meza I. CBD Reverts the mesenchymal invasive phenotype of breast cancer cells induced by the inflammatory cytokine IL-1β. International Journal of Molecular Sciences. 2020;21:2429. DOI: 10.3390/ijms21072429

[90] Elbaz M, Ahirwar D, Xiaoli Z, Zhou X, Lustberg M, Nasser MW, Shilo K, Ganju RK. TRPV2 is a novel biomarker and therapeutic target in triple negative breast cancer. Oncotarget. 2016; 9:33459-33470. DOI: 10.18632/oncotarget.9663.

[91] Fraguas-Sánchez AI, Fernández-Carballido A, Simancas-Herbada R, Martin-Sabroso C, Torres-Suárez AI. CBD loaded microparticles as a potential formulation to improve paclitaxel and doxorubicin-based chemotherapy in breast cancer. International Journal of Pharmaceutics.2020;574:118916. DOI: 10.1016/j.ijpharm.2019.118916

[92] Schoeman R, Beukes N, Frost C. Cannabinoid combination induces cytoplasmic vacuolation in mcf-7 breast cancer cells. Molecules. 2020; 25:4682. DOI: 10.3390/molecules25204682.

[93] Parihar V, Rogers A, Blain AM, Zacharias SRK, Patterson LL, Siyam MA. Reduction in tamoxifen metabolites Endoxifen and N-desmethyltamoxifen with chronic administration of low dose cannabidiol: A CYP3A4 and CYP2D6 Drug Interaction. Journal of Pharmacy Practice. 2020; 15:897190020972208. DOI: 10.1177/0897190020972208

[94] Tomko A, O'Leary L, Trask H, Achenbach JC, Hall SR, Goralski KB, Ellis LD, Dupré DJ. Antitumor activity of abnormal cannabidiol and its analog o-1602 in taxol-resistant preclinical models of breast cancer. Frontiers in Pharmacology. 2019; 10:1124. DOI: 10.3389/fphar.2019.01124.

[95] Blasco-Benito S, Seijo-Vila M, Caro-Villalobos M, Tundidor I, Andradas C, García-Taboada E, Wade J, Smith S, Guzmán M, Pérez-Gómez E, Gordon M, Sánchez C. Appraising the "entourage effect": Antitumor action of a pure cannabinoid versus a botanical drug preparation in preclinical models of breast cancer. Biochemical Pharmacology. 2018; 157:285-293. DOI: 10.1016/j.bcp.2018.06.025

[96] Kenyon J, Liu W, Dalgleish A. Report of objective clinical responses of cancer patients to pharmaceutical-grade synthetic cannabidiol. Anticancer Research. 2018; 38:5831-5835. DOI: 10.21873/anticanres.12924.

[97] Pellati F, Borgonetti V, Brighenti V, Biagi M, Benvenuti S, Corsi L. *Cannabis sativa* L. and Nonpsychoactive Cannabinoids: Their Chemistry and Role against Oxidative Stress, Inflammation, and Cancer. BioMed Research International. 2018; 4:1691428. DOI: 10.1155/2018/1691428

[98] Kisková T, Mungenast F, Suváková M, Jäger W, Thalhammer T. Future aspects for cannabinoids in breast cancer therapy. International Journal of Molecular Sciences. 2019; 20:1673. DOI: 10.3390/ijms20071673

Chapter 6

Structural Insight of the Anticancer Properties of Doxazosin on Overexpressing EGFR/HER2 Cell Lines

Martiniano Bello and Miguel Ángel Vargas Mejía

Abstract

The selective α1-adrenergic receptor antagonist doxazosin is used for the treatment of hypertension. More recently, an experimental report demonstrated that this compound exhibits antiproliferative activity in breast cancer cell lines with similar inhibitory activity to gefitinib, a selective inhibitor of EGFR in the active state ($EGFR_{AC}$). This experimental study provided evidence that doxazosin can be employed as an anticancer compound, however, the structural basis for its inhibitory properties is poorly understood at the atomic level. To gain insight about this molecule, molecular dynamics (MD) simulation with the molecular mechanics generalized Born surface area (MMGBSA) approach was employed to explore the structural and energetic features that guide the inhibitory properties of doxazosin and gefitinib in overexpressing EGFR/HER2 cell lines. Our result suggest that doxazosin exerts its inhibitory properties in breast cancer cell lines by targeting EGFR/HER2 but mainly HER2 in the inactive state ($HER2_{IN}$), whereas gefitinib by targeting mainly $EGFR_{AC}$, in line with previous literature. Decomposition of the binding affinity into individual contributions of $HER2_{IN\text{-}doxazosin}$ and $EGFR_{AC\text{-}gefitinib}$ systems detected hot spot residues but also showed polar interactions of Met801/Met793 with the quinazoline ring of both compounds. Principal component (PC) analysis revealed that the molecular recognition of the $HER2_{IN\text{-}doxazosin}$ system was linked to conformational changes but $EGFR_{AC\text{-}gefitinib}$ was not.

Keywords: HER2, EGFR, doxazosin, docking, MD simulations

1. Introduction

Human epidermal growth factor receptor 1 (EGFR) and 2 (HER2) form part of a family of human epidermal grown factor receptors (EGFRs), and whose phosphorylation impacts cell proliferation, differentiation, and migration [1]. The cytoplasmic tyrosine kinase domain (TKD) is considered one of the most studied receptors for developing new anticancer drugs [2]. Activation of EGFR starts the molecular recognition of endogenous growth factors at the extracellular domain that, at the time, promotes the formation of homo- and heterodimers among the different members of EGFR, with HER2 the preferred member of EGFRs to form heterodimers [3–5]. The transition from a monomeric to dimeric state in EGFR is coupled to a conformational change in the TKD from an inactive to active state [6–8], whereas that for

IntechOpen

HER2 transitions from inactive, intermediate, and inactive states [9–11]. Generally, the signaling activity regulated by EGFR/HER2 is under control, however, mutations in TKD give place to constitutive activation of these receptors, which results in the development of different types of cancer, such as lung [12] and breast cancer [13]. In addition, overexpression of EGFR/HER2 also happens with radiotherapy and chemotherapy resistance [14–16].

Based on the ability of tyrosine kinase inhibitors (TKIs) to inhibit EGFR, they can be divided in two types, those targeting the active state, such as Iressa, and those targeting the inactive state, such as erlotinib and lapatinib [17–20]. Lapatinib showed dual activity on EGFR/HER2 [21–26]. Despite the benefits of using these TKIs, the employment of them has been linked to severe side effects and drug resistance [27–30]. Therefore, it is necessary to identify new compounds, either through drug design or drug repurposing, that target EGFR and/or HER2 receptors and are effective for cancer therapy. In this context, the combination of docking and molecular dynamics (MD) simulations has been widely exploited to generate new information about the binding properties between natural or synthetic TKIs and EGFR/HER2 [10, 11, 19, 20, 31–36]. In a previous study, Hui et al. explored the inhibitory properties of doxazosin, an α-1 antagonist used for the treatment of hypertension, in two human breast cancer cell lines: BCC MDA-MB-231 and MCF-7 cells [37]. MDA-MB-231 and MCF-7 cells are estrogen receptor (ER) positive and ER negative, respectively [38], and both cell lines also expressed EGFR and HER2; however, MDA-MB-231 expressed both receptors in higher concentrations than MCF-7 [39]. Although EGFR and HER2 are important regulators for normal cellular processes, their dysregulation has been associated to protein overexpression that leads to the development of different types of cancer [1, 5]. They demonstrated that doxazosin induces apoptosis in breast cancer cell lines similar to Iressa (Gefitinib), reducing phosphorylated EGFR by a mechanism that does not involve the α1-adrenergic receptor, however, the structural and energetic basis for its inhibitory properties is poorly understood. In addition, Sharkawi et al. identified similar experimental antiproliferative activity of doxazosin in an MCF-7 cell line through the inhibition of EGFR [40]. Thus, more robust structural and energetic studies are required to provide structural insight into the affinity of doxazosin for EGFR/HER2 compared with gefitinib. Structural data, docking, and molecular dynamics (MD) simulations combined with the MMGBSA approach were used to elucidate the molecular mechanism through which doxazosin and gefitinib inhibit EGFR/HER2.

2. Methods

2.1 Structural modeling

The free forms of EGFR in the inactive ($EGFR_{IN}$) and active ($EGFR_{AC}$) states were taken from the crystallographic structures of $EGFR_{IN}$ (PDB entry 1XKK) and $EGFR_{AC}$ (PDB entry 1 M17) conformations. The free forms of HER2 in the inactive ($HER2_{IN}$) and active ($HER2_{AC}$) states were taken from previous MD simulation studies; $HER2_{IN}$ [10] and $HER2_{AC}$ [11] conformations. Amino acid residues missing in the electron density map of EGFR structures were built with MODELER Version 9.14 [41].

2.2 Docking studies

Docking calculations were carried out using AutoDock 4.2 and AutoDock Tools 1.5.6 software [42]. The ligand structures were built and optimized with the Gaussian package [43]. The initial geometries of ligands were optimized at the AM1 level. Hydrogen atoms were added to ligands and receptors, and

Kollman and Gasteiger partial charges were assigned for ligand and proteins, respectively. The affinity grid maps were constructed on the receptor using a grid size of 70 × 70 × 70 Å and 0.370 Å of spacing. Due to the stochastic nature of the Lamarckian algorithm, 20 runs were performed for each compound, and 30 conformations of the ligand (binding poses) were observed between ligand and protein. The best binding poses were selected using the criteria of having the lowest energetic conformations at the receptor binding site.

2.3 Molecular dynamics simulations

The protein-ligand results obtained by docking were checked through MD simulation studies. MD simulations were carried out using the AMBER16 package [44], in conjunction with the ff14SB force field [45]. The systems simulated were put into a space-filling dodecahedric box of 12 Å, solvated with TIP3P water model [46], and neutralized with sodium and chloride ions (0.10 M) to create a physiological concentration. The parameterizations of the ligands were performed assigning AM1-BCC atomic charges and matching the atoms with the general Amber force field (GAFF) [47]. Once the systems were constructed, they were minimized using steepest descent with position restraint of the ligands, followed by steepest descent without position restraint and conjugate gradients. The minimized systems were then submitted to 100 ns-long MD simulations using an NPT ensemble with the velocity rescaling arrangement to simulate a constant temperature at 310 K. A constant temperature and pressure (1 atm) were maintained using the weak-coupling algorithm [48], with coupling constants τ_T and τ_P of 1.0 and 0.2 ps, respectively. The electrostatic term was described by the PME method [49], and a 10 Å cut-off was selected for the van der Waals interactions. The time step for the MD simulations was set to 2.0 fs. The SHAKE algorithm [50] was employed to reset bonds to their right lengths after an unconstrained update. The conformations obtained from MD simulations at intervals of 20 picoseconds (ps) were analyzed using the cpptraj tool in Amber16. Plots of variation of root mean squared deviation (RMSD) and radius of gyration (R_G) were generated to evaluate convergence. Clustering analysis using a cutoff of 2.5 Å was performed to identify the most populated conformation in the simulation. Principal components (PC) analysis along the most essential eigenvectors was carried out to evaluate total flexibility. A map of interactions was generated using Maestro Version 10.1, 2015–1 [51].

2.4 Affinity prediction and per-residue decomposition

The binding free energy (ΔG_{bind}) and per residue contribution were determined using the MMGBSA method [52–55]. Analysis was carried out using a total of 500 protein-ligand conformers at intervals of 100 ps (over the last 50 ns of simulation), considering a salt concentration of 0.10 M and implicit solvent models [56]. The binding free energy (ΔG_{bind}) and per-residue decomposition for each complex was calculated as previously described [11] and were the average result of triplicate experiments.

3. Results and discussion

3.1 Convergence and equilibrium

The stability of the evaluated systems was observed by measuring two geometrical parameters. The root mean squared deviation (RMSD) and the radius of gyration (RG) were determined to identify the time at which the systems reached convergence (**Table 1**). RMSD analysis showed that free and bound EGFR/HER2 systems reached stability between 20 to 50 ns with RMSD values, which oscillated between 1.40 and 4.20 Å. RG examination revealed that free and bound EGFR/HER2 systems exhibited stability from 20 to 50 ns with values oscillating between 18.8 and 20.2 Å. Based on this result, further analysis was carried out discarding the first 50 ns.

System	RMSD	RG
$EGFR_{AC}$	2.1 ± 0.20	19.0 ± 0.12
$EGFR_{AC\text{-}doxazosin}$	1.7 ± 0.10	19.1 ± 0.10
$EGFR_{AC\text{-}gefitinib}$	2.2 ± 0.20	19.2 ± 0.10
$EGFR_{IN}$	1.8 ± 0.20	18.8 ± 0.10
$EGFR_{IN\text{-}doxazosin}$	2.2 ± 0.20	19.0 ± 0.10
$EGFR_{IN\text{-}gefitinib}$	2.7 ± 0.21	19.0 ± 0.10
$HER2_{AC}$	3.6 ± 0.17	20.0 ± 0.10
$HER2_{AC\text{-}doxazosin}$	1.7 ± 0.20	20.0 ± 0.14
$HER2_{AC\text{-}gefitinib}$	1.4 ± 0.20	19.9 ± 0.10
$HER2_{IN}$	3.9 ± 0.40	20.0 ± 0.01
$HER2_{IN\text{-}doxazosin}$	3.4 ± 0.40	20.2 ± 0.10
$HER2_{IN\text{-}gefitinib}$	4.2 ± 0.22	19.6 ± 0.13

Table 1.
Average geometrical values (Å) over the last 50 ns of 100-ns-long MD simulations.

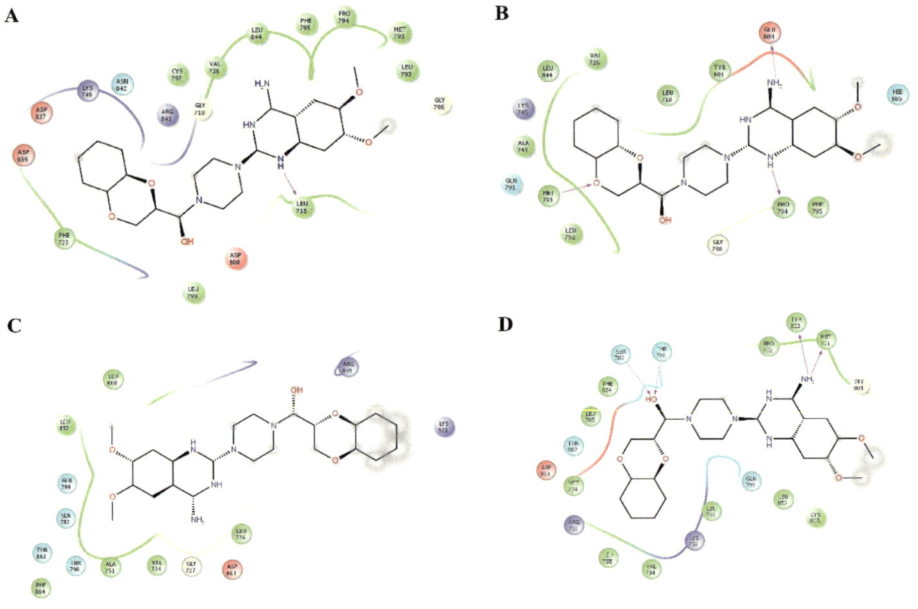

Figure 1.
Map of interactions for the most populated conformation of EGFR/HER2–doxazosin systems. Binding conformations and map of interaction for $EGFR_{AC\text{-}doxazosin}$ (A) $EGFR_{IN\text{-}doxazosin}$ (B) $HER2_{AC\text{-}doxazosin}$ (C) and $HER2_{IN\text{-}doxazosin}$ (D). The map of interactions was performed with maestro Schrödinger version 10.1.

3.2 Structural analysis of complexes between doxazosin and $EGFR_{AC}$/$EGFR_{IN}$

To explore the structural differences between doxazosin and gefitinib on EGFR/HER2, the most populated receptor-ligand conformations were retrieved over the equilibrated simulation time (the last 50 ns) through clustering analysis. Analysis of the complex between doxazosin and $EGFR_{AC}$ showed that the ligand was stabilized through van der Waals interactions with Phe723, Val726, Leu792, Met793, Pro794, Phe795, Cys797, Leu799, and Leu844, and polar interactions with Gly719, Lys745, Gly796, Asp800, Asp837, Arg841, Asn842, and Asp855 (**Figure 1A**). In contrast, Val718 formed both van der Waals interactions and a hydrogen bond with the quinazoline ring of doxazosin. In the complex with $EGFR_{IN}$, dozaxosin was bound through van der Waals interactions with Phe723, Val718, Val726, Ala743, Leu792, Phe795, Tyr801, and Leu844. The polar contact took place with Lys745, Gln791, Gly796, Glu804, and His805. Met793 formed both van der Waals interactions and one hydrogen bond with the benzodioxin moiety of doxazosin. Pro794 established both van der Waals contacts and one hydrogen bond with the quinazoline ring of doxazosin, whereas Glu804 formed hydrogen bonds with the quinazoline ring of doxazosin (**Figure 1B**). Stabilization of doxazosin did not establish interactions with Thr790 and Met766, two residues whose mutations have been linked to EGFR drug resistance [57, 58]. In addition, the characteristic interactions between Met793 and the quinazoline moiety were not observed, which has previously been observed for other TKIs of EGFR [10].

3.3 Structural analysis of complexes between doxazosin and $HER2_{AC}$/$HER2_{IN}$

Dozaxosin in complex with $HER2_{AC}$ was bound through van der Waals interactions with Leu726, Val734, Ala751, Phe864, Leu852, and Leu800 and polar interactions with Gly727, Ser783, Thr798, Gln799, Arg849, Thr862, Asp863, and Lys921 (**Figure 1C**). For the complex between doxazosin and $HER2_{IN}$, the ligand was stabilized by Val754, Leu755, Met774, Leu785, Leu796, Pro802, Cys805, Leu852, and Phe864 and polar contacts with Lys753, Arg756, Gln799, Thr862, and Asp863. Tyr803 and Met801 formed van der Waals and hydrogen bonds with polar groups of the quinazoline ring, whereas Ser783 and Thr798 formed polar contacts with the linker between piperazine and the benzodioxin moiety (**Figure 1D**). Structural comparison of the complexes of doxazosin with $HER2_{AC}$/$HER2_{IN}$ showed that doxazosin was better coordinated on $HER2_{IN}$ than $HER2_{AC}$ through more well-adjusted types of van der Waals and hydrogen bonds. In addition, the characteristic hinge hydrogen bond between Met801 and the polar atoms of the quinazoline moiety of several TKIs [31, 59] was present only in for the complex with doxazosin and $HER2_{IN}$.

3.4 Structural analysis of complexes between gefitinib and $EGFR_{AC}$/$EGFR_{IN}$

Analysis of complexes between gefitinib and $EGFR_{AC}$ illustrated that the ligand was bound through van der Waals interactions with Leu718, Val726, Ala743, Met766, Leu788, Ile789, Leu792, Pro794, Phe795, Cys797, Leu844, and Phe856. The polar interactions were through contacts with Gly719, Ser720, Gly721, Lys745, Glu762, Thr790, Gln791, Gly796, Arg803, Thr854, and Asp855. Met793 formed van der Waals interactions and one polar interaction with the quinazoline ring of gefitinib, whereas Asp800 formed a hydrogen bond with one of the substituents at the quinazoline ring (**Figure 2A**). In complex with $EGFR_{IN}$, gefitinib was stabilized by van der Waals contacts with Phe723, Val718, Val726, Ala743, Cys775, Leu792, and

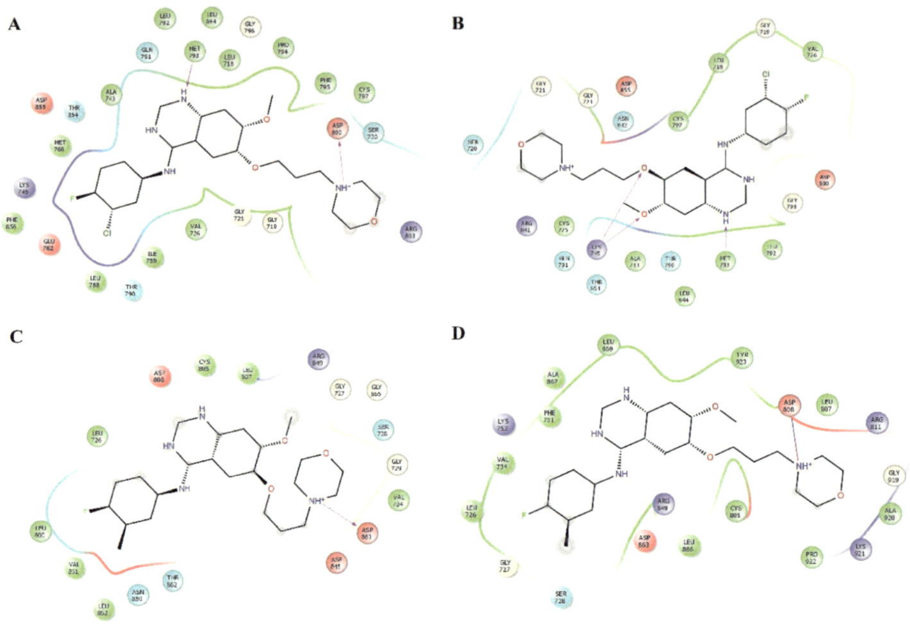

Figure 2.
Map of interactions for the most populated conformation of EGFR/HER2–gefitinib systems. Binding conformations and map of interaction for $EGFR_{AC\text{-}gefitinib}$ (A) $EGFR_{IN\text{-}gefitinib}$ (B) $HER2_{AC\text{-}gefitinib}$ (C) and $HER2_{IN\text{-}gefitinib}$ (D). The map of interactions was performed with maestro Schrödinger version 10.1.

Cys797. The polar contacts were through Gly719, Ser720, Gly721, Gly724, Thr790, Gln791, Arg841, Asn842, Thr854, and Asp 855. Met793 established both van der Waals interactions and one hydrogen bond with the quinazoline ring, whereas Lys745 made a hydrogen bond with one of the substituents of the quinazoline ring (**Figure 2B**). Comparison of the map of interactions of both complexes showed that gefitinib was better coordinated on $EGFR_{IN}$ than $EGFR_{AC}$. In both complexes, gefitinib established interactions with Thr790, a residue whose mutation is linked to EGFR drug resistance [57, 58]. In addition, in both complexes, the characteristic interactions between Met793 and the quinazoline moiety of ligand were observed, which has been reported elsewhere [10].

3.5 Structural analysis of complexes between gefitinib and $HER2_{AC}$/$HER2_{IN}$

Gefitinib in complex with $HER2_{AC}$ was bound through van der Waals interactions by Leu726, Val734, Leu800, Cys805, Leu807, Val851, and Leu852 (**Figure 2C**). Polar interactions were stabilized by Gly727, Ser728, Gly729, Asp808, Asp845, Arg849, Asn850, Thr862, and Gly865 residues, whereas Asp863 formed a hydrogen bond with one of the substituents of the quinazoline ring (**Figure 2C**). Gefitinib formed a complex with $HER2_{IN}$, coordinated by Leu726, Val734, Val731, Cys805, Leu807, Leu866, Ala867, Leu869, Tyr923, Ala920, and Pro922 residues through van der Waals interactions. Polar interactions took place by Gly727, Ser728, Lys753, Arg811, Arg849, Asp863, and Lys921 residues, whereas Asp808 formed a hydrogen bond with one of the quinazoline ring substituents (**Figure 2D**). Structural comparison of both systems depicted that gefitinib was better stabilized on $HER2_{IN}$ than $HER2_{AC}$. In addition, in both complexes, the characteristic polar interaction between Met801 and polar atoms of the quinazoline moiety of ligand was not observed [31, 59], as observed for the complex between doxasozin and $HER2_{IN}$ (**Figure 1C**).

3.6 Binding free energy

Determination of the ΔG_{bind} values was performed using the MMGBSA method. **Table 2** shows that all systems exhibited thermodynamically favorable ΔG_{bind} values. Nonpolar contributions formed by van der Waals energy (ΔE_{vdw}) and nonpolar desolvation ($\Delta G_{\text{npol,sol}}$) guided the binding of the complexes. Comparative analyses of the complexes between doxazosin or gefitinib on $HER2_{AC}$, $HER2_{IN}$, $EGFR_{AC}$, and $EGFR_{IN}$ showed that doxazosin reached more favorable ΔG_{bind} values on $HER2_{IN}$ than on $EGFR_{AC}$, $EGFR_{IN}$, and $HER2_{AC}$. Gefitinib showed a higher affinity for $EGFR_{IN}$ than $EGFR_{AC}$, $HER2_{AC}$, and HER_{IN}. Comparative analysis between the affinity of doxazosin and gefitinib for the four systems showed that doxazosin reached more favorable affinity for $HER2_{IN}$ than gefitinib, whereas gefitinib reached higher affinity for $EGFR_{AC}$ than doxazosin. The results suggested that the inhibitory activity of doxazosin in breast cancer cell lines is by mainly targeting $HER2_{IN}$, whereas that for gefitinib is mainly through inhibiting $EGFR_{AC}$, in line with previous studies where the selectivity of gefitinib toward $EGFR_{AC}$ was observed [60]. In addition, this analysis showed that the binding properties of doxazosin could be improved by exploring how changes in the binding affinity of new derivatives of doxazosin coupled on $HER2_{IN}$.

3.7 Decomposition of the per-residue free energy

This analysis identified the residues that contributed the most to the ΔG_{bind} value for each complex. **Table 3** shows that Leu718, Gly719, Phe723, Val726, Cys797, Leu799, Arg841, and Leu844 were the major contributors in the stabilization of the $EGFR_{AC\text{-doxazosin}}$ complex, from which Leu718 established hydrogen bonds with polar atoms of the quinazoline ring of doxazosin (**Figure 1A**). In the $EGFR_{IN\text{-doxazosin}}$ complex, Leu718, Val726, Ala743, Leu792, Met793, Pro794, Phe795, Gly796, Tyr801, Glu804, and Leu844 were the main stabilizers of this system. From these residues, Met793, Pro794, and Glu804 formed hydrogen bonds, stabilizing the quinazoline and benzodioxine rings of doxazosin (**Figure 1B**). In the $EGFR_{AC\text{-gefitinib}}$ complex, Leu718, Val726, Ala743, Lys745, Met766, Ile789, Thr790, Gln791, Leu792, Met793, Gly796, Cys797, and Thr854 were key residues in the affinity of gefitinib. Among these residues, the participation of Met793 through a hydrogen bond was appreciated (**Figure 2A**), whereas Leu718, Gly719, Val726, Ala743, Lys745, Leu792, Met793, Cys797, Asn842, Leu844, and Thr854 were the major contributors to the ΔG_{bind} value in the $EGFR_{IN\text{-gefitinib}}$ complex. Of these residues, the participation of Lys745

Systems	ΔE_{vdw}	ΔE_{ele}	$\Delta G_{ele,sol}$	$\Delta G_{npol,sol}$	ΔG_{bind}
$EGFR_{AC\text{-doxazosin}}$	−43.52 (5.13)	22.33 (4.91)	−2.69 (0.80)	−5.46 (0.50)	−29.33 (6.14)
$EGFR_{IN\text{-doxazosin}}$	−38.78 (3.90)	3.25 (0.91)	9.68 (2.80)	−4.62 (0.37)	−30.46 (4.20)
$HER2_{AC\text{-doxazosin}}$	−36.77 (6.0)	40.15 (12.0)	−21.06 (11.0)	−4.36 (0.55)	−22.05 (4.60)
$HER2_{IN\text{-doxazosin}}$	−48.93 (4.0)	23.99 (9.0)	−7.39 (1.50)	−5.99 (0.30)	−38.32 (4.0)
$EGFR_{AC\text{-gefitinib}}$	−55.01 (0.16)	−11.11 (0.65)	−25.40 (0.60)	−7.16 (0.01)	−47.88 (0.17)
$EGFR_{IN\text{-gefitinib}}$	−44.10 (0.15)	27.00 (0.69)	−16.48 (0.65)	−5.74 (0.01)	−39.32 (0.23)
$HER2_{AC\text{-gefitinib}}$	−34.76 (4.0)	38.46 (16.0)	−22.98 (5.0)	−4.90 (0.70)	−24.18 (5.0)
$HER2_{IN\text{-gefitinib}}$	−38.78 (5.7)	−31.92 (13.0)	49.70 (1.50)	−4.90 (0.50)	−25.91 (6.0)

Table 2.
Binding free energy components of protein-ligand systems (in units of kcal/Mol).

Residue	$EGFR_{AC\text{-}doxazosin}$	$EGFR_{IN\text{-}doxazosin}$	$EGFR_{AC\text{-}gefitinib}$	$EGFR_{IN\text{-}gefitinib}$
Leu718	−1.071	−2.243	−1.664	−1.261
Gly719	−0.532			−0.871
Phe723	−2.805			
Val726	−1.325	−0.674	−2.183	−1.705
Ala743		−0.548	−1.188	−0.592
Lys745			−0.782	−2.276
Met766			−0.727	
Ile789			−0.520	
Thr790			−1.190	
Gln791			−0.186	
Leu792		−1.257	−1.663	−1.897
Met793		−1.394	−2.045	−1.618
Pro794		−0.696		
Phe795		−2.053		
Gly796		−1.43	−1.122	
Cys797	−1.622		−1.015	−1.109
Leu799	−0.672			
Tyr801		−0.737		
Glu804		−1.064		
Arg841	−1.904			
Asn842				−0.504
Leu844	−0.935	−0.809		−2.063
Thr854			−0.839	−1.069

Table 3.
Per-residue free energy for complexes between doxazosin and gefitinib with $EGFR_{AC}$/$EGFR_{IN}$ (values kcal/Mol).

and Met793 were important in the stabilization of quinazoline and substitution at the quinazoline ring (**Figure 2B**).

Table 4 shows that Leu726, Gly727, Ser728, Val734, Asp863, and Phe864 contributed the most to the ΔG_{bind} value of the $HER2_{AC\text{-}doxazosin}$ complex. Met774, Ser783, Leu785, Leu796, Thr798, Met801, Tyr803, Gly804, Cys805, Leu852, Thr862, and Phe864 were the major residues stabilizing the $HER2_{IN\text{-}doxazosin}$ complex. The participation of Ser783, Thr798, Met801, and Tyr803 was visualized through the formation of hydrogen bonds with gefitinib (**Figure 1D**). Leu726, Cys805, Leu807, Arg849, Asn850, Leu852, and Thr862 were the main contributors in the $HER2_{AC\text{-}gefitinib}$ complex (**Table 4**). Leu726, Phe731, Val734, Cys805, Leu807, Arg849, Leu866, Pro922, and Tyr923 contributed the most to the ΔG_{bind} value in the $HER2_{IN\text{-}gefitinib}$ complex.

3.8 Principal component analysis

We evaluated the differences in mobility for the free and bound EGFR/HER2 systems via PC analysis. Evaluation of the quantification of the diagonalized covariance matrix based on covariance showed the following values: $HER2_{AC}$, 15.0 nm^2;

Residue	$HER2_{AC\text{-}doxazosin}$	$HER2_{IN\text{-}doxazosin}$	$HER2_{AC\text{-}gefitinib}$	$HER2_{IN\text{-}gefitinib}$
Leu726	−1.913		−0.67	−0.551
Gly727	−1.056			
Ser728	−0.756			
Phe731				−2.184
Val734	−1.163			−0.855
Met774		−0.56		
Ser783		−0.837		
Leu785		−1.414		
Leu796		−1.069		
Thr798		−1.122		
Met801		−2.045		
Tyr803		−1.854		
Gly804		−0.652		
Cys805		−1.1	−1.378	−0.531
Leu807			−0.844	−0.597
Arg849			−2.104	−2.011
Asn850			−0.559	
Leu852		−2.069	−1.026	
Thr862		−2.25	−0.757	
Asp863	−1.631			
Phe864	−0.828	−1.09		
Leu866				−0.822
Pro922				−1.358
Tyr923				−1.685

Table 4.
Per-residue free energy for complexes between doxazosin and gefitinib with $HER2_{AC}/HER2_{IN}$ (values kcal/Mol).

$HER2_{AC\text{-}doxazosin}$, 10.26 nm^2; $HER2_{AC\text{-}gefitinib}$, 8.83 nm^2; $HER2_{IN}$, 28.9 nm^2; $HER2_{IN\text{-}doxazosin}$, 18.21 nm^2; $HER2_{IN\text{-}gefitinib}$, 20.41 nm^2; $EGFR_{AC}$, 10.79 nm^2; $EGFRAC_{AC\text{-}doxazosin}$, 9.46 nm^2; $EGFR_{AC\text{-}gefitinib}$, 7.69 nm^2; $EGFR_{IN}$, 8.17 nm^2; $EGFR_{IN\text{-}doxazosin}$, 11.55 nm^2; and $EGFR_{AC\text{-}gefitinib}$, 10.0 nm^2. This result indicates that the molecular recognition of doxazosin or gefitinib on $HER2_{AC}$, $HER2_{IN}$, and $EGFR_{AC}$ decreased the number of conformational states compared to that of free $HER2_{AC}$, $HER2_{IN}$, and $EGFR_{AC}$ states. However, this conformational reduction was more significant for the free and bound $HER2_{IN}$ system. In contrast, a small increase in the conformational mobility was experienced upon the coupling of gefitinib by $EGFR_{IN}$. This indicated that doxazosin and gefitinib binding to $HER2_{IN}$ was linked with reduced heterogeneity, which suggests that this molecular recognition was associated with an unfavorable entropy contribution that could contribute to decrease the favorable ΔG_{bind} values for $HER2_{IN\text{-}doxazosin}$ and $HER2_{IN\text{-}gefitinib}$, as seen in **Table 2**.

4. Conclusion

In this chapter, we explored the structural and energetic features that guide the similar inhibitory properties of doxazosin with gefitinib in overexpressing

EGFR/HER2 cell lines combining docking and MD simulation with the MMGBSA approach. Based on these studies, we identified that doxazosin was able to target the active and inactive states of EGFR and HER2, however, its inhibitory activity against breast cancer cell lines was mainly by targeting $HER2_{IN}$. Similarly, although gefitinib was able to target the inactive and inactive states of EGFR and HER2, its activity mainly targeted $EGFR_{AC}$, in line with previous reports. Per-residue free energy analysis identified the key residues stabilizing $HER2_{IN\text{-}DOX}$ and $EGFR_{AC\text{-}GEF}$ systems, showing that in the stabilization of both systems, Met793 and Met801 were involved for EGFR and HER2, respectively. These residues stabilized $HER2_{IN\text{-}DOX}$ and $EGFR_{AC\text{-}GEF}$ systems through the formation of hydrogen bonds with the quinazoline ring, as reported for other TKIs. This study provides structural and energetic information that can be used to design new inhibitors for $HER2_{IN}$ or $EGFR_{AC}$ using doxazosin or gefitinib, respectively, as a pharmacophoric model.

Acknowledgements

This is an unpublished original article. The work was supported by grants from CONACYT (CB-A1-S-21278) and SIP/IPN (20201015).

Author details

Martiniano Bello[1]* and Miguel Ángel Vargas Mejía[2]

1 Laboratorio de Diseño y Desarrollo de Nuevos Fármacos e Innovación Biotecnológica de la Escuela Superior de Medicina, Instituto Politécnico Nacional, México

2 Departamento de Biomedicina Molecular, Centro de Investigación y de Estudios Avanzados del Instituto Politécnico Nacional (CINVESTAV-IPN), Ciudad de México, México

*Address all correspondence to: bellomartini@gmail.com and mbellor@ipn.mx

References

[1] M.A. Olayioye, R.M. Neve, H.A. Lane, N.E. Hynes, The ErbB signaling network: receptor heterodimerization in development and cancer, EMBO J. 19 (2000) 3159-3167.

[2] G. Lurje, H.-J. Lenz, EGFR signaling and drug discovery, Oncology 77 (6) (2009) 400-410.

[3] E. Tzahar, H. Waterman, X. Chen, G. Levkowitz, D. Karunagaran, S. Lavi, B.J. Ratzkin, Y. Yarden. A hierarchical network of interreceptor interactions determines signal transduction by Neu differentiation factor/neuregulin and epidermal growth factor. Mol. Cell. Biol. 16 (1996), pp. 5276-5287

[4] X. Qian, C.M. LeVea, J.K., Freeman, W. C. Dougall, M.I. Greene. Heterodimerization of epidermal growth factor receptor and wild-type or kinase-deficient Neu: a mechanism of interreceptor kinase activation and transphosphorylation. Proc. Natl. Acad. Sci. U. S. A., 91 (1994), pp. 1500-1504

[5] D. Graus-Porta, R.R. Beerli, J. M. Daly, N.E. Hynes. ErbB-2, the preferred heterodimerization partner of all ErbB receptors, is a mediator of lateral signaling. EMBO J., 16 (1997), pp. 1647-1655

[6] D.J. Riese 2nd, R.M. Gallo, J. Settleman, Mutational activation of ErbB family receptor tyrosine kinases: insights into mechanisms of signal transduction and tumorigenesis, BioEssays 29 (2007) 558-565.

[7] X. Zhang, J. Gureasko, K. Shen, P.A. Cole, J. Kuriyan, An allosteric mechanism for activation of the kinase domain of epidermal growth factor receptor, Cell 125 (2006) 1137-1149.

[8] S.R. Hubbard, W.T. Miller, Receptor tyrosine kinases: mechanisms of activation and signaling, Curr. Opin. Cell Biol. 19 (2007) 117-123.

[9] K. Aertgeerts, R. Skene, J. Yano, B.-C. Sang, H. Zou, G. Snell, A. Jennings, K. Iwamoto, N. Habuka, A. Hirokawa, T. Ishikawa, T. Tanaka, H. Miki, Y. Ohta, S. 15 Sogabe. Structural analysis of the mechanism of inhibition and allosteric activation of the kinase domain of HER2 protein. J. Biol. Chem., 286 (2011), pp. 18756-18765

[10] Bello, M., Guadarrama-García, C. & Rodriguez-Fonseca, R.A. Dissecting the Molecular Recognition of Dual Lapatinib Derivatives for EGFR/HER2. J Comput Aided Mol Des 2020 Mar; 34(3):293-303.

[11] Bello, Martiniano, et al. "Structural and energetic basis for the molecular recognition of dual synthetic vs. natural inhibitors of EGFR/HER2." International journal of biological macromolecules 111 (2018): 569-586.

[12] S.V. Sharma, D.W. Bell, J. Settleman, D.A. Haber, Epidermal growth factor receptor mutations in lung cancer, Nat. Rev. Cancer 7 (2007) 169-181.

[13] J.R.C. Sainsbury, J.R. Farndon, G.K. Needham, A.J. Malcolm, A.L. Harris, Epidermalgrowth-factor receptor status as predictor of early recurrence of and death from breast-cancer, Lancet 1 (1987) 1398-1402

[14] F. Ciardiello, G. Tortora. A novel approach in the treatment of cancer: targeting the epidermal growth factor receptor. Clin Cancer Res., 7(2001), pp. 2958-2970

[15] B.N. Rexer, R. Ghosh, A. Narasanna. Human breast cancer cells harboring a gatekeeper T798M mutation in HER2 overexpress EGFR ligands and are sensitive to dual inhibition of EGFR and HER2. Clin Cancer Res., 19(2013), pp. 5390-401

[16] I.M. Gonzaga, S.C. Soares-Lima, P.T. de Santos. Alterations in epidermal

growth factor receptors 1 and 2 in esophageal squamous cell carcinomas. BMC Cancer., 12(2012), pp. 56

[17] E.R. Wood, A.T. Truesdale, O.B. McDonald, D. Yuan, A. Hassell, S.H. Dickerson, B. Ellis, C. Pennisi, E. Horne, K. Lackey, K.J. Alligood, D.W. Rusnak, T.M. Gilmer, L. Shewchuk. A unique structure for epidermal growth factor receptor bound to GW572016 (Lapatinib): relationships among protein conformation, inhibitor off-rate, and receptor activity in tumor cells. Cancer Res., 64 (2004), pp. 6652-6659

[18] M.A. Seeliger, P. Ranjitkar, C. Kasap, Y. Shan, D.E. Shaw, N.P. Shah, J. Kuriyan, D.J. Maly. Equally potent inhibition of c-Src and Abl by compounds that recognize inactive kinase conformations. Cancer Res., 69 (2009), pp. 2384-2392

[19] M. Bello. Binding mechanism of kinase inhibitors to EGFR and T790M, L858R and L858R/T790M mutants through structural and energetic analysis. International journal of biological macromolecules, 118 2018, pp. 1948-1962

[20] L. Saldaña-Rivera, M. Bello, D. Méndez-Luna. Structural insight into the binding mechanism of ATP to EGFR and L858R, and T790M and L858R/T790 mutants. Journal of Biomolecular Structure and Dynamics, 1 (2019), pp. 1-14

[21] D.W. Rusnak, K. Lackey, K. Affleck. The effects of the novel, reversible epidermal growth factor receptor/ErbB-2 tyrosine kinase inhibitor, GW2016, on the growth of human normal and tumor-derived cell lines in vitro and in vivo. Mol. Cancer Ther., 1 (2001), pp. 85-9

[22] G.E. Konecny, M.D. Pegram, N. Venkatesan, R. Finn, G. Yang. Activity of the dual kinase inhibitor lapatinib (GW572016) against HER-2- overexpressing and trastuzumab-treated breast cancer cells. Cancer Res., 66 (2006), pp. 1630-1639

[23] S.R. Johnston, A. Leary. Lapatinib: a novel EGFR/HER2 tyrosine kinase inhibitor for cancer. Drugs Today Barc, 42 (2006), pp. 441-453

[24] Y. Zhou, S. Li, Hu YP, J. Wang, J. Hauser. Blockade of EGFR and ErbB2 by the novel dual EGFR and ErbB2 tyrosine kinase inhibitor GW572016 sensitizes human colon carcinoma GEO cells to apoptosis. Cancer Res., 66 (2006), pp. 404-411

[25] P.J. Medina, S. Goodin. Lapatinib: a dual inhibitor of human epidermal growth factor receptor tyrosine kinases. Clin. Ther., 30 (2008), pp. 1426-1447

[26] S.R. Johnston, A. Leary, Lapatinib: a novel EGFR/HER2 tyrosine kinase inhibitor for cancer, Drugs Today (Barc) 42 (2006) 441-453.

[27] B. Forsythe, K. Faulkner, Overview of the tolerability of gefitinib (IRESSA) monotherapy: clinical experience in non-small-cell lung cancer, Drug Saf. 27 (2004) 1081-1092.

[28] D.M. Jackman, V.A. Miller, L.A. Cioffredi, B.Y. Yeap, P.A. Jänne, G.J. Riely, M.G. Ruiz, G. Giaccone, L.V. Sequist, B.E. Johnson, Clin. Cancer Res. 15 (2009) 5267.

[29] W. Pao, V.A. Miller, K.A. Politi, G.J. Riely, R. Somwar, M.F. Zakowski, M.G. Kris, H. Varmus, Acquired resistance of lung adenocarcinomas to gefitinib or erlotinib is associated with a second mutation in the EGFR kinase domain, PLoS Med. 2 (2005), e73.

[30] C.H. Yun, K.E. Mengwasser, A.V. Toms, M.S. Woo, H. Greulich, K.K. Wong, M. Meyerson, M.J. Eck, The T790M mutation in EGFR kinase causes drug resistance by increasing the affinity for ATP, PNAS 105 (2008) 2070-2075.

[31] M. Ahmed, M. Sadek, K. A. Abouzid, F. Wang. In silico design: extended molecular dynamic simulations of a new series of dually acting inhibitors against EGFR and HER2. Journal of Molecular Graphics and Modelling, 44 (2013), pp. 220-231

[32] M.M. Sadek, R.A. Serrya, A.-H.N. Kafafy, M. Ahmed, F. Wang, K.A.M. Abouzid, Discovery of new HER2/EGFR dual kinase inhibitors based on the anilinoquinazoline scaffold as potential anticancer agents, J. Enzyme Inhib. Med. Chem. 1 (2013) 1-8.

[33] S.C. Yang, S.S. Chang, H.Y. Chen, C.Y.C. Chen, Identification of potent EGFR inhibitors from TCM database@Taiwan, PLoS Comput. Biol. 7 (10) (2011), e1002189.

[34] Y. Liu, N.S. Gray, Rational design of inhibitors that bind to inactive kinase conformations, Nat. Chem. Biol. 2 (2006) 358-364.

[35] C.N. Cavasotto, R.A. Abagyan, Protein flexibility in ligand docking and virtual screening to protein kinases, J. Mol. Biol. 337 (2004) 209-226.

[36] B. Chandrika, J. Subramanian, S.D. Sharma, Managing protein flexibility in docking and its applications, Drug Discov. Today 14 (2009) 394-400.

[37] Hui, Hongxiang, Manory A. Fernando, and Anthony P. Heaney. "The α1-adrenergic receptor antagonist doxazosin inhibits EGFR and NF-κB signalling to induce breast cancer cell apoptosis." *European journal of cancer* 44.1 (2008): 160-166.

[38] Ford, Christopher HJ, et al. "Reassessment of estrogen receptor expression in human breast cancer cell lines." *Anticancer research* 31.2 (2011): 521-527.

[39] Stanley, Aryan, et al. "Synergistic effects of various Her inhibitors in combination with IGF-1R, C-MET and Src targeting agents in breast cancer cell lines." *Scientific Reports* 7.1 (2017): 1-15.

[40] El Sharkawi, Fathia Zaky, Hany Abdelaziz El Shemy, and Hussein Moustafa Khaled. "Possible anticancer activity of rosuvastatine, doxazosin, repaglinide and oxcarbazepin." *Asian Pacific Journal of Cancer Prevention* 15.1 (2014): 199-203.

[41] A. Sali, T.L. Blundell, Comparative protein modelling by satisfaction of spatial restraints, J. Mol. Biol. 234 (3) (1993) 779-815.

[42] G.M. Morris, R. Huey, W. Lindstrom, M.F. Sanner, R.K. Belew, D.S. Goodsell, A.J. Olson, Computational, Chemistry 16 (2009) 2785-2791.

[43] M.J. Frisch, G.W. Trucks, H.B. Schlegel, G.E. Scuseria, M.A. Robb, J.R. Cheeseman, J.A. Montgomery, Jr., T. Vreven, K.N. Kudin, J.C. Burant, J.M. Millam, S.S. Iyengar, J. Tomasi, V. Barone, B. Mennucci, M. Cossi, G. Scalmani, N. Rega, G.A. Petersson, H. Nakatsuji, M. Hada, M. Ehara, K. Toyota, R. Fukuda, J. Hasegawa, M. Ishida, T. Nakajima, Y. Honda, O. Kitao, H. Nakai, M. Klene, X. Li, J.E. Knox, H.P. Hratchian, J.B. Cross, V. Bakken, C. Adamo, J. Jaramillo, R. Gomperts, R.E. Stratmann, O. Yazyev, A.J. Austin, R. Cammi, C. Pomelli, J.W. Ochterski, P.Y. Ayala, K. Morokuma, G.A. Voth, P. Salvador, J.J. Dannenberg, V.G. Zakrzewski, S. Dapprich, A.D. Daniels, M.C. Strain, O. Farkas, D.K. Malick, A.D. Rabuck, K. Raghavachari, J.B. Foresman, J.V. Ortiz, Q. Cui, A.G. Baboul, S. Clifford, J. Cioslowski, B.B. Stefanov, G. Liu, A. Liashenko, P. Piskorz, I. Komaromi, R.L. Martin, D.J. Fox, T. Keith, M.A. Al-Laham, C.Y. Peng, A. Nanayakkara, M. Challacombe, P.M.W. Gill, B. Johnson, W. Chen, M.W. Wong, C. Gonzalez, and J.A. Pople, Gaussian 03, Revision B.04, Gaussian, Inc., Wallingford, CT, 2004

[44] D.A. Case, T.E. Cheatham, T. Darden, H. Gohlke, R. Luo, K.M. Merz Jr., R.J. Woods, The Amber biomolecular simulation programs, J. Comput. Chem. 26 (2005) 1668-1688

[45] Y. Duan, C. Wu, S. Chowdhury, M.C. Lee, G. Xiong, W. Zhang, et al., Apoint-charge force field for molecular mechanics simulations of proteinsbased on condensedphase quantum mechanical calculations, J. Comput. Chem. 24 (16) (2003) 1999-2012

[46] W.L. Jorgensen, J. Chandrasekhar, J.D. Madura, R.W. Impey, M.L. Klein, Comparison of simple potential functions for simulating liquid water, J. Chem. Phys. 79 (1983) 926-935.

[47] J. Wang, R.M. Wolf, J.W. Caldwell, P.A. Kollman, D.A. Case, Development andtesting of a general amber force field, J. Comput. Chem. 25 (9) (2004) 1157-1174

[48] H.J.C. Berendsen, J.P.M. Postma, W.F. van Gunsteren, A. DiNola, J.R. Haak, Moleculardynamics with coupling to an external bath, J. Chem. Phys. 81 (8) (1984) 3684-3690.

[49] T. Darden, D. York, L. Pedersen, Particle mesh Ewald-an N. log(N) method forewald sums in large systems, J. Chem. Phys. 98 (1993) 10089-10092.

[50] W.F. Van Gunsteren, H.J.C. Berendsen, Algorithms for macromoleculardynamics and constraint dynamics, Mol. Phys. 34 (1977) 1311-1327.

[51] Maestro, version 10.1. Schrödinger, LLC; New York, NY, USA: 2015-1.

[52] B.R. Miller, T.D. McGee, J.M. Swails, N. Homeyer, H. Gohlke, A.E. Roitberg. MMPBSA.py: an efficient program for end-state free energy calculations. J.Chem. Theory Comput., 8 (2012), pp. 3314-3321

[53] H. Gohlke, C. Kiel, D. A. J. Case. Insights into protein-protein binding by binding free energy calculation and free energy decomposition for the Ras-Raf and Ras-RalGDS complexes. Mol. Biol., 330 (2003), pp. 891-913

[54] P.A. Kollman, I. Massova, C. Reyes, B. Kuhn, S. Huo, L. Chong. Calculating structures and free energies of complex molecules: combining molecular mechanics and continuum models. Acc. Chem. Res., 33 (2000), pp. 889-897

[55] J. M. Wang, T. J. Hou, X. J. Xu. Recent advances in free energy calculations with a combination of molecular mechanics and continuum model. Drug Des., 2 (2006), pp. 287-306

[56] A. Onufriev, V. Bashford, D. A. Case. Exploring protein native states and large-scale conformational changes with a modified generalized born model. Proteins., 55 (2004), pp. 383-394

[57] C.H. Yun, K.E. Mengwasser, A.V. Toms, M.S. Woo, H. Greulich, K.K. Wong, M. Meyerson, M.J. Eck. The T790M mutation in EGFR kinase causes drug resistance by increasing the affinity for ATP. PNAS, 105 (2008), pp. 2070-2075

[58] Z. Ruan, S. Katiyar, N. Kannan. Computational and Experimental Characterization of Patient Derived Mutations Reveal an Unusual Mode of Regulatory Spine Assembly and Drug Sensitivity in EGFR Kinase. Biochemistry, 56(2017), pp. 22-32

[59] Xing, L., Klug-Mcleod, J., Rai, B., & Lunney, E. A. (2015). Kinase hinge binding scaffolds and their hydrogen bond patterns. Bioorganic & medicinal chemistry, 23(19), 6520-6527.

[60] J.H. Park, Y. Liu, M.A. Lemmon, R. Radhakrishnan, Erlotinib binds both inactive and active conformations of the EGFR tyrosine kinase domain, Biochem. J. 448 (3) (2012) 417-423

Section 5

Breast Cancer Screening and Management

Chapter 7

Persistent Breast Cancer Pain

Sachin Sahni and James Khan

Abstract

Fortunately, with advances in screening and management, the prognosis of breast cancer has substantially improved. However, as patients with breast cancer are living much longer, consequences of management are becoming increasingly apparent, particularly persistent pain after breast cancer surgery. This pain disorder, referred to as Post-Mastectomy Pain Syndrome (PMPS) is common and typically presents as pain with neuropathic features around the surgical incision. This pain disorder is associated with negative effects on the patient's social and psychological well-being as well as increased healthcare expenditures. Despite the common occurrence of this disorder, it is vastly under-recognized with a lack of preventative and treatment options. This chapter aims to outline the management of persistent breast surgery pain. The pathophysiology and etiology will be reviewed, followed by tools that clinicians can implement in order to appropriately diagnose neuropathic pain. Pertinent risk factors that are commonly seen in practice will be outlined, followed by non-pharmacological, pharmacological, and interventional therapeutic options that can be offered.

Keywords: persistent pain, chronic pain, neuropathy, post-mastectomy pain syndrome, intercostobrachial neuralgia, intercostal neuralgia, psychological factors, axillary lymph node dissection, postoperative pain, pharmacological therapy, interventional therapy, nerve blocks, neuromodulation

1. Introduction

Breast cancer continues to be the most frequently diagnosed cancer in women worldwide [1] and cases in the United States are expected to rise by 64% between 2011 and 2030 [2]. Nonetheless, with significant progress in prevention and treatment over the past 30 years, survivorship has substantially increased [3], most notably in women ages 20–39 years [4]. The 5-year relative survival rate for breast cancer now approaches 90% [5] and while mortality rates have declined, it presents a unique challenge, as long-term complications of breast cancer management are becoming increasingly apparent, particularly persistent post-surgical pain.

Persistent pain has become a significant area of concern as it appears to afflict up to 50% of women after breast cancer surgery [6]. This pain disorder is typically neuropathic in nature and described as burning, spontaneous, electrical, numbness, tingling, and pinprick pain affecting the area of surgery in the chest, shoulder, axilla, and medial arm [7]. While the literature commonly refers to this presentation as post-mastectomy pain syndrome (PMPS), it is important to note that damage of nerves can occur after all types of breast cancer surgeries, including unilateral or bilateral surgeries, radical mastectomies, lumpectomies, and from axillary lymph node dissection. Thus, in 2016 Waltho et al. proposed the term post-breast surgery pain syndrome (PBSPS) which is not only a more inclusive term but may also help to decrease the wide variation in overall prevalence [8].

IntechOpen

The International Association for Study of Pain (IASP) also recently updated their definition to include all types of breast surgeries in the classification. Thus, the term "persistent pain after breast surgery" was chosen, and it is pain which persists for more than 3 months after a surgical incision to the anterolateral chest wall and in some cases in the ipsilateral axillary region [9].

Management of persistent pain after breast cancer surgery can be a challenging task with the lack of effective treatment options [10]. Furthermore, this pain disorder places a financial burden on both patients and the healthcare system with studies showing an estimated cost of approximately $1 billion USD annually to the US healthcare system [11]. Identifying perioperative risk factors associated with the development of persistent pain can help decrease the incidence and the need for ongoing healthcare services.

In this chapter we will provide an outline of the pathophysiology of persistent pain after breast cancer surgery, including a review of pertinent risk factors, clinical features, and various treatment options.

2. Pathophysiology

Pain can originate from a multitude of sources, such as from injury to the overlying skin, tissue, or nerves during surgical intervention, or from the effects of radiation and chemotherapy. Additionally, the origin is frequently multifactorial, with psychosocial factors also playing a role.

2.1 Nerve injury

Surgical factors can cause nerve injuries that contribute to persistent pain after breast cancer surgery. Direct nerve injury, for instance from skin incisions, surgical retractors, or extensive axillary lymph node dissection, can lead to direct nerve transections [12]. This can subsequently lead to the eventual formation of neuromas and scar adhesions. Nerve damage can also be due to indirect injury from postoperative inflammation, hematoma formation, or positioning during surgery (resulting in nerve stretching during the procedure) [12]. The nerves most commonly at risk for injury during breast cancer surgery are the intercostobrachial nerve (ICBN), the thoracic intercostal nerves, medial and lateral pectoral nerves, the thoracodorsal nerve, and the long thoracic nerve [13].

Intercostobrachial neuralgia is a well-known cause of persistent pain after breast cancer surgery and presents as neuropathic pain in the ipsilateral axilla and arm [14]. The ICBN is the lateral cutaneous branch of the second intercostal nerve (T2) and is pure sensory in nature [12]. It innervates areas of the axilla, lateral chest wall, and aspects of the medial arm (**Figure 1**), and due to its trajectory and close relation to the axillary lymph nodes, is at high risk of injury during axillary lymph node dissection and radical mastectomies [16]. Furthermore, a study by Zhu et al. demonstrated that identification, dissection, and preservation of the ICBN during surgery reduced the incidence of persistent pain and improved quality of life for patients after breast cancer surgery [17]. While this finding has been observed in additional studies [18, 19], it is important to note that while sensitivity was preserved, the incidence of reduced pain was not always obtainable [19].

Along with the ICBN, which is a branch of the T2 intercostal nerve, the T3-T6 intercostal nerves are also at high risk for injury and subsequent intercostal neuralgia. These nerves primarily innervate the skin of the breast, and major branches include the rami communicates, the muscular branches, the collateral branch, the lateral cutaneous branch, and the anterior cutaneous branch [20]. Involvement

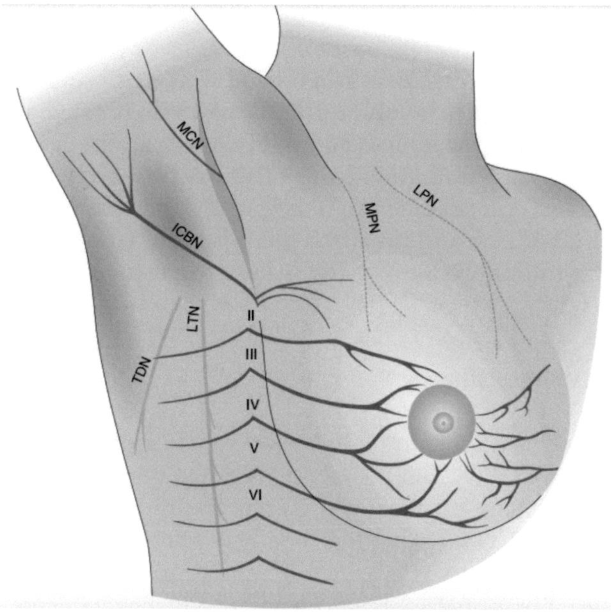

Figure 1.
*Peripheral nerves innervating the breast. *obtained with permission from Dr. Nelun Wijayasinghe from article [15] . II-VI – intercostal nerves II to VI; ICBN – intercostobrachial nerve; LPN – lateral pectoral nerve; LTN – long thoracic nerve; MPN – medial pectoral nerve; MCN – musculocutaneous nerve; TDN – thoracodorsal nerve;*

of intercostal nerves can present as pain originating at the posterior axillary line radiating anteriorly into the chest wall, in the distribution of the affected intercostal nerve. It is not uncommon to have multiple intercostal nerves involved in the presentation of persistent pain after breast cancer surgery.

Another nerve, albeit less commonly involved, is the medial cutaneous nerve of the arm. This nerve branches from the medial cord of the brachial plexus and can form a connection with the ICBN. Damage to this nerve results in sensory loss to the lower medial skin of the upper arm [14]. Additionally, neuromas can develop within the surgical scar and be a problematic source of persistent pain - scar neuromas are an elusive source of pain after any type of surgical procedure.

2.2 Phantom pain

As with other types of amputations, resection of breast tissue is susceptible to the development of phantom pain and sensations. Ahmed et al. enrolled eighty patients undergoing a modified radical mastectomy and at the one-year mark, 13.6% experienced phantom pain, while 17% experienced phantom sensation. Its lower incidence compared to phantom limb pain may be due to the fact that breasts do not involve kinesthetic sensory impulses in the same manner as limbs do [21]. Likewise, there may simply be a lack of widespread knowledge and education for this condition and thus it may be overlooked in clinical practice. Regardless, while less prevalent than neuropathic pain secondary to nerve injury, its importance may be greater as treatment options are even more limited [22].

2.3 Perioperative radiation

Radiation therapy can also lead to nerve damage, producing persistent peripheral neuropathy. While treatment is targeted, radiation therapy may still cause unavoidable injury to nearby nerves such as the brachial plexus, including proximal and distal branches. The onset and severity of radiation-induced pain can be proportional to the total dose received [23]. A meta-analysis by Wang et al. reviewing thirty studies involving 19,813 patients showed an increased likelihood of PMPS among women who underwent radiotherapy [24]. This is likely secondary to an increased incidence of tissue fibrosis, which can lead to local constriction and compression on nerves and subsequent neural entrapment. Furthermore, lymphedema and impaired glenohumeral motion are other sequelae that can arise after radiation therapy and lead to the formation of persistent pain and morbidity.

2.4 Perioperative chemotherapy

Several commonly used chemotherapy agents such as paclitaxel, vinblastine, and vincristine have all been identified as causing residual neuropathic symptoms [25]. Peripheral neuropathies are the most common presentation with patients experiencing sensations of numbness and tingling usually in a stocking and glove-like formation [25]. Unfortunately, those receiving both radiation and chemotherapy tend to experience enhanced neuropathic symptoms [26]. The mechanism of chemotherapy-induced peripheral neuropathy caused by common antineoplastic agents is multifactorial. For platinum-based drugs such as oxaliplatin and cisplatin, activation of glial cells causes nearby immune cells to release pro-inflammatory cytokines, and altered activity in Na^+ and K^+ ion channels can result in nociceptor sensitization and hyperexcitability of peripheral neurons [27]. Vinca alkaloids also cause the release of pro-inflammatory mediators and influence microtubule polymerization that inhibits axonal transport. This, along with Wallerian degeneration, leads to distal axonopathy [27].

3. Risk factors

PMPS is multifactorial in nature and several risk factors have been evaluated for their association in the development of persistent pain. Risk factors can be categorized broadly into patient demographics, psychological influence, and surgical and anesthetic factors. While an abundance of literature has evaluated risk factors for chronic pain, only some consensus exists. Nonetheless, identifying risk factors and modifying them early in the perioperative period could potentially help in decreasing the risk of persistent pain in high-risk patients.

3.1 Patient demographics

3.1.1 Age

Younger age has been strongly correlated with a higher pain burden index and relationship of younger age with persistent pain is well supported [28–31]. This finding may be secondary to the fact that younger patients usually present with more aggressive, estrogen-receptor negative disease, or higher tumor grade requiring more radical surgeries or adjuvant therapies [32]. Younger patients also tend to have greater levels of perioperative anxiety and a lower threshold to pain, when compared to older patient groups, thus increasing their overall risk [12]. While younger age has been one of the most consistent factors associated with PMPS, some reviews have not always found this to be the case [33].

3.1.2 Body Mass Index (BMI)

Literature also reports that patients with a higher BMI are more likely to experience persistent pain after breast cancer surgery. A study by Spivey et al. found that both a young age and higher BMI correlated with higher pain scores at the six month follow up [34], and Juhl et al. showed that a BMI $\geq$30 kg/m^2 was significantly associated with persistent pain in both univariate and multivariate models [14]. Surprisingly however, a systematic review and meta-analysis of thirty high-grade observational studies totaling 19,813 patients showed that BMI was not associated with persistent pain [24]. Thus, the correlation may be multifactorial in nature. Surgery in obese patients may be associated with more difficult axillary dissections due to larger breasts, thus placing them at a higher risk for greater tissue and nerve damage. Regardless, as with other surgical disciplines, the risks of perioperative complications such as impaired wound healing and increased blood loss remain higher in patients with a higher BMI [35, 36].

3.2 Psychological

Several studies have shown a significant correlation between high levels of preoperative anxiety [37], catastrophizing symptoms [38], and persistent breast pain following breast cancer surgery [34, 39, 40]. Furthermore, there is also a significant and independent association between PMPS and somatization, depressive symptoms, and sleep disturbance, regardless of the surgical or medical treatment a patient received [33]. Furthermore, pain catastrophizing has been found to intensify the experience of both pain and depression [23, 41]. Patients undergoing breast surgery may expect to have severe pain after the procedure, thus increasing their emotional distress and cause them to excessively focus on only negative aspects such as chronic pain. These negative emotions and beliefs may evolve into catastrophic thoughts and irrational patterns of thinking and become self-fulfilling in producing higher pain levels [42]. In contrast, patients who have a more positive mindset going into surgery, and lower levels of emotional distress, are more likely to experiences less acute pain [43] and therefore experience a lower incidence of PMPS [40].

3.3 Surgical type

With the advancement of surgical management, the association between surgical type and chronic pain development seems to vary in the literature. Both breast-conserving surgery (BCS), with or without lymph node dissection, and radical mastectomy have not consistently shown a positive relationship in the development of PMPS. A study of 475 patients found that patients who underwent breast-conserving surgery were at higher risks of developing moderate to severe chronic pain at rest (OR 2.0, 95% CI = 1.2–3.3) [30]. Some reports however, indicate that more extensive surgery (e.g. radical mastectomies, bilateral procedures, reconstruction) does lead to greater acute postoperative pain, which in turn is a risk factor in developing chronic pain [44]. A prospective, observational study by Spivey et al. with 216 patients, and a systematic review and meta-analysis of thirty observational studies of 19,813 patients by Wang, et al. both did not observe a significant relationship between surgical type and pain at three and six months, respectively [24, 34].

3.4 Axillary lymph node dissection (ALND)

Lymph node dissection can help with the staging and management of breast cancer [45]. Compared to sentinel lymph node biopsy, ALND has been an associated risk factor with PMPS in several studies [17, 34, 44, 46]. Fabro et al. analyzed ALND on persistent pain, and after controlling for confounding variables they reported that removal of more than fifteen lymph nodes resulted in two times the risk for developing persistent pain [47]. ALND involves more extensive damage to tissues in the axilla, and the intercostobrachial nerve is at most risk during the dissection [48]. As mentioned above, when possible, the ICBN should aim to be preserved during ALND. Abdullah et al. conducted a randomized controlled trial where the ICBN was preserved during ALND and found a decreased incidence of sensory deficits at the three-month follow up. Notably however, preservation could only be obtained in 65% of the patients.

3.5 Acute postoperative pain

Postoperative pain scores in the acute setting have been shown to be a significant risk factor associated with persistent pain across numerous surgical sub-groups, including breast surgeries. Acute surgical injury has been linked to central and peripheral pain sensitization, which can lead to the development of persistent chronic pain [49, 50]. Bruce et al. studied 362 post-mastectomy patients and found that higher levels of postoperative pain increased the odds of developing PMPS at four months (OR 1.34, 95% CI 1.12–1.60) and at nine months (OR 1.17, 95% CI 1.00–1.37) after surgery [51]. Wang et al. also concluded that for every point on a 10-point scale, the level of postoperative pain severity increased the likelihood of PMPS (OR 1.16, 95% CI 1.03–1.30) [24]. Extensive surgical reconstruction, axillary lymph node dissection, high levels of anxiety and pain catastrophizing, and presence of preoperative pain all increase the risk of severe acute postoperative pain [34]. Therefore, acute postoperative pain is a worthy indicator for the development of chronic pain [38] and emphasis should be placed on controlling it early in the postoperative course. Improved postoperative pain control is best managed using a multimodal strategy such as through the use of anti-inflammatories, N-methyl-D-aspartate (NMDA) inhibitors, interventions such as nerve or fascial plane blocks with local anesthetics, or by addressing preoperative psychological factors such as anxiousness or fear of the postsurgical path.

4. Presentation

There are a number of etiologies that can be responsible for pain after breast cancer surgery. Largely, persistent pain is due to neuropathic causes (**Table 1**) [7, 10], such as from trauma or injury to the intercostobrachial nerve and other local peripheral nerves (medial and lateral pectoral nerve, intercostal nerves, etc), but also due to phantom breast pain, scar neuroma formation, and chemotherapy/radiation induced peripheral neuropathy.

Neuropathic pain due to local peripheral nerve injuries typically present as pain in and around the surgical incision, but due to the peripheral nerve distribution, it can be felt as if it also involves the chest wall, medial arm, axilla, and shoulder [7]. Pain is associated with neuropathic pain features which include burning, paresthesia, tingling, as well as allodynia and hyperalgesia [46, 52]. Pain is also typically associated with sensory changes, such as numbness and hypoesthesia. Furthermore, the incision itself may be a source of spontaneous pain and mechanosensitivity, which may indicate the presence of a scar neuroma, which is more common after a lumpectomy than a mastectomy [53].

Other non-neuropathic etiologies can occur after breast cancer surgery and include musculoskeletal impairments such as rotator cuff dysfunction, adhesive

Neuropathic	Intercostobrachial neuralgia
	Phantom breast pain
	Neuroma formation
	Local peripheral nerve injuries - medial and lateral pectoral nerves, intercostal nerves, long thoracic, brachial plexopathy
	Chemotherapy-induced peripheral neuropathy
	Radiation-induced peripheral neuropathy
Musculoskeletal	Rotator cuff dysfunction
	Adhesive capsulitis
	Myofascial pain syndrome
	Aromatase inhibitor-associated arthralgia
Others	Axillary web syndrome
	Lymphedema

**from previously published article by Dr. James Khan: [10].*

Table 1.
Pain disorders after breast cancer surgery.

capsulitis of the glenohumeral joint, myofascial pain syndrome of the pectoral or intercostal muscles, and aromatase inhibitor-associated arthralgias (**Table 1**) [7, 10]. Other potential disorders include axillary web syndrome and lymphedema.

When patients present for evaluation of their pain, the first step involves diagnosing the type of pain being experienced. Origin of pain is broadly categorized as either nociceptive or neuropathic [54]. In the acute postoperative phase, pain after breast surgery is likely to be nociceptive in nature resulting from intraoperative injury and subsequent inflammation to tissue, ligaments, or muscles. In order to help diagnose the type of pain, and track its severity over time, routine use of questionnaire-based assessments are commonly implemented. One that is frequently used is the Douleur Neuropathique en 4 (DN4), which consists of two sections – a set of interview questions and examination findings [55]. The yes/no interview questions ask for the presence of burning, painful cold, or electric shocks, and one or more of tingling, pins and needles, numbness, and itching. The second section assesses if the patient experiences hypoesthesia to touch or pinprick, and if brushing provokes the pain. With each point valued at 1, a total score ≥ 4 signifies a 90% probability of neuropathic pain. The questionnaire is quick and reliable, with a sensitivity of 78.0% and specificity of 81.2% [56].

It is important that a thorough history and physical examination is conducted. History will include an evaluation of the patient's preoperative diagnosis and any adjuvant chemotherapy or radiation. Reviewing surgical records will be important to establish what type of procedure was conducted (mastectomy versus lumpectomy), whether axillary lymph nodes were resected, if ICBN nerve sparing surgery was performed, and if implants or expanders were placed. The anesthesia record will also include helpful information on whether perioperative regional anesthetic techniques (i.e., Serratus plane or Pectoralis blocks) or intravenous lidocaine infusions were administered — these techniques are known to be effective on reducing acute pain but also potentially helpful in preventing persistent pain [10, 57].

Physical examination will include a detailed evaluation of the surgical incision and surrounding area, documenting any sensory changes. An evaluation for upper extremity lymphedema and a comprehensive shoulder exam should also be performed.

5. Treatments

Approach to the treatment of persistent pain after breast surgery should be multimodal and include the use of both non-pharmacological and pharmacological therapeutic modalities. The involvement of a multidisciplinary team, including an oncologist, pain management specialist, physiotherapist, psychologist, palliative care specialist, and social worker should be implemented whenever possible. Furthermore, a preoperative comprehensive and patient-tailored pain management plan should be formulated in advance, which includes education on surgery sequelae, the nature and development of their symptoms, and available treatment options.

5.1 Non-pharmacological

Non-pharmacological interventions should always be included in the pain management plan, regardless of whether medications are employed or not. Moreover, patients should be aware that non-pharmacological treatments are only one part of the overall comprehensive treatment plan. Some patients may actually prefer non-pharmacological modalities to pharmacological, to avoid risks of drug side effects or costs [58].

5.1.1 Physical therapy

The initiation of physical therapy (PT) has repeatedly been shown to be beneficial to patients recovering from breast cancer surgery. Range of motion exercises and active stretching helps to improve upper extremity strength and function, maintain glenohumeral and scapular movement, and allow neuromuscular recruitment with the overall goal of minimizing dysfunction. A systematic review, which evaluated the effectiveness of PT after breast cancer surgery, showed that therapy involving active exercise and stretching was effective in not only improving range of motion but also decreasing postoperative pain [59].

Timing on when to initiate PT has also been studied. Most studies focus on implementing PT early in the postoperative period, with clinical practice guidelines recommending starting gentle range of motion exercises the day after surgery to reduce shoulder dysfunction and pain [60]. Active stretching, followed by strengthening, can then be introduced over the next 6–8 weeks [60]. Several studies however, do report an increase in complications when starting PT too soon after ALND, with Schultz et al. suggesting that a delay of one week can help reduce the incidence of postoperative seromas [61]. Fortunately, patients taking part in early PT after ALND still tend to recover sufficiently by the two-year mark [62].

Besides pain relief, PT has been shown to offer several added benefits to patients after breast surgery. A meta-analysis of 56 studies evaluating the effects of exercise interventions showed significant benefits in fatigue, depression, body image, and health-related quality of life in cancer survivors [63]. As psychological factors play a known role in the incidence of persistent pain [51], long-term benefits can be obtained if practitioners include a PT or exercise course with the hospital discharge plan.

5.1.2 Psychological therapies

As outlined earlier, psychological factors such as anxiety and catastrophizing play a crucial role in the development of persistent pain. Thus, implementing various psychological interventions into the treatment plan not only helps with pain control [64], but also allows patients to effectively cope during this challenging period in their life. Facing a cancer diagnosis, undergoing invasive treatments, and managing treatment sequelae can all add to the emotional suffering breast cancer patients are faced with. The effectiveness of psychological interventions for non-metastatic breast cancer in women was evaluated in twenty-eight randomized controlled trials involving 3940 patients. The study showed that psychological intervention, in particular cognitive behavioural therapy (CBT), produced favourable effects on anxiety, depression, and mood disturbance [65]. Mindfulness-based stress reduction (MBSR) has also been examined in breast cancer patients, with a recent meta-analysis by Haller et al. evaluating the effectiveness of MBSR in 1709 patients. MBSR was found to have a significant effect on improving health-related quality of life, fatigue, sleep, stress, anxiety, and depression [66].

Perioperative screening questionnaires evaluating psychological stressors, fears, and overall mood, such as the Pain Catastrophizing Scale (PCS) or the Amsterdam Preoperative Anxiety and Information Scale (APAIS) should be implemented both in the pre- and postoperative phase. From this, at-risk patients can be identified and the involvement of psychological interventions can be applied. Moreover, with the advancement of technology and involvement of virtual care into clinical practice, it now allows for easier access and for group therapies to support even larger number of participants per session.

5.2 Pharmacological therapy

Treatment with oral analgesics provides a non-invasive approach to treating pain, and most patients begin here as they transition from acute to chronic pain. Appropriate medication selection relies heavily on obtaining the correct diagnosis, patient comorbidities, drug side-effect profiles, and at times, cost. Furthermore, we must be cognizant of the chronicity of symptoms and the potential long-term consequences of certain therapies, such as with opioids.

A variety of mediation classes have shown to be effective in neuropathic pain, and these same classes are effective in patients with chronic neuropathic pain after breast cancer surgery. Several guidelines are also available to assist prescribers in selecting the most appropriate medication, and second or third line alternatives, if necessary [67–69]. Various medication choices by class are briefly outlined in this section.

5.2.1 Antidepressants

Treatment of neuropathic pain has benefitted from the analgesic properties provided by well-studied and familiar anti-depressants. Tricyclic antidepressants (TCAs) and serotonin-norepinephrine reuptake inhibitors (SNRIs) have become common medication choices when treating neuropathic pain [70], albeit usually at lower doses than that needed for anti-depressant effects.

Tricyclic antidepressants, such as amitriptyline and nortriptyline, inhibit norepinephrine, serotonin, and adenosine re-uptake at nerve terminals. While not fully understood, the increased concentration of these neurotransmitters plays a role in the analgesic effects [71]. Furthermore, TCAs also have an antagonistic action at the N-methyl-D-aspartate (NMDA) receptor [72], which further helps to reduce pain. Doses of TCAs for the treatment of neuropathic pain are much lower than those required for depression [73], and may be the reason that the analgesic properties of TCAs differ from their anti-depressant properties. The effect of amitriptyline was studied in a double-blinded randomized, placebo-controlled crossover trial involving 15 patients with PMPS [74]. A statistically significant improvement in pain, effect on daily life, and improved sleep was seen, particularly at the 100 mg daily dose. Initial starting dose was at 25 mg once daily, and most common adverse effects included tiredness, dry mouth, and constipation. While these effects may not be ideal, prescribing TCAs to be taken at bedtime may benefit patients who also have difficulty with sleep.

Serotonin-norepinephrine reuptake inhibitors, including duloxetine and venlafaxine, also work by inhibiting neurotransmitter reuptake, with venlafaxine slightly inhibiting the reuptake of dopamine as well [75]. Both medications have been used to treat neuropathic pain and beneficial effects have been reported in the literature [76]. Tasmuth et al. evaluated venlafaxine in neuropathic pain following breast cancer treatment in patients with pain and sensory disturbances in the anterior chest wall, and/or axilla, and/or the median upper arm. While the study only examined 15 patients, average pain relief and the maximum pain intensity were significantly lower with venlafaxine when compared with placebo [77]. When compared to TCAs, venlafaxine has minimal muscarinic and histaminergic activity, and the effect of the two medications has been comparable in some studies [78]. Furthermore, venlafaxine added to gabapentin has shown enhancement in neuropathic pain relief when the therapies are combined [79].

Along with providing benefit for post-surgical neuropathic pain, both duloxetine and venlafaxine also offer pain relief for patient's suffering from chemotherapy induced peripheral neuropathy [80, 81], and even decrease motor neuropathy symptoms [82]. Benefits of these two SNRIs has been their ability to target multiple concerns, such as depression, anxiety, musculoskeletal pain, and neuropathy [83] and thus should be strongly considered as an adjuvant when formulating a comprehensive pain management plan.

5.2.2 Gabapentinoids

Gabapentin and pregabalin are common medications used to treat neuropathic pain. While both have structural resemblance to the gamma-aminobutyric acid (GABA) neurotransmitter, neither acts as a GABA agonist. Gabapentin's primary mechanism of action is its high-affinity binding to the $\alpha_2\delta$ subunit of voltage-activated calcium channels, resulting in a reduction in nerve conduction [84]. A retrospective study of 89 patients with persistent breast cancer pain found a reduction in pain in 80% of patients with an average gabapentin dose of 1135 mg for 14 weeks [85]. Initiating gabapentin at 100-300 mg three times daily, and slowly escalating the dose as tolerated, can provide significant pain relief. While gabapentin continues to be a first line agent for neuropathic pain, certain drawbacks must be considered, such as drowsiness, weight gain, and three times a day dosing.

Pregabalin works similarly to gabapentin by inhibiting voltage-activated calcium channels. It was developed as a successor to gabapentin and has the added benefit of being almost completely absorbed in the body, unlike gabapentin. Thus, with absorption almost three times that of gabapentin, pregabalin reaches peak blood concentrations within one hour after ingestion [86]. Pregabalin has been shown to offer significant decrease in VAS pain scores in patients with PMPS [87, 88], along with significant improvement in quality of life [88].

5.2.3 Opioids

With the general shift away from prescribing narcotics in clinical practice, opioid therapy can still play an important role in pain management when used appropriately. The need for opioid therapy in the acute postoperative period is common and can help decrease nociceptive post-surgical pain. Unfortunately, limited data supports the use of opioids for neuropathic pain, especially in the long-term [89, 90]. Nonetheless, for cancer patients with continued pain and functional impairment, a trial of opioids in carefully selected patients can be beneficial. Local and national practice guidelines should be reviewed, risks of adverse effects should always be discussed, and signs of tolerance, abuse, addiction, and diversion should continually be assessed.

One major benefit of opioid therapy is its synergistic effect when combined with other medications. For instance, several studies have demonstrated greater pain relief when using gabapentin and an opioid, compared to opioid monotherapy, in the treatment of neuropathic pain [91–93]. Not only did combination therapy allow for greater reduction in overall pain scores, it also allowed for a decrease in the opioid dose. In turn, this helped to decrease the number of adverse effects that arise with chronic opioid therapy.

5.3 Interventional therapy

5.3.1 Nerve blocks

Several peripheral nerves can be directly targeted for perineural injections with local anesthetics, steroids, or even with neurolytic substances such as phenol or alcohol. Once the problematic nerves have been identified by a thorough history and physical exam, ultrasound guidance can help to visualize the nerves.

The intercostobrachial nerve (ICBN) and specific intercostal nerves can be specifically isolated on ultrasound, and medications can be administered under real-time visualization. The ICBN can be identified in the same approach as performing an axillary brachial plexus block - with the shoulder abducted 90° and externally rotated [94]. The ICBN can be seen posterior to the vessels and just deep to the superficial fascia. The medial cutaneous nerve of the arm can also be visualized just anterior to the ICBN [95]. It is important to note that patients experiencing pain in the anterior chest wall may not benefit from an ICBN block.

For chest wall pain, especially pain radiating laterally from the posterior to the anterior chest, intercostal nerve blocks should be considered. Each intercostal nerve branches from the anterior rami of the thoracic spinal nerves and travels on the underside of its corresponding rib [96]. Consecutive intercostal nerves can be blocked simultaneously under ultrasound guidance with the patient lying prone. While the actual nerve may not always be visible on ultrasound, the therapeutic solution can be deposited just inferior to the rib, posterior to the pleura, where the intercostal nerve resides with its corresponding artery and vein. Due to the location, the potential risk of pneumothorax should be explained to the patient, however the use of ultrasound decreases this risk [97].

When the pain is not consistent with a specific nerve, or involves a set of multiple interconnected nerves, various interfascial plane blocks can be an option for pain relief. Due to the complexity of innervation to the breast, the serratus anterior (SA) plane block helps to cover several small nerve branches altogether [98]. This block is approached in a similar manner as individual intercostal nerve blocks, and medication is injected in between the latissimus dorsi muscle and the SA muscle. Branches of the intercostal nerves can be found both above and below the SA [99] and thus some practitioners may choose to deposit additional medication below the SA muscle as well. The ICBN perforates the SA muscle in the mid-axillary line and can be indirectly captured with this plane block as well [10]. Zocca et al. performed the injection on eight patients suffering from PMPS, depositing 0.25% bupivacaine and 40 mg of methyl-prednisolone, and all patients had pain relief ranging from 25% to near complete relief [99].

Other nerve blocks commonly used for patients suffering from pain in the breast region include the thoracic paravertebral block and erector spinae plane block [100]. The true value of these blocks comes mainly in the perioperative period [101, 102]. As mentioned earlier, significant acute postoperative pain is a risk factor for the development of chronic pain. Thus, several studies have shown that the use of these blocks before surgical incision can help decrease the level of acute pain after surgery, and subsequently the prevalence of chronic pain at the six and twelve month follow ups [101, 103]. Furthermore, they have also shown to decrease postoperative opioid use [102, 104].

Regardless of the procedure chosen, the most optimal option should be one that is easy to perform, causes little discomfort to the patient, has reasonable low-risk complications, and allows adequate pain relief.

5.3.2 Neuromodulation

With increasing prevalence in the diagnosis of neuropathic pain, and a shift to decrease use of chronic opioid therapy, the use of neuromodulation has gained significant interest [105]. Both invasive and non-invasive mechanisms of neuromodulation exist and have been used in the treatment of PMPS. A conservative approach to PMPS with neuromodulation is with the use of a transcutaneous electrical nerve stimulation (TENS) unit. TENS has effects on the neurophysiological activities of receptors via the gate theory of pain and can induce the expression of endogenous opioids [106]. EEG changes with use of a TENS unit and decrease in overall pain have been observed particularly in patients with ICBN pain after breast cancer surgery [107]. Due to its low cost, non-invasiveness, and favourable side-effect profile, TENS units have gained attention in treating cancer pain [108].

Peripheral nerve stimulation (PNS) continues to gain growing recognition in the field of pain management due to its less invasive percutaneous approach [109]. PNS allows for direct electrical stimulation of a peripheral nerve to alleviate pain in the distribution of that nerve [110]. This offers targeted therapy and offers pain relief for patients suffering from ICBN or intercostal neuralgia [111]. PNS electrodes can be placed under ultrasound guidance alongside the nerve, avoiding the need for fluoroscopy, and the pulse generator can remain external to the body [112].

Spinal cord stimulators (SCS) are a better-known type of neuromodulation available for chronic neuropathic pain. Technological advancements in SCS throughout the years, such as high frequency SCS, burst stimulation, and dorsal root ganglion (DRG) stimulation, have helped tailor treatment to an individual's pain condition and target specific symptoms [105]. While SCS continues to play a major role in the relief of failed back surgery syndrome and complex regional pain syndrome, new literature has emerged considering SCS for the treatment of PMPS. A case report using DRG stimulation at the T3 nerve roots demonstrated effective pain relief in a patient with severe neuropathic pain [113], and another showed the effectiveness of SCS in treatment of chronic drug-resistant neuropathy in a patient with radiation-induced plexopathy [114]. While these cases are promising, larger studies still need to be conducted in order to evaluate the optimal spinal level for SCS electrode placement and the best neuromodulation programming.

6. Conclusion

Treatment of persistent pain after breast surgery continues to be a challenge and clinical vigilance is needed when caring for this patient population. Neuropathic pain features can affect nearly half the number of patients who undergo breast cancer surgery, and failure of diagnosis and treatment can lead to a long-term negative decline in mood, quality of life, and overall functioning. While effective treatments still remain areas of active research, identifying patients at risk allows for the implementation of an early multidisciplinary therapeutic approach. Prospective studies on larger populations of breast cancer survivors continue to be performed, and these will help to fill gaps in knowledge and uncover novel therapeutic measures.

Author details

Sachin Sahni* and James Khan
Department of Anesthesia, University of Toronto, Toronto, ON, Canada

*Address all correspondence to: sachin.sahni@uhn.ca

References

[1] Ferlay J, Soerjomataram I, Dikshit R, et al. Cancer incidence and mortality worldwide: sources, methods and major patterns in GLOBOCAN 2012. Int J Cancer. 2015;136(5):E359-E386.

[2] Smith BD, Smith GL, Hurria A, Hortobagyi GN, Buchholz TA. Future of cancer incidence in the United States: burdens upon an aging, changing nation. J Clin Oncol. 2009;27(17):2758-2765.

[3] Noone AM, Howlader N, Krapcho M, Miller D, Brest A, Yu M, Ruhl J, Tatalovich Z, Mariotto A, Lewis DR, Chen HS, Feuer EJ, Cronin KA (eds). SEER Cancer Statistics Review, 1975-2015, National Cancer Institute. Bethesda, MD, https://seer.cancer.gov/csr/1975_2015/, based on November 2017 SEER data submission, posted to the SEER web site, April 2018.

[4] DeSantis CE, Fedewa SA, Goding Sauer A, Kramer JL, Smith RA, Jemal A. Breast cancer statistics, 2015: Convergence of incidence rates between black and white women. CA Cancer J Clin. 2016;66(1):31-42.

[5] Siegel RL, Miller KD, Jemal A. Cancer statistics, 2019. CA Cancer J Clin. 2019;69(1):7-34.

[6] Gärtner R, Jensen MB, Nielsen J, Ewertz M, Kroman N, Kehlet H. Prevalence of and factors associated with persistent pain following breast cancer surgery [published correction appears in JAMA. 2012 Nov 21;308(19):1973]. JAMA. 2009;302(18):1985-1992.

[7] Jung BF, Ahrendt GM, Oaklander AL, Dworkin RH. Neuropathic pain following breast cancer surgery: proposed classification and research update. Pain. 2003;104(1-2):1-13.

[8] Waltho D, Rockwell G. Post-breast surgery pain syndrome: establishing a consensus for the definition of post-mastectomy pain syndrome to provide a standardized clinical and research approach - a review of the literature and discussion. Can J Surg. 2016;59(5):342-350.

[9] Schug SA, Lavand'homme P, Barke A, et al. The IASP classification of chronic pain for ICD-11: chronic postsurgical or posttraumatic pain. Pain. 2019;160(1):45-52.

[10] Khan JS, Ladha KS, Abdallah F, Clarke H. Treating Persistent Pain After Breast Cancer Surgery. Drugs. 2020;80(1):23-31.

[11] Visnjevac O, Matson B. Postmastectomy pain syndrome: An unrecognized annual billion dollar national financial burden. The Journal of Pain. 2013;14(4).

[12] Smith WC, Bourne D, Squair J, Phillips DO, Chambers WA. A retrospective cohort study of post mastectomy pain syndrome. Pain. 1999 Oct;83(1):91-95.

[13] Larsson IM, Ahm Sørensen J, Bille C. The Post-mastectomy Pain Syndrome-A Systematic Review of the Treatment Modalities. Breast J. 2017 May;23(3):338-343. doi: 10.1111/tbj.12739. Epub 2017 Jan 30.

[14] Juhl AA, Christiansen P, Damsgaard TE. Persistent Pain after Breast Cancer Treatment: A Questionnaire-Based Study on the Prevalence, Associated Treatment Variables, and Pain Type. J Breast Cancer. 2016;19(4):447-454.

[15] Wijayasinghe, N., Andersen, K.G. and Kehlet, H., 2014. Neural blockade for persistent pain after breast cancer surgery. Regional Anesthesia & Pain Medicine, 39(4), pp.272-278

[16] Kumar P, Meena RN, Sheikh BA, Belliappa V and Pais AV. Intercostobrachial Nerve - Anatomical Considerations and its Importance in Carcinoma Breast of Female Patients. Ann Surg Perioper Care. 2016; 1(2):1013.

[17] Zhu JJ, Liu XF, Zhang PL, Yang JZ, Wang J, Qin Y, Zhang GL, Ren DQ, Cui CL, Guo XG. Anatomical information for intercostobrachial nerve preservation in axillary lymph node dissection for breast cancer. Genet Mol Res. 2014 Jan 24;13(4):9315-9323.

[18] Salmon RJ, Ansquer Y, Asselain B. Preservation versus section of intercostal-brachial nerve (IBN) in axillary dissection for breast cancer--a prospective randomized trial. European Journal of Surgical Oncology: the Journal of the European Society of Surgical Oncology and the British Association of Surgical Oncology. 1998 Jun;24(3):158-161.

[19] Ivanović N, Granić M, Randelović T, et al. Functional effects of preserving the intercostobrachial nerve and the lateral thoracic vein during axillary dissection in breast cancer conservative surgery Vojnosanit Pregl. 2007;64(3):195-198.

[20] Haam S, Kim D, Hwang J, Paik H, Lee D. An anatomical study of the relationship between the sympathetic trunk and intercostal veins of the third and fourth intercostal spaces during thoracoscopy. Clin Anat. 2010;23(6):702-706.

[21] Simmel ML. A study of phantoms after amputation of the breast. Neuropsykologica. 1966;4:331-250.

[22] Ahmed A, Bhatnagar S, Rana SP, Ahmad SM, Joshi S, Mishra S. Prevalence of phantom breast pain and sensation among post-mastectomy patients suffering from breast cancer: a prospective study. Pain Pract. 2014;14(2):E17-E28.

[23] Habib AS, Kertai MD, Cooter M, Greenup RA, Hwang S. Risk factors for severe acute pain and persistent pain after surgery for breast cancer: a prospective observational study. Reg Anesth Pain Med. 2019;44(2):192-199.

[24] Wang L, Guyatt GH, Kennedy SA, Romerosa B, Kwon HY, Kaushal A, Chang Y, Craigie S, de Almeida CPB, Couban RJ, Parascandalo SR, Izhar Z, Reid S, Khan JS, McGillion M, Busse JW. Predictors of persistent pain after breast cancer surgery: a systematic review and meta-analysis of observational studies. CMAJ. 2016 Oct 4;188(14):E352-E361.

[25] Cioroiu C., Weimer L.H. Update on Chemotherapy-Induced Peripheral Neuropathy. Curr. Neurol. Neurosci. Rep. 2017;17:47.

[26] Johnstone PA, DeLuca AM, Bacher JD, et al. Clinical toxicity of peripheral nerve to intraoperative radiotherapy in a canine model. Int J Radiat Oncol Biol Phys. 1995;32(4):1031-1034.

[27] Zajączkowska R, Kocot-Kępska M, Leppert W, Wrzosek A, Mika J, Wordliczek J. Mechanisms of Chemotherapy-Induced Peripheral Neuropathy. Int J Mol Sci. 2019;20(6):1451.

[28] Macdonald L, Bruce J, Scott NW, Smith WC, Chambers WA. Long-term follow-up of breast cancer survivors with post-mastectomy pain syndrome. Br J Cancer. 2005;92(2):225-230.

[29] Johnstone PA, DeLuca AM, Bacher JD, et al. Clinical toxicity of peripheral nerve to intraoperative radiotherapy in a canine model. Int J Radiat Oncol Biol Phys. 1995;32(4):1031-1034.

[30] Andersen KG, Duriaud HM, Jensen HE, Kroman N, Kehlet H. Predictive factors for the development of persistent pain after breast cancer surgery. Pain. 2015;156(12):2413-2422.

[31] Alves Nogueira Fabro E, Bergmann A, do Amaral E Silva B, et al. Post-mastectomy pain syndrome: incidence and risks. Breast. 2012;21(3):321-325.

[32] Kroman N, Jensen M, Wohlfahrt J, Mouridsen HT, Andersen PK, Melbye M. Factors influencing the effect of age on prognosis in breast cancer: population based study. Br Med J 2000;320:474-479.

[33] Krøner K, Krebs B, Skov J, Jørgensen HS. Immediate and long-term phantom breast syndrome after mastectomy: incidence, clinical characteristics and relationship to pre-mastectomy breast pain. Pain. 1989;36(3):327-334.

[34] Spivey TL, Gutowski ED, Zinboonyahgoon N, et al. Chronic Pain After Breast Surgery: A Prospective, Observational Study. Ann Surg Oncol. 2018;25(10):2917-2924.

[35] Tjeertes EK, Hoeks SE, Beks SB, Valentijn TM, Hoofwijk AG, Stolker RJ. Obesity--a risk factor for postoperative complications in general surgery? BMC Anesthesiol. 2015;15:155.

[36] Galyfos G, Geropapas GI, Kerasidis S, Sianou A, Sigala F, Filis K. The effect of body mass index on major outcomes after vascular surgery. J Vasc Surg. 2017;65(4):1193-1207.

[37] Kehlet H, Jensen TS, Woolf CJ. Persistent postsurgical pain: risk factors and prevention. Lancet. 2006;367(9522):1618-1625.

[38] Tait RC, Zoberi K, Ferguson M, et al. Persistent Post-Mastectomy Pain: Risk Factors and Current Approaches to Treatment. J Pain. 2018;19(12):1367-1383.

[39] Belfer I, Schreiber KL, Shaffer JR, et al. Persistent postmastectomy pain in breast cancer survivors: analysis of clinical, demographic, and psychosocial factors. J Pain. 2013;14(10):1185-1195.

[40] Miaskowski C, Cooper B, Paul SM, et al. Identification of patient subgroups and risk factors for persistent breast pain following breast cancer surgery. J Pain. 2012;13(12):1172-1187.

[41] Sullivan MJ, D'Eon JL. Relation between catastrophizing and depression in chronic pain patients. J Abnorm Psychol. 1990;99(3):260-263.

[42] Ellis A, Grieger R. Handbook of Rational Emotive Therapy. New York, NY: Springer Publishing; 1977.

[43] Bruce J, Thornton AJ, Scott NW, Marfizo S, Powell R, Johnston M, Wells M, Heys SD, Thompson AM. Chronic preoperative pain and psychological robustness predict acute postoperative pain outcomes after surgery for breast cancer. Br J Cancer. 2012 Sep 4;107(6):937-946.

[44] Vilholm OJ, Cold S, Rasmussen L, Sindrup SH. The postmastectomy pain syndrome: an epidemiological study on the prevalence of chronic pain after surgery for breast cancer. Br J Cancer. 2008;99(4):604-610.

[45] Petrelli F, Lonati V, Barni S. Axillary dissection compared to sentinel node biopsy for the treatment of pathologically node-negative breast cancer: a meta-analysis of four randomized trials with long-term follow up. Oncol Rev. 2012;6(2):e20.

[46] Andersen KG, Kehlet H. Persistent pain after breast cancer treatment: a critical review of risk factors and

strategies for prevention. J Pain. 2011;12(7):725-746.

[47] Alves Nogueira Fabro E, Bergmann A, do Amaral E Silva B, et al. Post-mastectomy pain syndrome: incidence and risks. Breast. 2012;21(3):321-325.

[48] Vecht CJ, Van de Brand HJ, Wajer OJ. Post-axillary dissection pain in breast cancer due to a lesion of the intercostobrachial nerve. Pain. 1989 Aug;38(2):171-176.

[49] Gilron I, Vandenkerkhof E, Katz J, Kehlet H, Carley M. Evaluating the Association Between Acute and Chronic Pain After Surgery: Impact of Pain Measurement Methods. Clin J Pain. 2017;33(7):588-594.

[50] Fassoulaki A, Melemeni A, Staikou C, Triga A, Sarantopoulos C. Acute postoperative pain predicts chronic pain and long-term analgesic requirements after breast surgery for cancer. Acta Anaesthesiol Belg. 2008;59(4):241-248.

[51] Bruce J, Thornton AJ, Powell R, et al. Psychological, surgical, and sociodemographic predictors of pain outcomes after breast cancer surgery: a population-based cohort study. Pain. 2014;155(2):232-243.

[52] Peuckmann V, Ekholm O, Rasmussen NK, et al. Chronic pain and other sequelae in long-term breast cancer survivors: nationwide survey in Denmark. Eur J Pain. 2009;13(5):478-485.

[53] Rosso R, Scelsi M, Carnevali L. Granular cell traumatic neuroma: a lesion occurring in mastectomy scars. Arch Pathol Lab Med. 2000;124(5):709-711.

[54] Merskey H, Bogduk N. Classification of chronic pain: descriptions of chronic pain syndromes and definitions of pain terms, 2nd ed. Seattle:IASP Press; 1994.

[55] Timmerman H, Steegers MAH, Huygen FJPM, et al. Investigating the validity of the DN4 in a consecutive population of patients with chronic pain. PLoS One. 2017;12(11):e0187961.

[56] Bouhassira D, Attal N, Alchaar H, et al. Comparison of pain syndromes associated with nervous or somatic lesions and development of a new neuropathic pain diagnostic questionnaire (DN4). Pain. 2005;114(1-2):29-36.

[57] Khan JS, Hodgson N, Choi S, et al. Perioperative Pregabalin and Intraoperative Lidocaine Infusion to Reduce Persistent Neuropathic Pain After Breast Cancer Surgery: A Multicenter, Factorial, Randomized, Controlled Pilot Trial. J Pain. 2019;20(8):980-993.

[58] McCracken LM, Hoskins J, Eccleston C. Concerns about medication and medication use in chronic pain. J Pain. 2006;7:726-734.

[59] De Groef A, Van Kampen M, Dieltjens E, et al. Effectiveness of postoperative physical therapy for upper-limb impairments after breast cancer treatment: a systematic review. Arch Phys Med Rehabil. 2015;96(6):1140-1153.

[60] Harris SR, Schmitz KH, Campbell KL, McNeely ML. Clinical practice guidelines for breast cancer rehabilitation: syntheses of guideline recommendations and qualitative appraisals. Cancer. 2012;118(8 Suppl):2312-2324.

[61] Schultz I, Barholm M, Gröndal S. Delayed shoulder exercises in reducing seroma frequency after modified radical mastectomy: a prospective randomized study. Ann Surg Oncol. 1997;4(4):293-297.

[62] Bendz I, Fagevik Olsén M. Evaluation of immediate versus delayed shoulder exercises after breast cancer surgery including lymph node dissection--a randomised controlled trial. Breast. 2002;11(3):241-248.

[63] Duijts SF, Faber MM, Oldenburg HS, van Beurden M, Aaronson NK. Effectiveness of behavioral techniques and physical exercise on psychosocial functioning and health-related quality of life in breast cancer patients and survivors--a meta-analysis. Psychooncology. 2011;20(2):115-126.

[64] Veehof MM, Trompetter HR, Bohlmeijer ET, Schreurs KM. Acceptance- and mindfulness-based interventions for the treatment of chronic pain: a meta-analytic review. Cogn Behav Ther. 2016;45(1):5-31.

[65] Jassim GA, Whitford DL, Hickey A, Carter B. Psychological interventions for women with non-metastatic breast cancer. Cochrane Database Syst Rev. 2015;(5):CD008729.

[66] Haller H, Winkler MM, Klose P, Dobos G, Kümmel S, Cramer H. Mindfulness-based interventions for women with breast cancer: an updated systematic review and meta-analysis. Acta Oncol. 2017;56(12):1665-1676.

[67] Finnerup NB, Attal N, Haroutounian S, McNicol E, Baron R, Dworkin RH, Gilron I, Haanpää M, Hansson P, Jensen TS, Kamerman PR, Lund K, Moore A, Raja SN, Rice AS, Rowbotham M, Sena E, Siddall P, Smith BH, Wallace M. Pharmacotherapy for neuropathic pain in adults: a systematic review and meta-analysis. Lancet Neurol. 2015 Feb;14(2):162-173.

[68] Moulin D, Boulanger A, Clark AJ, et al. Pharmacological management of chronic neuropathic pain: revised consensus statement from the Canadian Pain Society. Pain Res Manag. 2014;19(6):328-335.

[69] Attal N, Cruccu G, Baron R, et al. EFNS guidelines on the pharmacological treatment of neuropathic pain: 2010 revision. Eur J Neurol. 2010;17(9):1113-1e88.

[70] Jackson KC 2nd, St Onge EL. Antidepressant pharmacotherapy: considerations for the pain clinician. Pain Pract. 2003;3(2):135-143.

[71] Yokogawa F, Kiuchi Y, Ishikawa Y, Otsuka N, Masuda Y, Oguchi K, Hosoyamada A. An investigation of monoamine receptors involved in antinociceptive effects of antidepressants. Anesth Analg 2002;95:163-168.

[72] Watanabe Y, Saito H, Abe K. Tricyclic antidepressants block NMDA receptor-mediated synaptic responses and induction of long-term potentiation in rat hippocampal slices. Neuropharmacology. 1993;32(5):479-486.

[73] Glassman AH, Perel JM, Shostak M, Kantor SJ, Fleiss JL. Clinical Implications of Imipramine Plasma Levels for Depressive Illness. Arch Gen Psychiatry. 1977;34(2):197-204.

[74] Eija K, Tiina T, Pertti JN. Amitriptyline effectively relieves neuropathic pain following treatment of breast cancer. Pain. 1995;64:293-302.

[75] Wellington K, Perry CM. Venlafaxine extended-release: a review of its use in the management of major depression. CNS Drugs. 2001;15(8):643-669.

[76] Jann MW, Slade JH. Antidepressant agents for the treatment of chronic pain and depression. Pharmacotherapy. 2007;27(11):1571-1587.

[77] Tasmuth T, Härtel B, Kalso E. Venlafaxine in neuropathic pain following treatment of breast cancer. Eur J Pain. 2002; 6(1):17-24.

[78] Holliday SM, Benfield P. Venlafaxine: a review of its pharmacology and therapeutic potential in depression. Drugs. 1995;49:280-294.

[79] Simpson DA. Gabapentin and venlafaxine for the treatment of painful diabetic neuropathy. J Clin Neuromusc Dis 2001;3:53-62.

[80] Kus T, Aktas G, Alpak G, et al. Efficacy of venlafaxine for the relief of taxane and oxaliplatin-induced acute neurotoxicity: a single-center retrospective case-control study. Support Care Cancer. 2016;24(5):2085-2091.

[81] Song SY, Ko YB, Kim H, et al. Effect of serotonin-norepinephrine reuptake inhibitors for patients with chemotherapy-induced painful peripheral neuropathy: A meta-analysis. Medicine (Baltimore). 2020;99(1):e18653.

[82] Farshchian N, Alavi A, Heydarheydari S, Moradian N. Comparative study of the effects of venlafaxine and duloxetine on chemotherapy-induced peripheral neuropathy. Cancer Chemother Pharmacol. 2018 Nov;82(5):787-793.

[83] Fishbain DA, Detke MJ, Wernicke J, Chappell AS, Kajdasz DK. The relationship between antidepressant and analgesic responses: findings from six placebo-controlled trials assessing the efficacy of duloxetine in patients with major depressive disorder. Curr Med Res Opin. 2008;24(11):3105-3115.

[84] Sindrup SH, Jensen TS. Pharmacologic treatment of pain in polyneuropathy. Neurology 2000;55:915-920.

[85] e Miguel-Jimeno JM, Forner-Cordero I, Zabalza-Azparren M, Matute-Tobias B. Sindrome de dolor posmastectomia en nuestro medio: caracteristicas, tratamiento y experiencia con gabapentina [Postmastectomy pain syndrome in our region: characteristics, treatment, and experience with gabapentin]. Rev Neurol. 2016;62(6):258-266.

[86] Bockbrader HN, Wesche D, Miller R, Chapel S, Janiczek N, Burger P. A comparison of the pharmacokinetics and pharmacodynamics of pregabalin and gabapentin. Clin Pharmacokinetics. 2010;49(10):661-669.

[87] Reyad RM, Omran AF, Abbas DN, et al. The Possible Preventive Role of Pregabalin in Postmastectomy Pain Syndrome: A Double-Blinded Randomized Controlled Trial [published correction appears in J Pain Symptom Manage. 2019 Jun;57(6):e11]. J Pain Symptom Manage. 2019;57(1):1-9.

[88] Kaur N, Kumar A, Saxena AK, Grover RK. Pregabalin in the treatment of postmastectomy chronic pain: Results of an open label, single-arm clinical study. Breast J. 2019;25(3):465-468.

[89] Paice JA, Portenoy R, Lacchetti C, et al. Management of Chronic Pain in Survivors of Adult Cancers: American Society of Clinical Oncology Clinical Practice Guideline. J Clin Oncol. 2016;34(27):3325-3345.

[90] Arnér S, Meyerson BA. Lack of analgesic effect of opioids on neuropathic and idiopathic forms of pain. Pain. 1988;33(1):11-23.

[91] Keskinbora K, Pekel AF, Aydinli I. Gabapentin and an opioid combination versus opioid alone for the management of neuropathic cancer pain: a randomized open trial. J Pain Symptom Manage. 2007;34(2):183-189.

[92] Li, Xm., Liu, Dq., Wu, Hy. et al. Controlled-release oxycodone alone or combined with gabapentin for management of malignant neuropathic pain. Chin. J. Cancer Res. 2010;22:80-86.

[93] Takahashi H, Shimoyama N. A prospective open-label trial of gabapentin as an adjuvant analgesic with opioids for Japanese patients with neuropathic cancer pain. Int J Clin Oncol. 2010;15(1):46-51.

[94] Kim ED, Baek JW, Kim JS, Oh SA, Kim YH. Ultrasound-Guided Block of the Axillary Nerve: A Prospective, Randomized, Single-Blind Study Comparing Interfascial and Perivascular Injections. Pain Physician. 2019;22(4):369-376.

[95] Loukas M, Hullett J, Louis RG Jr, Holdman S, Holdman D. The gross anatomy of the extrathoracic course of the intercostobrachial nerve. Clin Anat. 2006;19(2):106-111.

[96] Glenesk NL, Rahman S, Lopez PP. Anatomy, Thorax, Intercostal Nerves. [Updated 2020 Jul 27]. In: StatPearls [Internet]. Treasure Island (FL): StatPearls Publishing; 2020 Jan-.

[97] Shanti CM, Carlin AM, Tyburski JG. Incidence of pneumothorax from intercostal nerve block for analgesia in rib fractures. J Trauma. 2001;51(3):536-539.

[98] Blanco R, Parras T, McDonnell JG, Prats-Galino A. Serratus plane block: a novel ultrasound-guided thoracic wall nerve block. Anaesthesia. 2013;68(11):1107-1113.

[99] Zocca JA, Chen GH, Puttanniah VG, Hung JC, Gulati A. Ultrasound-Guided Serratus Plane Block for Treatment of Postmastectomy Pain Syndromes in Breast Cancer Patients: A Case Series. Pain Pract. 2017;17(1):141-146.

[100] Uchida K. Radiofrequency treatment of the thoracic paravertebral nerve combined with glucocorticoid for refractory neuropathic pain following breast cancer surgery. Pain Physician. 2009;12(4):E277-E283.

[101] Kairaluoma PM, Bachmann MS, Rosenberg PH, Pere PJ. Preincisional paravertebral block reduces the prevalence of chronic pain after breast surgery. Anesth Analg. 2006;103(3):703-708.

[102] Piraccini E, Calli M, Taddei S, Maitan S. Erector spinae plane block and rhomboid intercostal block for the treatment of post-mastectomy pain syndrome. Saudi J Anaesth. 2020;14(4):517-519.

[103] Qian B, Fu S, Yao Y, Lin D, Huang L. Preoperative ultrasound-guided multilevel paravertebral blocks reduce the incidence of postmastectomy chronic pain: a double-blind, placebo-controlled randomized trial. J Pain Res. 2019;12:597-603.

[104] El Ghamry MR, Amer AF. Role of erector spinae plane block versus paravertebral block in pain control after modified radical mastectomy. A prospective randomised trial. Indian J Anaesth. 2019;63(12):1008-1014.

[105] Grider JS, Manchikanti L, Carayannopoulos A, Sharma ML, Balog CC, Harned ME, et al. Effectiveness of spinal cord stimulation in chronic spinal pain: a systematic review. Pain Physician. 2016;19:E33–E54.

[106] Robb KA, Newham DJ, Williams JE. Transcutaneous electrical nerve stimulation vs. transcutaneous spinal electroanalgesia for chronic pain associated with breast cancer treatments. J Pain Symptom Manage. 2007;33(4):410-419.

[107] Silva JG, Santana CG, Inocêncio KR, Orsini M, Machado S, Bergmann A. Electrocortical Analysis of Patients with Intercostobrachial Pain Treated with TENS after Breast Cancer Surgery. J Phys Ther Sci. 2014;26(3):349-353.

[108] Hurlow A, Bennett MI, Robb KA, Johnson MI, Simpson KH, Oxberry SG. Transcutaneous electric nerve stimulation (TENS) for cancer pain in adults. Cochrane Database Syst Rev. 2012;2012(3):CD006276. Published 2012 Mar 14.

[109] Chakravarthy K, Nava A, Christo PJ, Williams K. Review of Recent Advances in Peripheral Nerve Stimulation (PNS). Curr Pain Headache Rep. 2016;20(11):60.

[110] Banks GP, Winfree CJ. Evolving Techniques and Indications in Peripheral Nerve Stimulation for Pain. Neurosurg Clin N Am. 2019;30(2):265-273.

[111] Mainkar O, Solla CA, Chen G, Legler A, Gulati A. Pilot Study in Temporary Peripheral Nerve Stimulation in Oncologic Pain. Neuromodulation. 2020;23(6):819-826. doi:10.1111/ner.13139

[112] Gupta S, Clendenen S, Ferreira-Dos-Santos G, Hurdle MF. Ultrasound-Guided Intercostal Peripheral Nerve Stimulator Implantation: Technique Report and Feasibility Study in a Cadaver. Pain Med. 2020;21(Suppl 1): S32-S37.

[113] Morgalla MH. Dorsal Root Ganglion Stimulation for the Treatment of Persistent Post-Mastectomy Pain: Case Report. Neuromodulation. 2019;22(1):117-118.

[114] Dorokhov EV, Isagulyan ED, Isaev PA, Semin DY, Polkin VV. Vopr Onkol. 2016;62(4):524-528.

Chapter 8

Breast Cancer Screening

Mohammed Tareq Mutar, Mustafa Majid Hameed, Mohammed Saleh Goyani, Aqeel Shakir Mahmood and Abo-Alhasan Hammed Obaid

Abstract

Breast cancer is a common malignancy worldwide. It is considered top cancer in women and about 13% of women in the general population will develop breast cancer sometimes during their lives, with a gradual increase in incidence as survival increases. Primary prevention of breast cancer is directed toward promoting a healthy lifestyle and reversing modifiable risk factors; these factors include smoking cessation, physical activity, alcohol, and dietary modification. Imaging plays an important role in the diagnosis and management of breast cancer, it is also considered the most valuable tool in screening breast cancer. Mammogram is the most widely used method; it is recommended by many societies and committees as a useful method for early detection of breast cancer. False-positive and over-diagnosis constitute a problem in using screening mammogram. The implementation of a screening program faces many issues that may adversely affect its success such as personal factors, social factors, and accessibility issues. These issues should be identified as the initial step in program implementation. The role of Magnetic Resonance Imaging and Ultrasound is mainly in high-risk patients. The introduction of Artificial Intelligence in Mammogram may add beneficial effects in time and efforts improving its efforts.

Keywords: breast cancer, screening, mammogram, breast self-examination, breast ultrasound

1. Introduction

Breast cancer is a common malignancy worldwide. It is considered top cancer in women and about 13% of women in the general population will sometimes develop breast cancer during their lives, with gradual increase in incidence as survival increases [1]. That is the reason why Breast cancer prevention is the core of many researches and trials worldwide. The World health organization has recommended breast self-examination, mammography as an effective screening tool since 2007. As in conclusion, early detection of breast cancer (secondary prevention) remains the cornerstone for breast cancer control [2].

Educating the population about eliminating modifiable risk factors (e.g. smoking, obesity) remains essential in the primary prevention of breast cancer [3].

1.1 Age

As a rule of thumb, breast cancer shows an increase in incidence as the age increases, about 8 in 10 cases of breast cancer occurs in women aged 50 or above [4].

However, this may not be applicable for all countries, as a study done by Mutar et al. shows that 45% percent of breast cancer patients were younger than 50 years [5].

The disease is extremely rare before the 20s, and it is as highly prevalent as 20% at age of 80 [6]. It is important to mention that the age may be the only risk factor present in a woman who develops breast cancer [7].

1.2 Hormonal factors

It is proposed that the longer a woman is exposed to cycling reproductive hormones, the higher the risk of breast cancer disease [8].

1.2.1 Time of menarche and menopause

In a large meta-analysis study done in 2012 [9]. An apparent association was found between the early age of menarche and the late age of menopause and breast cancer development, with the first factor being a stronger independent factor for breast cancer development.

In addition to that, these two factors seem to play a more complex role; they favor the development of estrogen-receptor positive disease & lobular histological type of breast cancer.

1.2.2 Parity, breastfeeding and age of having a first child

Breast cancer is more common in nulliparous women and breastfeeding, in particular, appears to be a protective factor. Also, having the first child at an early age seems to be protective [6].

Increasing parity was associated with a pronounced decrease in the risk of breast cancer, with each extra birth granting about 10 percent reduction of breast cancer risk, and the disease is 13 times more common for each five years increment in the age of having the first child [10].

And just like the effect of menarche & menopause, these factors not merely affect the duration of hormonal exposure but also the hormonal receptor status of breast cancer; for example, breastfeeding is inversely associated with hormone receptor-negative breast cancers and parous women were shown to have a lower risk of estrogen-positive breast cancer [11].

1.2.3 Contraceptive pills

Current or recent use of oral contraceptive pills increases the relative risk of breast cancer [12].

Post-menopausal hormonal replacement therapy (HRT) was associated with an increased risk for breast cancer [13]. Vaginal estrogens are considered an exception [4].

1.2.4 Obesity

Breast cancer is more common in obese women [6]. Obesity also affects breast cancer management; obese patients have lower treatment efficacy, more complications and higher recurrence rates [14].

Again, this supports the theory of linking breast cancer to the high estrogen states.

1.3 Lifestyle

1.3.1 Physical activity

A study held among Chinese women showed evidence that physical activity decreases breast cancer incidence; this is maybe due to the proposed effect of exercise on estrogen & insulin [15]. Education about this aspect seems reasonable for breast cancer prevention in high-risk groups.

1.3.2 Smoking

Both passive & active smoking are associated with an increased risk of breast cancer [16].

Also, women who were smoking at the time of their diagnosis have weaker outcomes and poorer survival [17]. However, there are inconclusive results about the smoking risk for the recurrence of the disease.

1.3.3 Alcohol

Just like smoking, it does increase the risk for breast cancer even in light to moderate intake in all ethnicities & with no association to estrogen hormonal status [18].

1.3.4 Dietary factors

Meat, caffeine, high fat diet, Low phytoestrogen all appear to increase the risk of breast cancer, in contrast to increment in vitamin D and calcium levels [6, 19].

1.3.5 Others

Living in stressful life/personality may appear to increase the breast cancer risk [20].

1.4 Drugs and radiation

- Non-steroidal anti-inflammatory drugs may appear to protect against breast cancer, although the evidence is not strong [21].

- Digoxin carries more pronounced research evidence to increase the risk of breast cancer, and all women should be informed about this relative risk before starting treatment [20, 22, 23]. This usually describes its use for more than four years and the risk is elevated by 21 to 40%.

- Radiation: patient's receiving radiotherapy as part of their treatment of Hodgkin lymphoma appeared to have an increased risk for breast cancer [6]. Routine chest X-ray and Computed tomography scans only have a little contribution to the risk [4].

2. Imaging in oncology

The first imaging modality to be discovered was X-ray by the German physicist Roentgen in 1895, the first use in oncology was to obtain a picture of sarcoma in an amputated leg by German Surgeon Konig. the second imaging modality involved in oncology was ultrasonography, which was used for brain tumors, it Dussik used and called (hyper phonography) [24, 25]. The ultrasonography was then used in bowel, breast and obstetrics.

The history of mammography in breast cancer began in 1913 by Salomon who used it to evaluate 3000 mastectomies specimens [26]. He evaluated the role of radiological assessment correlated with the macrocalcifications and microscopic assessment of breast in order to differentiate between benign and malignant diseases [27].

The use of Xeromammography in 1960s shows improvement in mammogram diagnostic ability, the 1970s and 80s were the time to establish of screening mammography. In 1996 the Food and Drug Administration (FDA) established guidelines for commercializing digital mammography equipment [27].

Offering a screening mammography started in different times according to each country, for example, Australia had started screening by mammography every 2 years for women aged 50–69 years since 1991, while in Europe it started in 1986 [28, 29].

3. Screening

Screening is applied to many types of cancer, including mainly breast, colorectal, prostate, cervical and lung cancer. Breast cancer screening includes three main types screening mammography, clinical examination and ultrasound [30, 31].

Mammography is the most common screening modality for detecting breast cancers in asymptomatic women. The age and the frequency for screening mammogram is the subject of ongoing debate [32]. There is a considerable disagreement between guidelines regarding the recommendation for the age and frequency this might results from the wide variation in studies as found by Raichand et al. [32]. In a meta-analysis of 11 randomized clinical trials, the relative risk RR of breast cancer mortality for screening compared with controls was 0·80 (95% CI 0·73–0·89), with a 20% relative risk reduction [33].

The starting of 'Europe against Cancer' program in 1986, has led the committee of experts to start systematic population-based screening for cancer that shows decreased mortality with implementation. The effectiveness and benefits of mammography screening have been evaluated in randomized trials that showed decreased mortality by 20–35% in women 50–69 year [34].

If breast cancer is not diagnosed, the screening result is considered false-positive resulting in distress and anxiety among women [35]. The rates of false-positive results depend on many factors including screening interval, single versus double reading, sensitivity of the performance, participation patterns, equipment, and characteristics of the screening population [36]. Women who had false-positive results had a twofold increased risk of a later screen-detected cancer and might cause a reduced likelihood of reattendance [36, 37]. A recent meta-analysis had shown that a previous false-positive test does not influence participation in subsequent screening program [38].

It might better to encourage women with false-positive results to participate in regular screening, as the potential benefit is higher than in women who had negative tests [36].

The elements suggestive of a successful screening program are substantial reduction in cancer-related mortality, good participants' compliance, acceptability among participants, coverage, and high reattendance rate [37, 39].

Box 1 conditions required for successful mammogram screening.

1. It requires sufficient health system as well as financial resources to achieve a sustainable program with effective diagnostic and treatment capabilities including equipment, infrastructure, quality assurance, and monitoring processes.
2. It requires an administrative facilities responsible for the process of implementation and evaluation.
3. It requires validated protocols for screening steps, including recognizing the target population, inviting women who are eligible to be screened, applying screening tests, referral mechanism and its regulations, and management of each case accordingly.
4. It requires a good Communication and education of eligible women using culturally appropriate, objective information about the benefits and harms of breast cancer screening.
5. Ensuring good adherence to the guidelines for screening, diagnosis and treatment which are evidence based.
6. Information system for recording data of the screening process like calling the participants for follow up if abnormality was detected on screening.
7. Continuous regular monitoring, assessment and reporting of program performance and impact depending on reliable indicators like women's safety and satisfaction [40].

Box 1.
According to WHO, conditions for successful mammography screening.

3.1 Barriers to participating in mammogram

3.1.1 Personal beliefs

Fear of a positive result, pain and embarrassment related to the procedure, lack of knowledge about breast cancer and its screening, absence of trust in doctors and hospitals, lack of knowledge regarding mammography and its advantages, perception of being healthy, and fear of radiation exposure.

3.1.2 Accessibility and associated factors

Low-income population and lack of resources and health insurance, cost of mammogram, language barrier for minorities, lack of time required for mammogram, lack of transportation including personal and public transport, registration difficulties, and lower educational level.

3.1.3 Social factors

Lack of medical recommendation and advice regarding mammogram and discouragement from other people.

Other factors that affect participation include Age, Religiosity, family and personal history, and role of responsibility [41, 42].

3.2 Benefits and harms of breast cancer screening

Breast cancer mortality is generally reduced with mammography screening, although the magnitudes of effect are small. Advanced cancer is reduced with screening for women aged 50 years or older [43].

The detection of breast cancer in Australia increased in 2004 and mortality decreased [28]. On the other hand, possible harms of breast cancer screening may be related to false-positive results. According to a study published in 2011, most abnormal mammograms are actually false-positive. Follow-up testing adds additional cost [44].

3.3 Breast cancer overdiagnosis

The effectiveness of screening is mainly dependent on detecting cancer at early stage to promote early detection and better outcome, however, screening yields malignancies that may not have progressed during lifetime [45]. the lead time is the period between detection of cancer at screening and when it might be presented clinically, with stopping screening, the cancer incidence must fall, and at the end of screening time plus lead time, the cumulative incidence of the controlled and the screened populations should be the same. During the screening, some cancer detected might never progress throughout woman's life and might die from another cause before cancer becomes clinically detected. In another word overdiagnosis is defined as "detection of cancers that would never have been found without screening" [46–51] (**Tables 1** and **2**).

3.4 Clinical Breast examination (CBE)

Benefits: The current evidence does not support additional benefits and harms of CBE due to lack of evidence. CBE accuracy in the community screening might be lower than in the RCT [53].

Harms:

- False positives with additional testing and anxiety.
- False negatives with potential false reassurance and delay in cancer diagnosis.

3.5 Breast self-examination (BSE)

Benefits: BSE has been compared with no screening and has been shown to have no benefit in reducing breast cancer mortality [53].

Harms: There is solid evidence that formal instruction and encouragement to perform BSE leads to more breast biopsies and more diagnoses of benign breast

Risk stratification	Criteria
Low (L) risk	Category 1 breast density without or with only one risk factor (family history or breast biopsy) or Category 2 breast density with no risk factors
Medium-Low (ML) risk	Category 1 breast density with two additional risk factors, Category 2 breast density with only one risk factor, or Categories 3 or 4 breast density with no additional risk factors
Medium-High (MH) risk	Category 2 breast density with two additional risk factors, or Categories 3 or 4 breast density with only one risk factor
High (H) risk	Categories 3 or 4 breast density with two additional risk factors

Table 1.
Risk stratification for breast cancer screening. It is adopted from Yamamuro et al. [47].

Ages (Years)	U.S. Preventive Services Task Force [52]	American Cancer Society	American College of Obstetricians and Gynecologists	The Canadian Task Force	International Agency for Research on Cancer	European Commission Initiative for Breast Cancer Screening and Diagnosis guidelines (European Breast Guidelines)	American College of Radiology	American College of Physicians	American Academy of Family Physicians
Prior to 50	The decision should be individualized. Women who place a higher benefit than harms can start biennial screening between 40 and 49 years	Women have the choice of screening from age 40 to 44 once a year. Women should be screened from age 45 to 49 years.	If the individual prefers to screen and after taking consultation, mammography may be done once a year or once every two years with clinical breast exams once a year. Those choices should be taken after shared doctor with patient decisions.	For women aged 40–49 we recommend not routinely screening with mammography. (Weak recommendation; moderate quality evidence)	There is limited evidence that screening with mammography reduces breast cancer mortality in women 40–49 years of age.	For asymptomatic women aged 40 to 44 years with an average risk for breast cancer, the ECIBC's GDG suggests not implementing organized mammography screening	Screening with mammography is recommended once per year.	The choice of whether or not to screen with mammography before 50 years should be discussed by clinicians, taking into consideration the potential the benefit and harms and a woman's preferences. The potential risks outweigh benefits in most women between 40 to 49 years.	The decision to start screening with mammography should be an individual one. Women who place a higher value on the potential benefit than the potential harms may choose to begin screening.
50–74	Biennial screening mammography for women aged 50 to 74 years	Between 50 and 54, women should be screened with annual	Mammography is recommenced once a year or every two years. Decisions should	For women aged 50–69 years we recommend routinely screening with	There is sufficient evidence that screening with mammography	For asymptomatic women aged 50 to 69 years with an average risk for breast cancer, the	Screening with mammography is recommended once a year.	Clinicians should offer screening with mammography once every two	Screening with mammography is recommended once every two years.

Ages (Years)	U.S. Preventive Services Task Force [52]	American Cancer Society	American College of Obstetricians and Gynecologists	The Canadian Task Force	International Agency for Research on Cancer	European Commission Initiative for Breast Cancer Screening and Diagnosis guidelines (European Breast Guidelines)	American College of Radiology	American College of Physicians	American Academy of Family Physicians
		mammography, While after 55 years, mammography is recommended once every one or two years. After 55 years, individuals should be transitioned to biennial screening or continue to screen annually.	be made after shared patient with doctor discussion Clinical breast examination can be done annually. .	mammography every 2 to 3 years. (Weak recommendation; moderate quality evidence) For women aged 70–74 we recommend routinely screening with mammography every 2 to 3 years. (Weak recommendation; low quality evidence)	reduces breast-cancer mortality to the extent that its benefits substantially outweigh the risk of radiation-induced cancer from mammography. There is inadequate evidence that clinical breast examination reduces breast cancer mortality. There is sufficient evidence that clinical breast examination shifts the stage distribution of tumors detected toward a lower stage.	ECIBC's GDG recommends mammography screening over no mammography screening, in the context of an organized screening program (strong recommendation, moderate certainty of evidence;		years. In average-risk women of all ages, clinicians should not use clinical breast examination to screen for breast cancer.	Current evidence is insufficient to assess the benefits and harms of clinical breast exams.

Ages (Years)	U.S. Preventive Services Task Force [52]	American Cancer Society	American College of Obstetricians and Gynecologists	The Canadian Task Force	International Agency for Research on Cancer	European Commission Initiative for Breast Cancer Screening and Diagnosis guidelines (European Breast Guidelines)	American College of Radiology	American College of Physicians	American Academy of Family Physicians
75 and older	The current evidence is insufficient to assess the balance of benefits and harms of screening mammography in women aged 75 years or older	Women should continue screening with mammography as long as their overall health is good and they have a life expectancy of 10 years or more.	The decision to stop screening should be based on a shared decision-making process. The decision-making process should include a discussion of the woman's health status and longevity.	—	—	For asymptomatic women aged 70 to 74 years with an average risk for breast cancer, the ECIBC's GDG suggests mammography screening over no mammography screening, in the context of an organized screening program (conditional recommendation, moderate certainty of evidence	The age to stop screening with mammography should be based on each woman's health status rather than an age-based determination.	Screening should be discontinued for average-risk women of 75 years or older, also in women of life expectancy of 10 years or less	Current evidence is insufficient to assess the balance of benefits and harms of screening with mammography.
Women with dense breast	Current evidence is insufficient to assess the balance of benefits and harms of	Evidence is insufficient to recommend for or against yearly MRI screening.	No routine use of other alternative tests is recommended, other than	—	There is inadequate evidence that ultrasonography as an adjunct to	—	In addition to mammography, contrast-enhanced breast MRI is also	There is insufficient evidence on the beneficial and harmful effects	Current evidence is insufficient to assess the balance of benefits and harms of

Ages (Years)	U.S. Preventive Services Task Force [52]	American Cancer Society	American College of Obstetricians and Gynecologists	The Canadian Task Force	International Agency for Research on Cancer	European Commission Initiative for Breast Cancer Screening and Diagnosis guidelines (European Breast Guidelines)	American College of Radiology	American College of Physicians	American Academy of Family Physicians
	adjunctive screening for breast cancer using breast ultrasonography, magnetic resonance imaging (MRI), digital breast tomosynthesis (DBT), or other methods in women identified to have dense breasts on an otherwise negative screening mammogram.		screening mammograph. State laws may require disclosure to women of their breast density as recorded in a mammogram report.		mammography reduces breast cancer mortality. There is limited evidence that ultrasonography as an adjunct to mammography increases the breast cancer detection rate. There is sufficient evidence that ultrasonography as an adjunct to mammography increases the proportion of false positive screening outcomes		recommended. After weighing benefits and risks, ultrasound can be considered for those who cannot undergo MRI	of screening for women with dense breast	adjunctive screening for breast cancer using breast ultrasonography, MRI, DBT, or other methods. Women

U.S: United state, ECIBC, GDG: The European Commission Initiative on Breast Cancer Guidelines Development Group.

Table 2.
Guidelines and recommendations for breast cancer screening mammogram. The references are enlighten between parentheses.

lesions. The biopsy rate was 1.8% among the study population compared with 1.0% among the control group.

3.6 Magnetic resonance imaging (MRI)

MRI has the greatest sensitivity of all imaging techniques, and it is considered a problem-solving modality, as a negative breast MRI can exclude malignancy. Only microcalcification seen on mammography cannot be excluded sufficiently by MRI and mammography in such case should be used to judge for biopsy indications. The role of MRI in screening high-risk patients is established, the sensitivity of MRI in high risk patients is between 71 and 100% compared with 16–40% in mammography, while specificity ranges 81–99% for MRI and 93–99% in mammography [54].

The American Cancer Society Guidelines recommends annual breast MRI screening starting from 25 to 30 years in women with a first-degree relative with a BRCA mutation, patients with a BRCA gene mutation, and women with 25% or greater lifetime risk of cancer [55].

European Society of Breast Imaging also advises annual screening with MRI for patients with breast cancer diagnosed under 50 years of age who have a 20% lifetime risk of recurrence and for patients who received radiation to the chest in their second or third decade of life and for patients with inherited syndromes, like Cowden and LiFraumeni syndrome, and their first-degree relatives [54].

Starting Screening at age 40 years may provide some benefits in average-risk populations, but offer higher levels of harm than strategies initiated at age 50 years. The age for cessation of screening can be based on the Comorbidity levels. Biennial screening strategies can be used and considered as the most efficient, but annual screening might be indicated from 40 to 74 years of age in groups with have a 2- to 4-fold higher risk than average [56].

3.7 Ultrasound (US)

Until the early 1990's, breast ultrasound was used primarily to distinguish solid from cystic lesions and image-guided interventions [57]. Ultrasound can be added to mammography in women with dense breasts so that, to increase the sensitivity of detecting the cancer. Ultrasound has relatively good specificity and sensitivity as a follow up tool in women with dense breast and negative mammogram, for that reason, ultrasound can be considered as an adjunct to mammography in screening women with dense breasts [58]. One meta-analysis results suggest the addition of US to mammography of women with dense breasts improves the sensitivity of detecting breast cancer, despite a slightly decreased specificity. Follow-up US also had good diagnostic sensitivity and specificity [59].

Ultrasound, when compared to mammography, is radiation-free, cheaper and less strenuous modality [60].

Using mammography alone for screening has been shown to have poorer diagnostic performance for high-risk women than when used for the general population. For high-risk women, mammography has lower sensitivity and a higher interval cancers rate that might be spread to the lymph nodes. Many factors described in the literature may be responsible for that; like higher breast density, younger age of onset, and increased tumor growth, breast cancer associated with genetic mutation may also be invisible on screening mammography. Supplemental screening with (MRI) significantly improves the detection rate of breast cancer in high-risk populations, compared to mammography alone. Ultrasound may be used instead in patients with a contraindication of MRI due to anxiety or severe claustrophobia, or metallic implants, or patients allergic to the contrast agents [61].

3.8 Artificial intelligence in breast screening

Computer-aided detection software for mammography was intimated in 1990s and since that improvement had been made to improve outcomes. The use of artificial intelligence in screening mammogram has been shown to provide an absolute reduction of 1.2–5.7% in false positives and 2.7–9.4% in false negatives [62]. Artificial intelligence use in screening has the potential advantages of reducing the interval cancer rate without any additional modality, the reduction in interval cancer risk is an important indicator for screening program efficacy [63]. The use of AI in screening requires acceptance to participate and trust in their results, many people as shown by Ongena et al. [64] do not supply the use of AI alone in screening.

4. Conclusions

As breast cancer is among the most common cancer in women, prevention represents an important step to decrease morbidity and mortality. Prevention can be applied on three levels primary, secondary, and tertiary. Screening mammogram has the main advantage of early detection leading to better management and decreased mortality.

Acknowledgements

Authors want to thank their family and friends, particularly Tareq Mutar, Seemaa Albahrani, Zahraa Mutar, Reem Alsaad, Majid Hameed, Akhlass Al-naiemi, Saleh Goyani, Siham Jalal, Hamed Obaid, Fatima Khadem, Batool Ali Ghalib.

Conflict of interest

The authors declare no conflict of interest.

Notes/thanks/other declarations

Place any other declarations, such as "Notes", "Thanks", etc. in before the References section. Assign the appropriate heading. Do NOT put your short biography in this section. It will be removed.

Author details

Mohammed Tareq Mutar[1*], Mustafa Majid Hameed[1], Mohammed Saleh Goyani[1], Aqeel Shakir Mahmood[1] and Abo-Alhasan Hammed Obaid[2]

1 Department of Surgery, College of Medicine, University of Baghdad, Iraq

2 Department of Surgery, College of Medicine, Almustansrya University, Iraq

*Address all correspondence to: muhammed.tariq64@gmail.com

References

[1] Howlader N, Noone AM, Krapcho M, et al. SEER Cancer Statistics Review, 1975–2017, National Cancer Institute. Bethesda, MD. Available at https://seer.cancer.gov/csr/1975_2017.

[2] Breast cancer prevention and control: Early Detection. Available at: https://www.who.int/cancer/detection/breastcancer/en/

[3] Edward R. Sauter. Breast Cancer Prevention: Current Approaches and Future Directions.Eur J Breast Health. 2018 Apr; 14(2): 64–71. doi: 10.5152/ejbh.2018.3978

[4] National health service (NHS), available at: https://www.nhs.uk/conditions/breast-cancer/causes/.

[5] Mutar MT, Goyani MS, Had AM, Mahmood AS. Pattern of Presentation of Patients With Breast Cancer in Iraq in 2018: A Cross-Sectional Study. J Glob Oncol. 2019 Nov;5:1-6. doi: 10.1200/JGO.19.00041. PMID: 31721627; PMCID: PMC6882514.

[6] Bailey and Love's Short Practice of Surgery; 27th edition. N. S. Williams, C. J. K. Bulstrode and P. R. O' Connell. Boca Raton, FL: CRC Press, 2018.

[7] Center for disease control,breast cancer risk factors, available at https://www.cdc.gov/cancer/breast/basic_info/risk_factors.htm

[8] Kara Britt, Menarche, menopause, and breast cancer risk The Lancet Oncology, 2012:13(11): 1071-1072 avaipable at :https://www.thelancet.com/journals/lanonc/article/PIIS1470-2045(12)70456-4/fulltext.

[9] Collaborative Group on Hormonal Factors in Breast Cancer.Menarche, menopause, and breast cancer risk: individual participant meta-analysis, including 118 964 women with breast cancer from 117 epidemiological studies. Lancet Oncol. 2012 Nov; 13(11): 1141–1151. doi: 10.1016/S1470-2045(12) 70425-4

[10] Lambe M, Hsieh CC, Chan HW, Ekbom A, Trichopoulos D, Adami HO. Parity, age at first and last birth, and risk of breast cancer: a population-based study in Sweden. Breast Cancer Res Treat. 1996;38(3):305-311. doi: 10.1007/BF01806150. PMID: 8739084.

[11] Fortner, R.T., Sisti, J., Chai, B. et al. Parity, breastfeeding, and breast cancer risk by hormone receptor status and molecular phenotype: results from the Nurses' Health Studies. Breast Cancer Res 21, 40 (2019). https://doi.org/10.1186/s13058-019-1119-y

[12] Bhupathiraju SN, Grodstein F, Stampfer MJ, et al. Exogenous hormone use: Oral contraceptives, postmenopausal hormone therapy, and health outcomes in the Nurses' Health Study. American Journal of Public Health 2016; 106(9):1631-1637

[13] Vinogradova Y, Coupland C, Hippisley-Cox J. Use of hormone replacement therapy and risk of breast cancer: nested case-control studies using the QResearch and CPRD databases. BMJ. 2020 Oct 28;371:m3873. doi: 10.1136/bmj.m3873.

[14] Kyuwan Lee, Laura Kruper, Christina M. Dieli-Conwright, and Joanne E. Mortimer. The Impact of Obesity on Breast Cancer Diagnosis and Treatment. 2019. Curr Oncol Rep. 2019; 21(5): 41. doi: 10.1007/s11912-019-0787-1

[15] Gao Y, Huang YB, Liu XO, Chen C, Dai HJ, Song FJ, et al. Tea consumption, alcohol drinking and physical activity associations with breast cancer risk among Chinese females: a systematic review and meta-analysis. Asian Pacific journal of cancer prevention : APJCP. 2013;14(12):7543–50. Epub 2014/01/28

[16] Rosenberg L, Boggs DA, Bethea TN, Wise LA, Adams-Campbell LL, Palmer JR. A prospective study of smoking and breast cancer risk among African-American women. Cancer causes & control : CCC. 2013;24(12):2207–2215. Epub 2013/10/03.

[17] Berube S, Lemieux J, Moore L, Maunsell E, Brisson J. Smoking at time of diagnosis and breast cancer-specific survival: new findings and systematic review with meta-analysis. Breast cancer research : BCR. 2014;16(2):R42. Epub 2014/04/22.

[18] Park SY, Kolonel LN, Lim U, White KK, Henderson BE, Wilkens LR. Alcohol consumption and breast cancer risk among women from five ethnic groups with light to moderate intakes: the Multiethnic Cohort Study. International journal of cancer Journal international du cancer. 2014;134(6): 1504–1510. Epub 2013/09/17.

[19] Seyed Hesam Bani Hashemi, Samieh Karimi, and Hamidreza Mahboobi. Lifestyle changes for prevention of breast cancer Electron Physician. 2014 Jul-Sep; 6 (3): 894–905. doi: 10.14661/2014.894-905

[20] Butow PN, Hiller JE, Price MA, Thackway SV, Kricker A, Tennant CC. Epidemiological evidence for a relationship between life events, coping style, and personality factors in the development of breast cancer. Journal of psychosomatic research. 2000;49(3): 169–181. Epub 2000/12/09

[21] Zhao YS, Zhu S, Li XW, Wang F, Hu FL, Li DD, et al. Association between NSAIDs use and breast cancer risk: a systematic review and meta-analysis. Breast cancer research and treatment. 2009;117(1):141–50. Epub 2008/11/04.

[22] Ahern TP, Tamimi RM, Rosner BA, Hankinson SE. Digoxin use and risk of invasive breast cancer: evidence from the Nurses' Health Study and meta-analysis. Breast cancer research and treatment. 2014;144(2):427–435. Epub 2014/02/28.

[23] Mathur P, Sathishkumar K, Chaturvedi M, Das P , Sudarshan KL, Santhappan S Cancer Statistics, 2020: Report From National Cancer Registry Programme, India. J Glob Oncol. 2020;6: 1063-1075. DOI: 10.1200/GO.20.00122

[24] Shampo, Marc A.; Kyle, Robert A. (1995). Karl Theodore Dussik—Pioneer in Ultrasound. , 70(12), 1136–. doi: 10.4065/70.12.1136.

[25] DUSSIK KT, DUSSIK F, WYT L. Auf dem Wege zur Hyperphonographie des Gehirnes [Towards hyperphonography of the brain]. Wien Med Wochenschr. 1947 Oct 4;97 (38-39):425-9. German. PMID: 18911482.

[26] Picard JD. Histoire de la mammographie [History of mammography]. Bull Acad Natl Med. 1998;182(8):1613-20. French. PMID: 10188307.

[27] Kalaf JM. Mammography: a history of success and scientific enthusiasm. *Radiol Bras*. 2014;47(4):VII-VIII. doi: 10.1590/0100-3984.2014.47.4e2

[28] Trevena L. Cancer screening Pros, cons, choice, and the patient. Australian Family Physician. 2009;30(4):189. Available at: https://pubmed.ncbi.nlm.nih.gov/19350066/

[29] Biesheuvel C, Weige S, Heindel W. Mammography Screening: Evidence, History and Current Practice in Germany and Other European Countries. Breast Care. 2011;6(2): 104-109.

[30] https://www.ncbi.nlm.nih.gov/pmc/articles/PMC5009951/#__ffn_sectitle

[31] Geisel J, Raghu M, Hooley R. The Role of Ultrasound in Breast Cancer

Screening: The Case for and Against Ultrasound. Semin Ultrasound CT MR. 2018 Feb;39(1):25-34. doi: 10.1053/j.sult.2017.09.006. Epub 2017 Sep 22. PMID: 29317037.

[32] Raichand, S., Dunn, A.G., Ong, MS. et al. Conclusions in systematic reviews of mammography for breast cancer screening and associations with review design and author characteristics. Syst Rev 6, 105 (2017). https://doi.org/10.1186/s13643-017-0495-6

[33] The Independent UK Panel on Breast Cancer Screening. The benefits and harms of breast cancer screening: an independent review. Lancet. 2012;380 (9855):1778–1786. doi:10.1016/S0140-6736(12)61611-0.

[34] Biesheuvel C, Weigel S, Heindel W. Mammography Screening: Evidence, History and Current Practice in Germany and Other European Countries. Breast Care (Basel). 2011;6(2):104-109. doi:10.1159/000327493.

[35] Román, M., Hofvind, S., von Euler-Chelpin, M. *et al.* Long-term risk of screen-detected and interval breast cancer after false-positive results at mammography screening: joint analysis of three national cohorts. *Br J Cancer* 2019; 120, 269–275 . https://doi.org/10.1038/s41416-018-0358-5

[36] Henderson LM, Hubbard RA, Sprague BL, Zhu W, Kerlikowske K. Increased Risk of Developing Breast Cancer after a False-Positive Screening Mammogram. *Cancer Epidemiol Biomarkers Prev*. 2015;24(12): 1882-1889. doi:10.1158/1055-9965.EPI-15-0623

[37] McCann, J., Stockton, D. & Godward, S. Impact of false-positive mammography on subsequent screening attendance and risk of cancer. *Breast Cancer Res* 4, R11 (2002). https://doi.org/10.1186/bcr455.

[38] Seigneurin, A., Exbrayat, C., Labarère, J. *et al.* Association of diagnostic work-up with subsequent attendance in a breast cancer screening program for false-positive cases. *Breast Cancer Res Treat. 2011;* 127, 221–228 #https://doi.org/10.1007/s10549-010-1118-2

[39] Lynge E, Olsen AH, Fracheboud J, Patnick J. Reporting of performance indicators of mammography screening in Europe. Eur J Cancer Prev. 2003 Jun; 12(3):213-222. doi: 10.1097/00008469-200306000-00008. PMID: 12771560.

[40] World Health Organization. WHO Position Paper on Mammography Screening, 2014. Available at: www.paho.org/cancer

[41] Alexandraki I, Mooradian AD. Barriers related to mammography use for breast cancer screening among minority women. J Natl Med Assoc. 2010 Mar;102(3):206-218. doi: 10.1016/s0027-9684(15)30527-7. PMID: 20355350.

[42] Orji CC, Kanu C, Adelodun AI, Brown CM. Factors that Influence Mammography Use for Breast Cancer Screening among African American Women. J Natl Med Assoc. 2020 Dec; 112(6):578-592. doi: 10.1016/j.jnma.2020.05.004. Epub 2020 Jul 5. PMID: 32641257.

[43] Nelson H, Fu R, Cantor A, Pappas M, Daeges M, Humphrey L. Effectiveness of Breast Cancer Screening: Systematic Review and Meta-analysis to Update the 2009 U.S. Preventive Services Task Force Recommendation. Annals of Internal Medicine. 2016;164(4):244. doi: 10.7326/M15-0969

[44] Fletcher S. Breast Cancer Screening: A 35-Year Perspective. Epidemiologic Reviews. 2011;33(1):165-175. DOI: 10.1093/epirev/mxr003

[45] Houssami N. Overdiagnosis of breast cancer in population screening: does it make breast screening worthless?. Cancer Biol Med. 2017;14(1):1-8. doi: 10.20892/j.issn.2095-3941.2016.0050

[46] Marmot MG, Altman DG, Cameron DA, Dewar JA, Thompson SG, Wilcox M. The benefits and harms of breast cancer screening: an independent review. *Br J Cancer*. 2013;108(11): 2205-2240. doi:10.1038/bjc.2013.177

[47] Puliti D, Miccinesi G, Paci E. Overdiagnosis in breast cancer: design and methods of estimation in observational studies. Prev Med. 2011 Sep;53(3):131-133. doi: 10.1016/j.ypmed.2011.05.012. Epub 2011 Jun 2. PMID: 21658405.

[48] Puliti D, Duffy SW, Miccinesi G, de Koning H, Lynge E, Zappa M, Paci E; EUROSCREEN Working Group. Overdiagnosis in mammographic screening for breast cancer in Europe: a literature review. J Med Screen. 2012;19 Suppl 1:42-56. doi: 10.1258/jms.2012.012082. PMID: 22972810.

[49] Yamamuro M, Asai Y, Hashimoto N, Yasuda N, Ozaki Y, Ishii K, Lee Y. The effect of breast density on the missed lesion rate in screening digital mammography determined using an adjustable-density breast phantom tailored to Japanese women. PLoS One 2021. DOI: 10.1371/journal.pone.0245060

[50] Ekpo EU, Alakhras M, Brennan P. Errors in Mammography Cannot be Solved Through Technology Alone. Asian Pac J Cancer Prev. 2018;19(2): 291-301. Published 2018 Feb 26. doi: 10.22034/APJCP.2018.19.2.291

[51] Vilaprinyo E, Forné C, Carles M, et al. Cost-effectiveness and harm-benefit analyses of risk-based screening strategies for breast cancer. PLoS One. 2014;9(2):e86858. Published 2014 Feb 3. doi:10.1371/journal.pone.0086858

[52] Siu A. Screening for Breast Cancer: U.S. Preventive Services Task Force Recommendation Statement. Annals of Internal Medicine. 2016;164(4):279.

[53] Breast Cancer Screening (PDQ®)–Health Professional Version [Internet]. National Cancer Institute. 2021 [cited 10 February 2021]. Available from: https://www.cancer.gov/types/breast/hp/breast-screening-pdq#_15_toc

[54] Menezes GL, Knuttel FM, Stehouwer BL, Pijnappel RM, van den Bosch MA. Magnetic resonance imaging in breast cancer: A literature review and future perspectives. World J Clin Oncol. 2014;5(2):61-70. doi:10.5306/wjco.v5.i2.61

[55] Mann RM, Kuhl CK, Kinkel K, Boetes C. Breast MRI: guidelines from the European Society of Breast Imaging. Eur Radiol. 2008;18(7):1307-1318. doi: 10.1007/s00330-008-0863-7

[56] Mandelblatt JS, Stout NK, Schechter CB, van den Broek JJ, Miglioretti DL, Krapcho M, Trentham-Dietz A, Munoz D, Lee SJ, Berry DA, van Ravesteyn NT, Alagoz O, Kerlikowske K, Tosteson AN, Near AM, Hoeffken A, Chang Y, Heijnsdijk EA, Chisholm G, Huang X, Huang H, Ergun MA, Gangnon R, Sprague BL, Plevritis S, Feuer E, de Koning HJ, Cronin KA. Collaborative Modeling of the Benefits and Harms Associated With Different U.S. Breast Cancer Screening Strategies. Ann Intern Med. 2016 Feb 16;164(4):215-225. doi: 10.7326/M15-1536.

[57] Nothacker M, Duda V, Hahn M, et al. Early detection of breast cancer: benefits and risks of supplemental breast ultrasound in asymptomatic women with mammographically dense breast tissue. A systematic review. BMC Cancer. 2009;9:335. Published 2009 Sep 20. doi:10.1186/1471-2407-9-33

[58] Yuan, WH., Hsu, HC., Chen, YY. et al. Supplemental breast

cancer-screening ultrasonography in women with dense breasts: a systematic review and meta-analysis. Br J Cancer 123, 673–688 (2020). https://doi.org/10.1038/s41416-020-0928-1

[59] Wang J, Zheng S, Ding L, et al. Is Ultrasound an Accurate Alternative for Mammography in Breast Cancer Screening in an Asian Population? A Meta-Analysis. Diagnostics (Basel). 2020;10(11):985. Published 2020 Nov 21. doi:10.3390/diagnostics1011098

[60] Yuan, WH., Hsu, HC., Chen, YY. *et al.* Supplemental breast cancer-screening ultrasonography in women with dense breasts: a systematic review and meta-analysis. Br J Cancer **123,** 673–688 (2020). https://doi.org/10.1038/s41416-020-0928-1

[61] Health Quality Ontario. Ultrasound as an Adjunct to Mammography for Breast Cancer Screening: A Health Technology Assessment. Ont Health Technol Assess Ser. 2016;16(15):1-71. Published 2016 Jul 1

[62] McKinney, S.M., Sieniek, M., Godbole, V. et al. International evaluation of an AI system for breast cancer screening. Nature 577, 89–94 (2020). https://doi.org/10.1038/s41586-019-1799-6

[63] Lång, K., Hofvind, S., Rodríguez-Ruiz, A. et al. Can artificial intelligence reduce the interval cancer rate in mammography screening?. Eur Radiol (2021). https://doi.org/10.1007/s00330-021-07686-3

[64] Ongena Y., Yakar D, Haan M., & KweeT. Artificial intelligence in screening mammography: A population survey of women's preferences. *Journal of* the American College of Radiology. *2021, 18*(1), 79-86. doi:10.1016/j.jacr.2020.09.042

Section 6

Breast Cancer Diagnostic Imaging

Chapter 9

Microwave Imaging for Breast Cancer Detection

Yoshihiko Kuwahara

Abstract

Microwave imaging (MI) is characterized by no exposure, stronger contrast between soft tissues than X-rays and ultrasound, and a smaller device scale. This chapter describes the electrical properties of the breast tissue that underlie MI, and then outlines the MI hardware configuration and three imaging algorithms: confocal imaging, scattering tomography, and near-field holography. After that, we will introduce the actual equipment and experimental results using the three imaging algorithms. Finally, we will summarize the challenges of realizing a medical imaging device using MI.

Keywords: microwave imaging, complex permittivity, confocal imaging, scattering tomography, near-field holography

1. Introduction

Breast cancer begins in the late 20s, but the mammary glands are well developed in the 20s and 30s, making initial diagnosis by X-ray mammography, which is a general examination, difficult. There is an ultrasonic diagnostic device (US) as an alternative method, but the reliability of the diagnosis depends on the skill of the inspector, the reproducibility of the data is poor, and continuous tomographic images cannot be obtained [1]. On the other hand, magnetic resonant image (MRI) and positron emission tomography (PET) are not candidates for examination equipment because of their large scale, long examination time, and high cost. Microwave imaging (MI) has a stronger contrast between soft tissues than X-rays and ultrasound. MI is not exposed to radiation, and has the characteristics of being small in scale and inexpensive. However, there are problems to be solved and it has not yet been put into practical use.

There are two types of MI, scattering tomography (ST), which solves the inverse scattering problem and reconstructs the relative permittivity and conductivity distribution in the breast, and confocal imaging (CI), which reconstructs the scattered power distribution [2]. In principle, the former can reconstruct the shape of intramammary tissue and is suitable as a diagnostic device. However, the inverse scattering problem is a non-linear ill-posed problem with more unknowns (relative permittivity / conductivity distribution in the breast) than the number of equations (measurement data), and is susceptible to modeling, manufacturing, and measurement errors. The latter has been clinically imaged by several research groups, including the author, and strong scattering has been confirmed around the cancer [3–6]. However, even in breasts without lesions, meaningless scattered images (artifacts) appear due to multiple reflections in the breast, so how to identify the presence or absence of cancer is an issue.

In recent years, as a third method, research on near field holographic imaging (NFHI), which can reconstruct the shape of intramammary tissue, is also in progress [7, 8]. Since the principle of image reconstruction of NFHI is based on the principle of Fourier transform, the time required for image reconstruction is short. However, there are still problems that a huge amount of observation data is required to increase the resolution and that images cannot be reconstructed correctly with high-contrast objects.

In this chapter, we first explain the electrical properties of breast tissue, which is the basis of MI, based on large-scale measurement data [9]. Next, the basic device configuration of MI, three imaging algorithms, and the features of CI, ST, and NFHI are described. Next, we will introduce the equipment that implements these algorithms and the experimental results. Finally, the issues of MI and future prospects will be described.

2. Electrical properties of breast tissue

Living tissue has different electrical properties depending on the tissue, and when electromagnetic waves are incident, reflection occurs at the boundary. The basis of MI is to detect reflections that occur at tissue boundaries. This section describes the electrical properties of breast tissue.

2.1 Complex permittivity and Debye model

Living tissue is a lossy dielectric, and when an electromagnetic wave is incident, its wavelength is shortened and propagates while being attenuated. When an electromagnetic wave having a main polarization in the x-axis direction propagates in the z-axis direction through a dielectric having a loss, the electric field at an arbitrary distance z is expressed by the following equation.

$$E_x = E_0 e^{-\alpha z} e^{-j\beta z} \tag{1}$$

Here, E_0 is the electric field at z = 0, α and β are the attenuation constant and the phase constant, and are expressed as follows using the relative permittivity ε_r, conductivity σ, and angular frequency ω = 2πf of the propagation medium.

$$\alpha = \frac{\omega}{c_0}\sqrt{\frac{\varepsilon_r}{2}}\left[\sqrt{1+\left(\frac{\sigma}{\omega\varepsilon_0\varepsilon_r}\right)^2} - 1\right]^{1/2} \tag{2}$$

$$\beta = \frac{\omega}{c_0}\sqrt{\frac{\varepsilon_r}{2}}\left[\sqrt{1+\left(\frac{\sigma}{\omega\varepsilon_0\varepsilon_r}\right)^2} + 1\right]^{1/2} \tag{3}$$

Here, c_0 is the speed of light propagating in the vacuum, and ε_0 is the permittivity of the vacuum.

The dielectric material with loss is represented by the complex permittivity.

$$\varepsilon(\omega) = \varepsilon_r\varepsilon_0 + \frac{\sigma}{j\omega} \tag{4}$$

It can be seen that the imaginary part of the complex permittivity changes with frequency. By the way, it is known that the real part of the complex permittivity of a living body changes depending on the frequency. The property of such a material is called dispersibility. The complex relative permittivity of dispersible materials can be modeled by the following equation [10].

$$\frac{\varepsilon(\omega)}{\varepsilon_0} = \varepsilon_\infty + \frac{\sigma_s}{j\omega\varepsilon_0} + \frac{\Delta\varepsilon}{1 + j\omega\tau} \quad (5)$$

The curve of the complex relative permittivity represented by Eq. (5) is called the Debye model. **Figure 1** shows the result of measuring the complex relative permittivity of the mammary gland tissue by the probe method [11] (solid line) and the approximate curve (dotted line) modeled by Eq. (5). Here, ε_∞, $\Delta\varepsilon$, σ_s, and τ are estimated by the simplex method [12] so that the squared norm of the difference between the measured value and the frequency characteristic of the complex permittivity expressed in Eq. (5) is minimized. When the respective values are −1.22, 59.1, 0.92, 10.4 ps, the frequency characteristics of the measurement and the Debye model are almost the same. Since wideband electromagnetic waves are often used in confocal imaging, it is desirable to model objects using ε_∞, $\Delta\varepsilon$, σ_s, and τ when performing propagation analysis.

2.2 Complex permittivity measuring device

The electrical constants of breast tissue can be measured using a dielectric probe [9, 11]. Ref. [11] shows that a cylindrical region with a depth of 1.5 mm and a radius of 3.75 mm is required to achieve a measurement error of 10% using a 2.2 mm diameter dielectric probe. In our study, we measure the complex permittivity of breast tissue

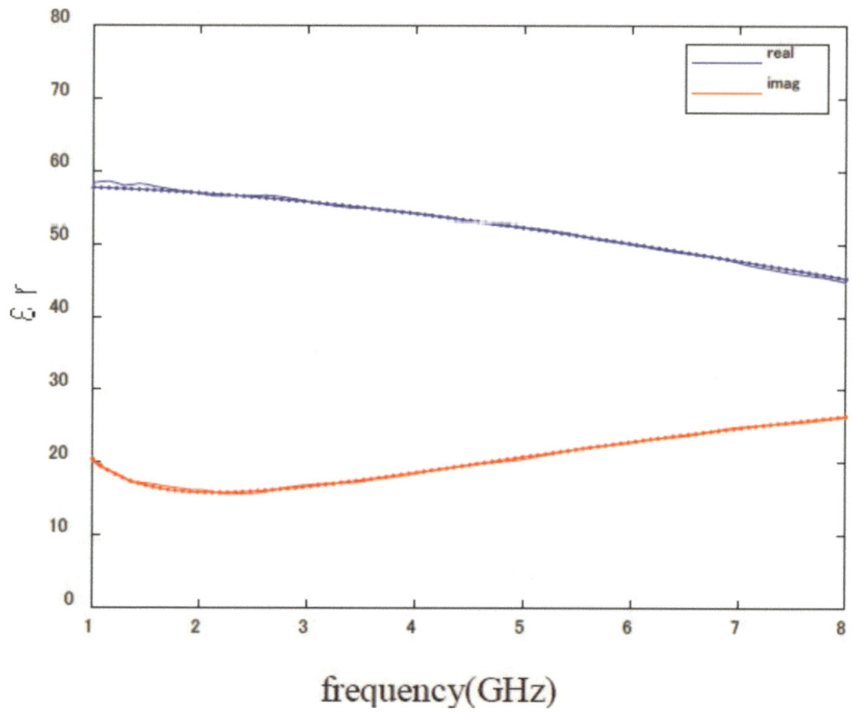

Figure 1.
Complex dielectric constant of glandular tissue and approximation by Debye model.

using a 2.2 mm diameter dielectric probe in the dielectric measurement kit Keysight 85070E and a vector network analyzer, E5071C. The measurement range is 1–8 GHz.

In recent year, since breast cancer is often detected at an early stage, the size of the tumors removed by surgery has become smaller. To investigate the minimum required volume of a specimen, the dielectric constant was measured by placing ketchup in containers of various volumes. Ketchup is readily available and has about the same electrical constant as cancer. The container, apart from the petri dish, was created using a 3D printer. The material of the container is ABS resin. **Figure 2** illustrates the appearance of the container and measurement system.

In the preliminary measurement using ketchup, for a container measuring $0.5 \times 0.5 \times 0.5$ cm, an error of 3% occurred with respect to the measurement result of the petri dish. However, in a container measuring $1 \times 1 \times 0.5$ cm, the error reduces to 1% or lower. We selected the $1 \times 1 \times 0.5$ cm container for analysis. Samples removed by surgery were cut into fats, mammary glands, and cancerous tumor tissues. Each tissue was placed in a container and the probe was pressed downwards to measure the complex permittivity. **Figure 3** shows a photograph of the tissue put in a container.

2.3 Measurement

2.3.1 Population of measurements

During the breast cancer surgery performed at Aichi Medical University from May 2018 to July 2020, breast tissue specimens were collected from 140 patients who consented to the specimen collection [9]. **Table 1** shows the number of samples and the average age of the patients classified by case. Here, mammary gland tissues of the highest possible density were collected from every patient.

In recent years, there have been many stage 0 and stage 1 (tumors less than 2 cm) surgery, and it has not been possible to collect tumor tissues that can withstand measurement from all patients. X-ray mammography findings of mammary gland density revealed that nearly half of the patients had dense mammary glands. Due to the disappearance of mammary gland tissue at an older age, it was not possible to obtain mammary gland tissue that could be used for measurement from all patients.

Invasive ductal carcinoma accounts for 84%, of which more than half are scirrhous type. Fibroadenoma is more common in young women, with a minimum age of onset of 15 in this study. Five patients in their 30s with invasive ductal carcinoma account for 4% of all patients with invasive ductal carcinoma. All of the patients were at stage 2. Women in their 30s are not eligible for breast cancer screening in Japan. When cancer grows, it is said that necrosis and calcification occur in the center of the cancer. X-ray mammography detects this calcification. In the pathological findings, there were necrosis in 6 cases and calcification in 11 cases.

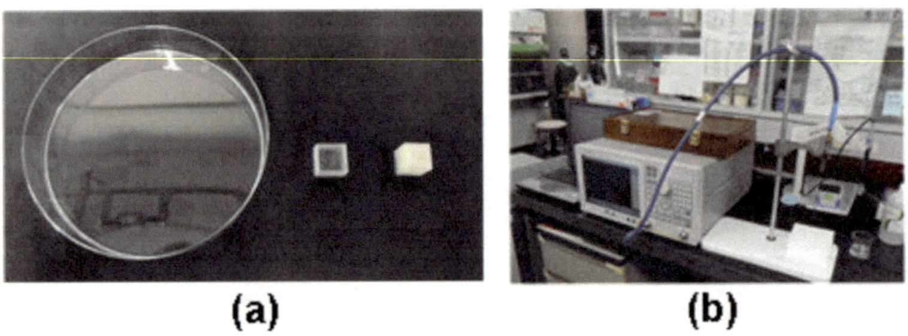

Figure 2
(a) Containers of various volumes, petri dish 1×1×0.5 cm, 0.5×0.5×0.5 cm container. (b) Measurement equipment for complex permittivity.

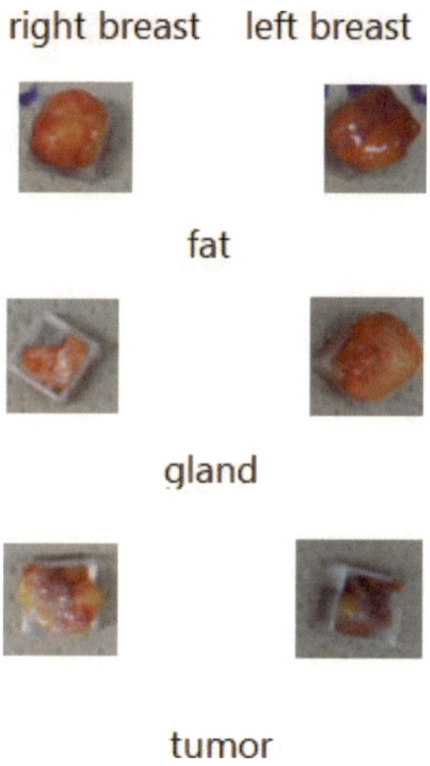

Figure 3.
Tissue samples.

Histological classification		Patient	Tumor	Gland	Fat	Age (years)
Invasive ductal carcinoma	Tuble forming	7	6	6	6	59.6
	Solid	38	35	23	36	63.3
	Scirrhous	64	52	46	58	61
	Others	9	8	6	9	59.9
Special	Invasive lobular carcinoma	4	4	4	4	63.6
	Mucinous carcinoma	6	6	4	5	66.8
	Others	5	0	5	5	49.4
Mixed connective tissue and epithelial tumors	Fibroadenoma	5	5	4	2	31.1
	Phyllodes tumor	2	2	0	1	54.2
Total		140	118	98	126	60.3

Table 1.
Number of samples taken out by surgery.

2.3.2 Measurement results

Figure 4 shows a typical example of the complex relative permittivity of the sample measured using the measurement system shown in **Figure 2**. The measurement result that we expect is that the relative permittivity of tumor tissue is considerably higher than that of mammary tissue, as shown in **Figure 4a**. However,

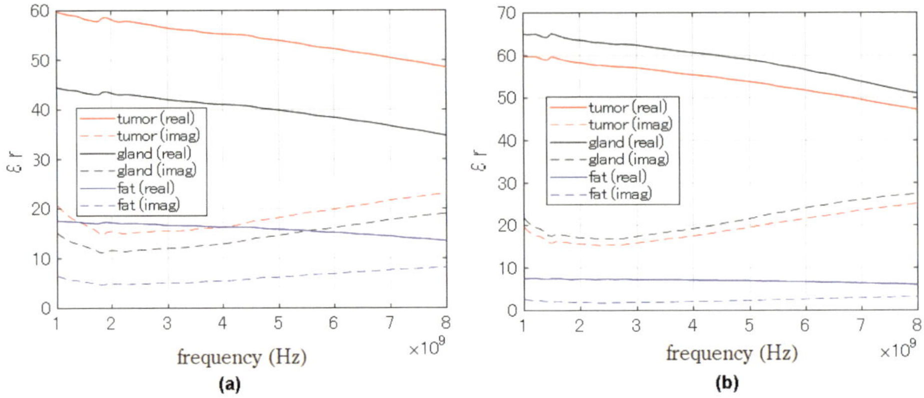

Figure 4.
(a) Measurement example of the complex permittivity, solid tubular carcinoma (Age 49, dense breast). (b) Measurement example of the complex permittivity, Scirrhous carcinoma (Age 49, dense breast).

as shown in **Figure 4b**, there were 8 cases in the scirrhous type and 1 case in the solid type in which the relative permittivity of the mammary gland tissue was higher than that of the tumor tissue. The reason for the opposite properties may be that, as noted in the Ref. [13], not all areas of the tumor sample are filled with tumor tissue.

Table 2 shows the average of relative permittivity ε_r and conductivity σ of tumor and mammary gland at 1.6 GHz by pathology. On average, the relative permittivity of cancer is 17.5% higher than that of mammary gland tissue, and the conductivity is 16.2% higher.

Fibroadenoma has the lowest contrast between the relative permittivity and conductivity of cancer and mammary gland. Fibroadenoma is common in women in their teens and 20s, has well-defined lump boundaries, and is often classified as a benign tumor. The disease is not a tumor, but is made up of an excessive amount of normal cells (anaplasia), so there is almost no difference in contrast with the mammary gland. Among the invasive cancers, tumors that are said to be a special type have a large contrast between the mammary gland and the cancer, and good

Histological classification		**Tumor**		**Mammary gland**	
		ε_r	σ [S/m]	ε_r	σ [S/m]
Invasive ductal carcinoma	Tuble forming	60.5	1.66	50.1	1.4
	Solid	58.6	1.59	49.8	1.39
	Scirrhous	58.9	1.65	52.4	1.47
	Others	59.6	1.63	41.6	1.15
Special	Invasive lobular carcinoma	58.4	1.63	43.0	1.19
	Mucinous carcinoma	65.3	1.93	45.9	1.3
	Others	—	—	53.4	1.5
Mixed connective tissue and epithelial tumors	Fibroadenoma	62.7	1.74	60.2	1.73
	Phyllodes tumor	61.7	1.61	—	—
Total		59.5	1.65	50.6	1.45

Table 2.
Averaged permittivity and conductivity.

detection by microwave imaging can be expected. The scirrhous type is the most common type of invasive ductal carcinoma, but the contrast between the relative permittivity and the conductivity of the cancer and mammary gland tissue is 12%, which is relatively small. Therefore, MI requires the ability to identify objects with a contrast of about 10%.

Table 3 shows the average Debye parameters for tumor and mammary gland by pathology. The Debye parameter is a parameter considering dispersibility (frequency characteristic). Relaxation time τ does not differ significantly between

Histological classification		Tumor				Mammary gland			
		ε_∞	$\Delta\varepsilon$	σ_s	τ [ps]	ε_∞	$\Delta\varepsilon$	σ_s	τ [ps]
Invasive ductal carcinoma	Tuble forming	5.63	55.9	0.94	11.6	1.25	49.7	0.77	11.5
	Solid	3.91	55.5	0.90	11.2	1.56	49.0	0.81	10.7
	Scirrhous	4.59	55.2	0.95	11.4	0.59	52.5	0.85	10.5
	Others	3.39	57.0	0.97	10.3	1.81	40.4	0.64	10.3
Special	Invasive lobular carcinoma	5.28	53.9	0.97	11.0	−0.45	44.0	0.70	9.9
	Mucinous carcinoma	−1.76	66.2	0.98	10.3	−4.71	47.0	0.68	9.8
	Others	—	—	—	—	−1.88	55.9	0.90	9.7
Mixed connective tissue and epithelial tumors	Fibroadenoma	1.46	61.8	0.96	11.1	1.99	56.3	0.96	11.8
	Phyllodes tumor	−0.45	63.0	0.89	10.3	—	—	—	—
total		3.87	56.3	0.94	11.2	0.64	50.5	0.81	10.6

Table 3.
Debye parameters.

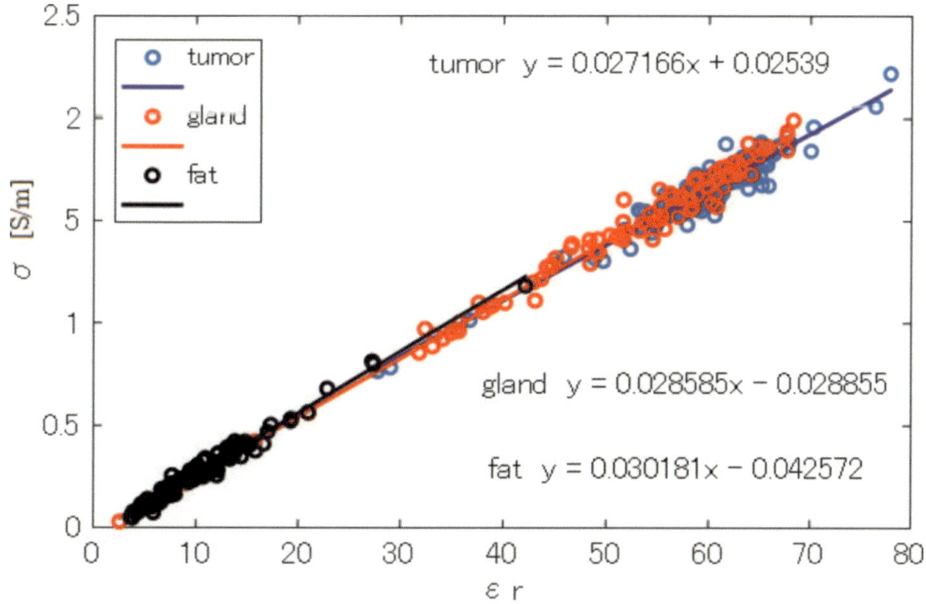

Figure 5.
Linear relationship between relative permittivity and conductivity.

tumor tissue and mammary gland tissue. This is an important prior knowledge of ST for solving the inverse scattering problem [14]. Among the Debye parameters, ε_∞ has an extremely high contrast between cancer and mammary gland. By utilizing this feature, it will become easy to distinguish between the mammary gland and cancer in microwave imaging.

Figure 5 is a plot showing the relationship between relative permittivity ε_r and conductivity σ of breast tissue at 1.6 GHz, It shows that there is a strong correlation between ε_r and σ. This is also important priori information for ST to solve the inverse scattering problem [15].

3. Microwave imaging

This chapter gives an overview of the configuration of an imaging device using microwaves and the algorithm for reconstructing images. The details of the reconstruction algorithm are omitted due to space limitations. For details of the reconstruction algorithm, refer to the related literature.

3.1 Equipment configuration

Figure 6 shows the hardware configuration of the MI system. Multiple antennas are placed around the object. One antenna is selected to transmit electromagnetic waves, and all antennas including the antenna used for transmission receive and record scattered waves from the imaging target. The observation data group X_{nn} (n = 1, .., N) is collected by changing the antenna used for transmission one after another. The first digit of the subscript of X_{nn} indicates the transmission condition number, and the second digit indicates the reception condition number. When transmitting and receiving using 18 antennas, N = 18 and 18 × 18 = 324 observation data groups can be obtained. If multiple signals are received at the same time, the hardware configuration becomes complicated, so a changeover switch is used for time-division reception. A commercially available vector network analyzer (VNA) can be used as the transmitter / receiver. Since short pulses are equivalent to wideband frequency sweep signals, VNA can be used even with radars that use pulses.

3.2 Imaging algorithm

Table 4 shows typical image reconstruction methods.

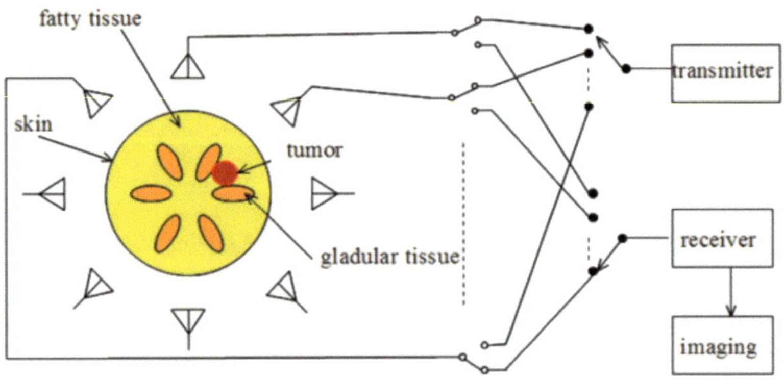

Figure 6.
Hardware of the MI system.

	CI	NFHI	MT
Reconstructed Image	Scattered power distribution	Reflection coefficients distribution	Complex permittivity distribution
Reproduction of tissue shape	Impossible	Possible	Possible
Processing time	Short	Very short	Long
Installation	Easy	difficult	difficult
Problems	• Identification of abnormal tissue	• Means for acquiring a large amount of observation data. • Investigating the effects of multiple reflections between objects	• Accuracy / resolution • Establishment of calibration method. • Design of high sensitivity antenna
Reference	[3–6, 16–19]	[7, 8, 20]	[14, 15, 21–25, 28]

Table 4.
Image reconstruction method.

The principle of image reconstruction of CI is the same as that of ultrasonic diagnostic equipment. That is, while shifting the focal point set in the imaging region, the magnitude of the scattered wave at the focal point is calculated and the magnitude distribution is visualized. Electromagnetic waves are more attenuated in the body than ultrasonic waves, and objects embedded in the high contrast tissue cannot accurately reproduce the tissue image due to the multiple reflections. Reconstructed images of breasts of breast cancer patients have been reported by the author and several other research institutes [3–6]. In all reports, large reflection images were observed around the cancer, but the shape and size of the cancer could not be accurately reconstructed. In addition, meaningless images are reconstructed even in cancer-free breasts. Doctors make a diagnosis from the reconstructed image, but it is not possible to make an accurate diagnosis because the tissue shape is not accurately reconstructed.

NFHI reconstructs the reflection coefficients' distribution in the imaging region, and the reconstructed image reflects the shape of the tissue [20]. Since the image reconstruction is based on the Fourier transform of the spatial region, the reconstruction time is extremely short and real-time display will be possible. The problem is that the resolution is governed by the sampling theorem, so a huge amount of observation data is required to obtain a high-definition reconstructed image, and it is difficult to realize a practical data acquisition system. For example, in order to obtain a spatial resolution of 2 mm, observation data for each 2 mm is required on the projection surface of the imaging region, and observation data at 2500 positions is required assuming an observation surface of 100 mm × 100 mm. Data can be acquired by mechanical scanning of the antenna, but the observation time will be significantly longer. If the antenna is an array to save time, 2500 transmitters and receivers are required, which increases the cost and limits the aperture length of one antenna to 2 mm or less. In this case, millimeter waves should be used, but the attenuation is extremely large in the body, which is not practical. Another issue is that the currently proposed 3D reconstruction algorithm does not take into account the effects of multiple reflections within the imaging region, making reconstructed images of object with a large size or a complicated structure difficult.

Research by the authors has shown that NFMI can, in principle, reconstruct the tissue image precisely [8]. In addition, Manitoba University has developed an experimental device that collects observation data by moving up and down while mechanically rotating two wideband horns, and showed that it can detect foreign matter in the phantom even in the air interface between the phantom and the antenna [7]. However, clinical imaging with NFMI has not yet been reported.

In ST, which solves the inverse scattering problem, the complex permittivity distribution in the imaging region is reconstructed and the structure shape can be reproduced. However, the processing time is long because it is necessary to repeat the full-wave electromagnetic field analysis. In our research, even workstations with the latest GPUs take hours for a single analysis and days for image reconstruction. The biggest problem is that the phenomenon of radio wave propagation in the imaging region cannot be faithfully reproduced on a computer. It is extremely difficult to completely match the results of experiments with computer simulations that model microwave equipment with current numerical analysis technology for electromagnetic waves. The key to the realization of this technology is how to calibrate the experimental results and match them with the computer simulation. In this method, the breast is treated as a set of small hexahedrons or tetrahedra (called voxels), and the complex permittivity of each voxel is estimated. To improve the resolution is to make the voxels smaller, and the number of complex permittivity to be estimated increases on the order of the third power. In the inverse scattering problem, the governing equations are Born approximated and solved by replacing them with linear simultaneous equations, but this is an ill-posed problem with many unknowns (complex dielectric constant of each voxel) with respect to the number of equations. In this case, the reconstructed image looks like a defocused photograph because the sudden change in contrast between voxels cannot be reproduced. In addition, a highly sensitive antenna that can capture small changes in the complex permittivity of small voxels is required.

A group at Dartmath University has prototyped an imaging device with a structure in which 18 monopoles are submerged together with the breast in a matching fluid, and is performing clinical imaging [21]. The monopole array is moved up and down to acquire several observation data. For the imaging algorithm, forward analysis by Discrete Dipole Assumption (DDA) and inverse analysis by iterative method are adopted. Reconstructed images of scattered mammary glands accurately capture the location and size of the cancer, but the results of imaging the dense breast are not shown, and it seems that they have not reached the stage of practical use.

4. Imaging device

This section introduces the MI device and imaging results developed by the author. Only the equipment using CI was performed up to clinical imaging, but the equipment of ST and NFHI is in the stage of basic experiment.

4.1 CI for clinical test

4.1.1 System configuration

A schematic diagram and photographs of the developed microwave mammography equipment are shown in **Figure** 7 [5]. The equipment comprised a sensor, an aspirator, an antenna switch, a network analyzer, a PC for control, and a workstation (WS) for data processing.

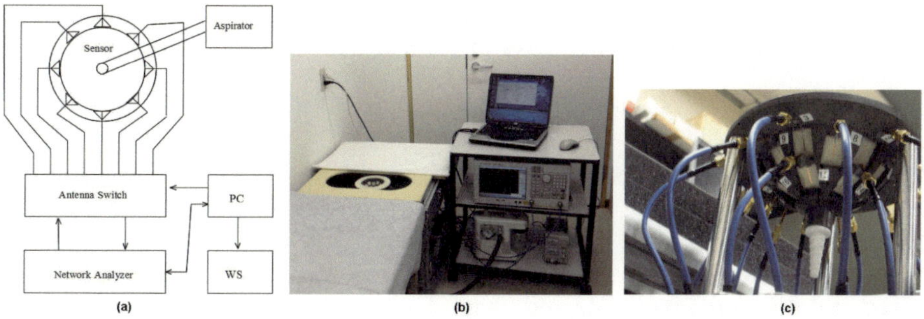

Figure 7.
(a) Schematic diagram of the microwave mammography. (b) Overview of the microwave mammography. (c) Overview of the sensor.

4.1.2 Sensor

Figure 8 shows the concept of the proposed sensor. It consists of several stacked patch antennas fed by the slot. The number of antennas depends on the breast size. The antennas are embedded in a cup made by Sumitomo Electric Industries, Ltd., the material of which has almost the same electromagnetic parameters as those of the adipose tissue (ε_r = 6.3, σ = 0.15, 6 GHz). The elements are designed so as to match impedance over the bandwidth of 4 to 9 GHz when the aperture touches the breast. When the pressure in the sensor is reduced by the aspirator, the breast is fixed to the inside of the sensor. Therefore, we need not know the breast shape for the image reconstruction process.

As shown in **Figure 8**, we prepared three different sensor types for various breast sizes: a 30-element sensor with a diameter of 13 cm and a depth of 5.4 cm

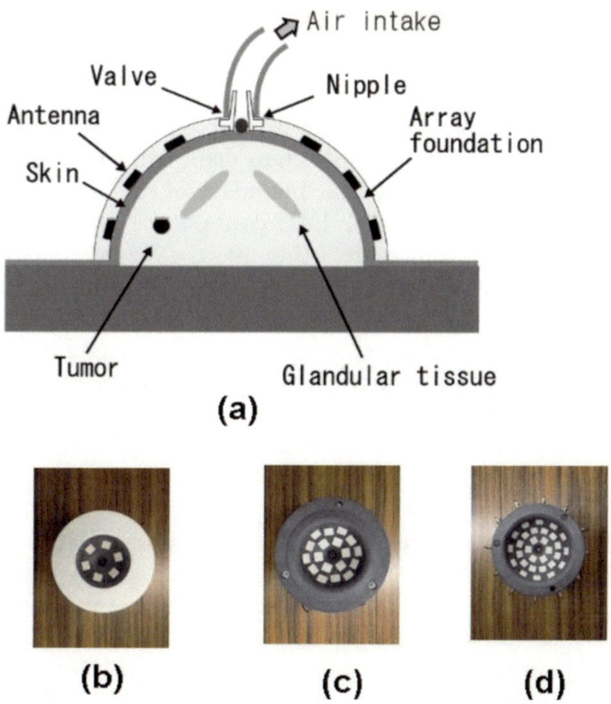

Figure 8.
(a) Sensor (longitudinal section). (b) Sensor (6-element). (c) Sensor (18 element). (d) Sensor (30-element).

(large), a 18-element sensor with a diameter of 10 cm and a depth of 4 cm (middle), and a 6-element sensor with a diameter of 8 cm and a depth of 2 cm (small).

4.1.3 Antenna switch and control

The antenna switch selects one or two antennas connected to the input/output port of the network analyzer (Agilent E5071C), and can correspond with the three sensor types. It consists of 42 single port double transfer (SPDT) switches and 6 single port 6 transfer (SP6T) switches. The total insertion loss is less than 5 dB at 6.5 GHz, and the peak amplitude and phase deviation are less than 0.2 dB and 10°, respectively. The antenna switch and network analyzer are automatically controlled by the PC.

4.1.4 Clinical inspection

The size of the microwave mammography equipment is 600 (width) × 600 (length) × 500 (height) mm. It is designed to align and connect lengthwise with a bed in the consulting room. Before inspection, a sensor with the proper size must be selected. Using a transparent cup that has the same size as the sensor on the breast and then by decompressing, one can confirm that the breast touches all elements by observation. Then, patient lies facedown on the bed and places her breast in the sensor and suction begins. S_{11} when the breast is placed in the sensor is compared with S_{11} when no breast is present. If S_{11} is not sufficiently reduced, an alarm is activated. In this case, the inspector aligns the position or inclination of the sensor. The inspection time is approximately 5, 30, and 200 s for 6, 18, and 30 sensor elements, respectively. An array rotation technique was used for artifact removal [16]. Additional inspection when the sensor is mechanically rotated by 20° was carried out.

4.1.5 Imaging results

We imaged the breasts of an elderly woman with fatty tissue. Referring MRI Image shown in **Figure 9a**, her right breast is infected with early breast cancer of 9 mm in diameter at lower inside near the chest wall, while no pathological changes can be seen in her left breast. In this case, boundary of the cancer is comparatively clear, and it isolates from the fibro-glandular tissue.

Figure 9b shows the imaging results using microwave mammography. In this case, the small-sized sensor was used. The reflection strength is normalized by the peak reflection field where it is generated around the cancer. Then, areas where the back-scattered energy is more than 80% of the peak scattered power are shown. In addition, estimated position and size from MRI image are shown as green circle. We can see a large scattering near the cancer.

4.1.6 Findings

Six breast cancer patients were clinically imaged and a strong scattering image was confirmed around the cancer. The location of the cancer can also be detected by confocal imaging. However, if the cancer is large, its shape cannot be reproduced. In the experiment, the scattering intensity distribution is standardized by the peak value of the response in the breast with the cancer with the largest scattering power. For this reason, the scattering intensity in cancer-free breasts is low. However, assuming cancer screening, it is predicted that scattered images will appear in such standardized processing because of the difference in mammary gland density

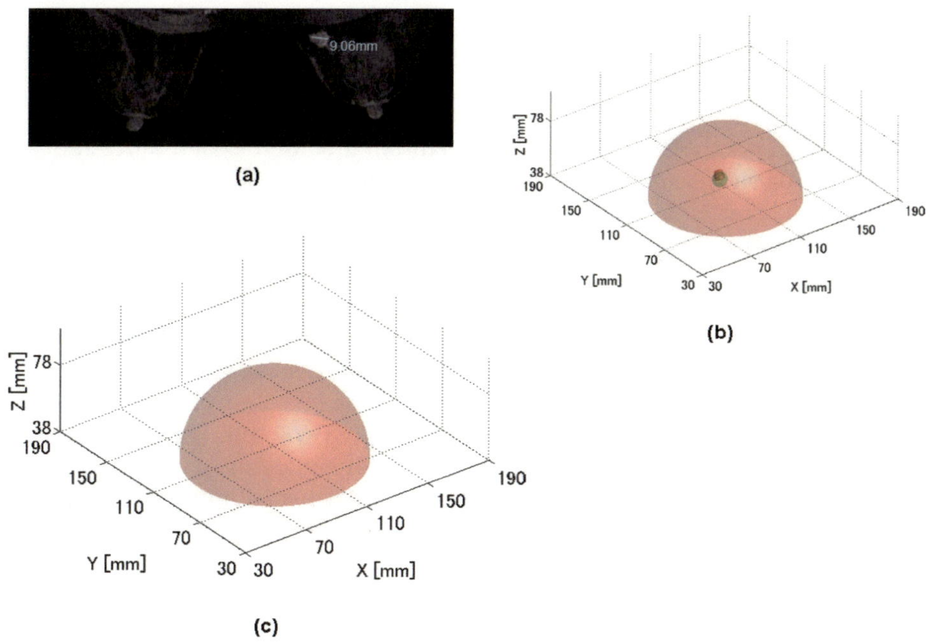

Figure 9.
(a) MRI image of the right breast with cancer and healthy left breast. (b) Imaging results by the microwave mammography (right breast). (c) Imaging results by the microwave mammography.

between the left and right breasts even without cancer. In addition to cancer, the breast has other diseases such as cysts and mastitis. The cyst is a bag of water, and it is predicted that a scattered image stronger than that of cancer will appear. Since it is necessary for medical devices to be able to accurately reproduce the shape of cancer and to distinguish between cancer and diseases such as cysts, the use of tumor markers in Ref. [17] is a realistic solution for confocal imaging.

4.2 ST

Since UWB radar could not reconstruct diagnostic images with the tissue structure, we are working on scattering tomography to solve the inverse scattering problem. A simple imaging sensor with a printed board dipole inserted in a dielectric block was prototyped and evaluated. However, if the rough position and size of the target were not used as preliminary knowledge, a reconstructed image with sufficient quality could be not obtained [5]. This was due to a modeling error issue as well as a lack of sensitivity. It was necessary to investigate a highly sensitive antenna with a structure with small modeling error.

In [24], the evaluation results of radar imaging using a circular array with a structure in which a folded quasi self- complementary antenna (FQSCA) composed of a printed board is pressed vertically against a cylindrical dielectric block containing the target are demonstrated. We evaluated the image reconstruction of an image sensor constructed by pressing FQSCA against a rectangular dielectric block by computer simulation compared with a printed dipole. As a result, it was found that the imaging sensor using FQSCA has higher image reconstruction capability than the printed dipole.

In this section, high sensitivity with FQSCA is first confirmed by computer simulation using the sensor structure in [22]. Next, FQSCA is applied to a sensor for clinical imaging, and it is confirmed that high-quality diagnosis image is reconstructed using a numerical phantom.

4.2.1 Printed dipole and FQCSA

4.2.1.1 Simulation model and method

Figure 10 shows the image sensor and phantom used in the computer simulation [25]. **Figure 10a** shows an imaging sensor in which two printed board dipoles arranged in an inverted L shape are inserted on the side of a dielectric block. **Figure 10b** shows an image sensor with a structure in which two FQSCAs arranged in an inverted L shape are pressed against the side surface of a dielectric block.

In this model, an imaging area of 40×40×40 mm is provided in the center of the dielectric block. The imaging area is modeled by cubic voxels with a side length of 10 mm or 5 mm. The number of voxels in the imaging area is 64 when the resolution is 10 mm and 512 when the resolution is 5 mm. In the image reconstruction using one frequency, the number of observation data is ${}_8C_2 = 28$, so it is an ill-posed problem with unknowns greater than the number of equations for any resolution. The distance between the imaging area and the antenna is 30 mm. The relative permittivity and conductivity of the dielectric block are 6.5 and 0.036 S/m.

Figure 11 shows photographs of the printed board dipole and FQSCA. The printed board dipole is mounted on a substrate with a thickness of 0.8 mm, relative dielectric constant of 3.8, and $\tan\delta = 0.003$. FQSCA is mounted on a substrate with a thickness of 1.6 mm, relative permittivity of 4, and $\tan\delta = 0.011$.

In order to evaluate image reconstruction quantitatively, the voxel number of the imaging area is determined as shown in **Figure 12**. As shown in **Figure 12**, the target of relative permittivity 39.6 and conductivity 1 S/m is set to 8 voxels in the center of the imaging area. The algorithm used for reconstruction is Distorted Born Iterative Method (DBIM) [14], the forward problem is solved with CST-Studio Suite [26], and the inverse problem is solved with MATLAB [27]. The frequency used for image reconstruction is 1.85 GHz for printed dipoles and 1.5 GHz for FQSCA. These are the frequencies of the lowest resonance point of each antenna.

4.2.1.2 Evaluation of image reconstruction

Figure 13 shows the results of reconstruction of the dielectric constant after 10 iterations assuming a resolution of 10 mm. Both the printed dipole and FQSCA show good reconstruction results. Note that the reconstruction result of the conductivity is omitted due to space limitations, but a reconstruction result equivalent to the relative dielectric constant has been confirmed.

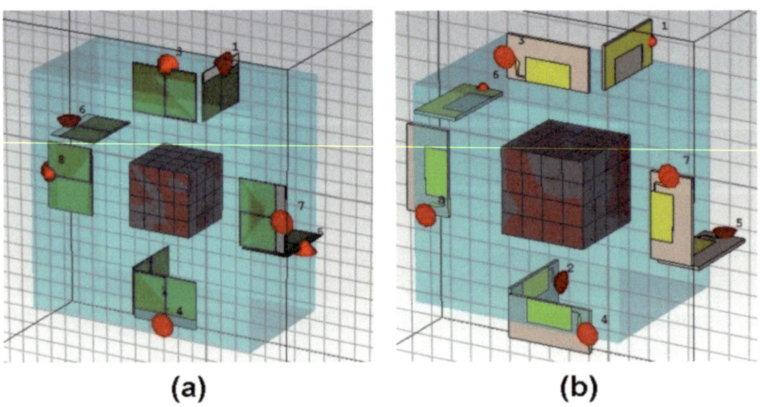

Figure 10.
(a) Simulated imaging sensor (printed dipole). (b) Simulated imaging sensor (FQSCA).

DOI: http://dx.doi.org/10.5772/intechopen.97313

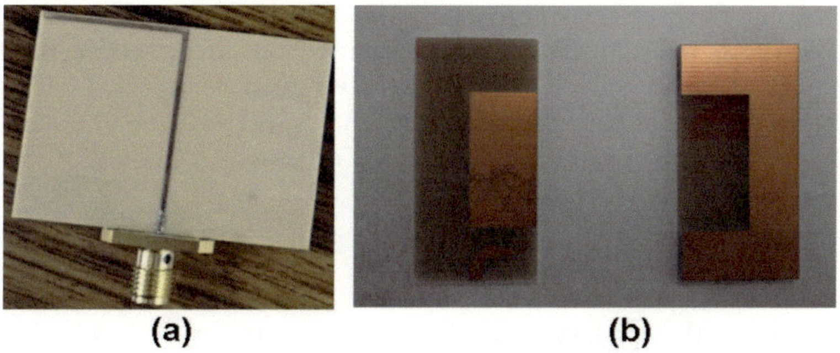

Figure 11.
(a) Printed dipole. (b) FQSCA.

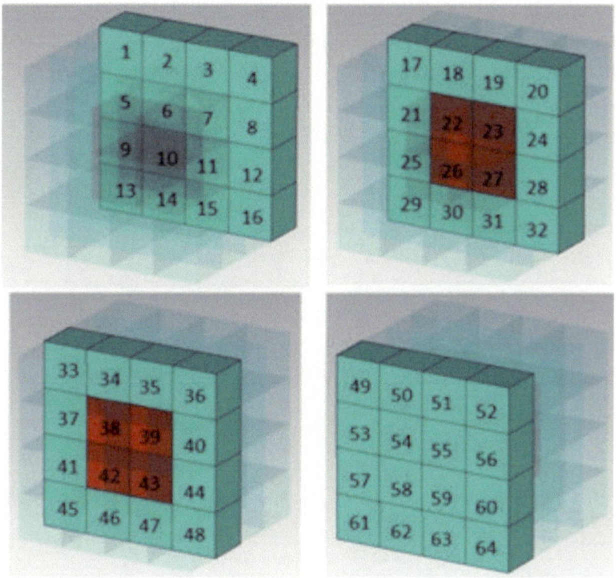

Figure 12.
Voxel number.

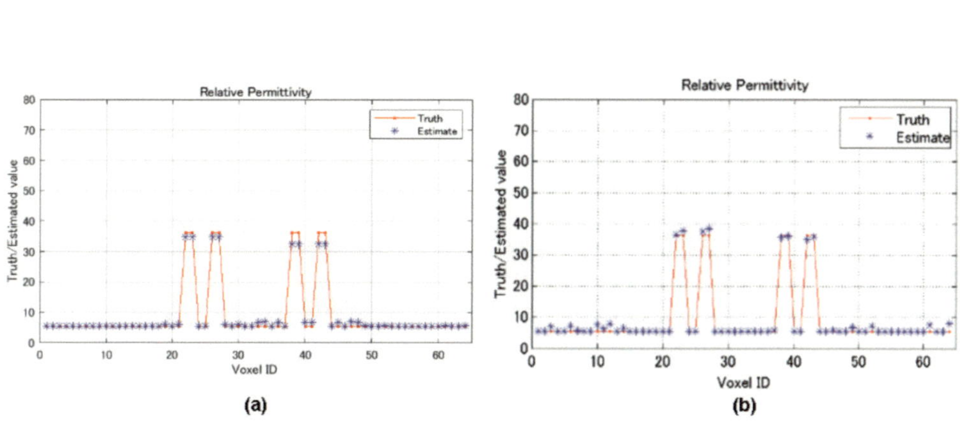

Figure 13.
(a) Reconstructed relative permittivity (resolution of 10 mm, printed dipole is used). (b) Reconstructed relative permittivity (resolution of 10 mm, FQSCA is used).

Figure 14 shows the results of reconstruction of the relative permittivity after 10 iterations, assuming a resolution of 5 mm, a relative permittivity of 39.6, and a conductivity of 1 S/m for only one voxel. Targets cannot be detected with printed dipoles, but targets can be detected with FQSCA.

4.2.2 Imaging sensor for clinical equipment

4.2.2.1 Design

Figure 15 shows the appearance of an imaging sensor for clinical trials using FQSCA and a breast modeled with hexahedral voxels. In this sensor, six FQSCA are arranged on the side of a 140×140×50 mm dielectric block, and 12 FQSCA are arranged on the upper surface with different polarization.

4.2.2.2 Simulation result

Figure 16a shows 3D distribution of permittivity and conductivity of the numerical breast phantom. **Figure 16b** shows the reconstructed 3D distribution of

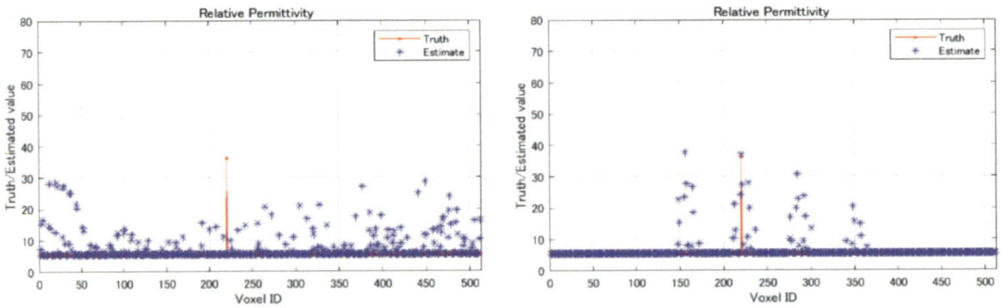

(a) (b)

Figure 14.
(a) Reconstructed relative permittivity (resolution of 5 mm, printed dipole is used). (b) Reconstructed relative permittivity (resolution of 5 mm, FQSCA is used).

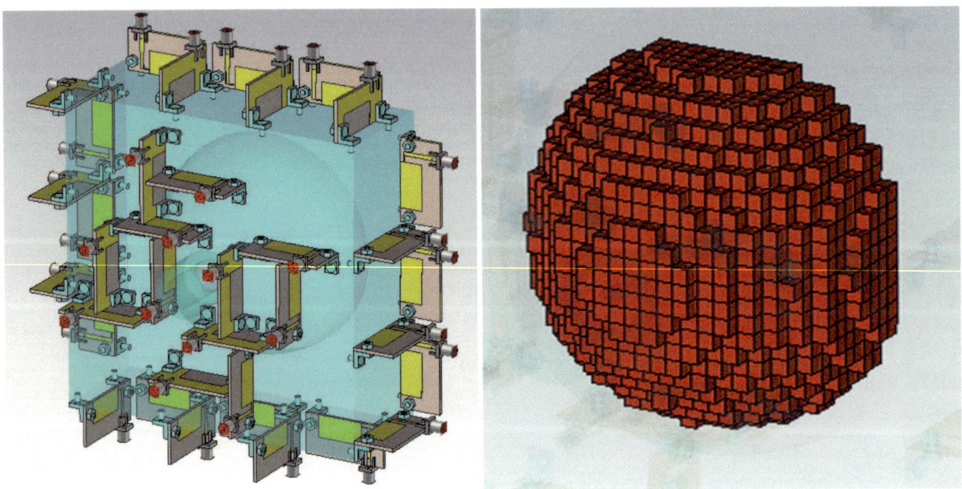

(a) (b)

Figure 15.
(a) Imaging sensor for clinical test. (b) Breast model.

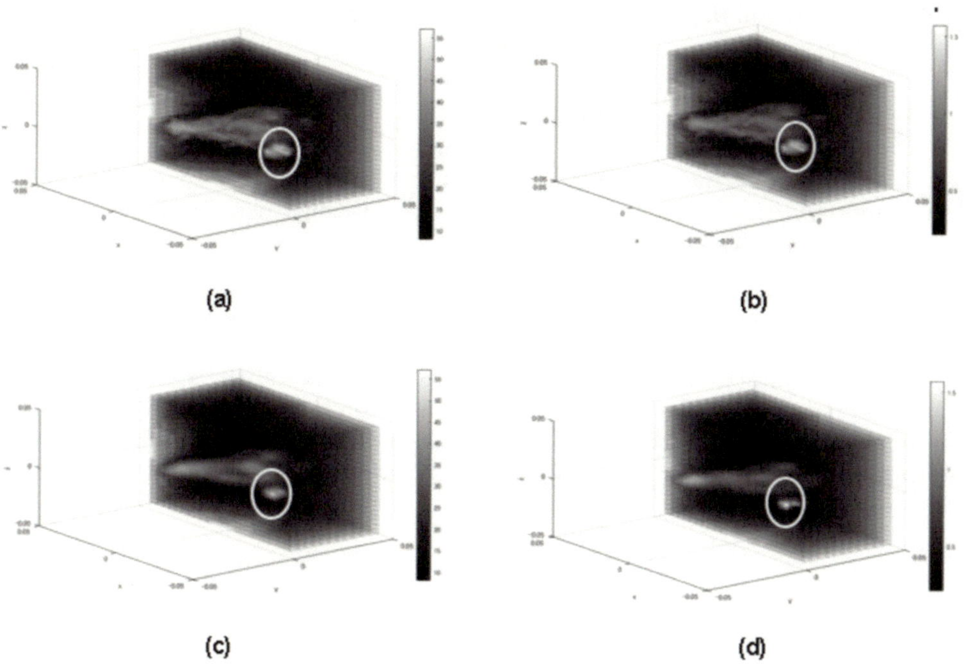

Figure 16.
(a) Set relative permittivity distribution. (b) Set conductivity. (c) Reconstructed relative permittivity distribution. (d) Reconstructed conductivity distribution.

permittivity and conductivity. The resolution is 4 mm and the frequency used is 1.5GHz. Circles indicate the cancer site. With the proposed sensor, mammary gland structure and cancer shape can be accurately reconstructed. The quality factor [28] evaluated by the complex dielectric constant was 0.96.

4.2.3 Manufacturing model

The sensor shown in **Figure 15** was prototyped and mounted on the system shown in **Figure 7**. **Figure 17** shows the prototype ST. The transmission characteristics of the antenna were measured with nothing in the cup that holds the breast, but as expected, they do not match the analysis results of CST Studio Suite. Therefore, we plan to adapt the measurement results to the simulation results by

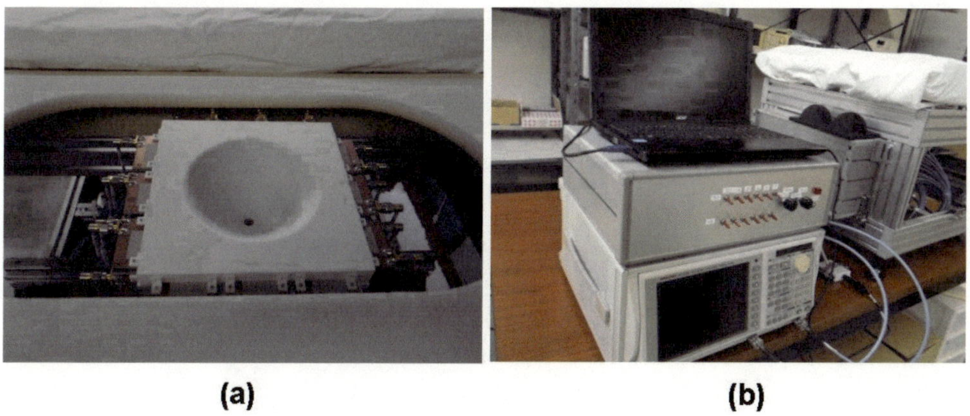

Figure 17.
(a) Sensor for the manufacturing model. (b) Overview of the manufacturing model.

calibration based on the measurement of the reference object in [23], and proceed to clinical imaging.

4.3 NFHI

First, we confirm by computer simulation that NFHI can reconstruct intramammary tissue. Next, a simple image system is constructed and experimental verification is performed.

4.3.1 Simulation

Computer simulations were performed to confirm that NFHI can reconstruct intramammary tissue. **Figure 18** shows the simulation model, and **Table 5** shows the simulation conditions. Similar to X-ray mammography imaging, imaging is performed with a model in which the breast is sandwiched between two glass plates

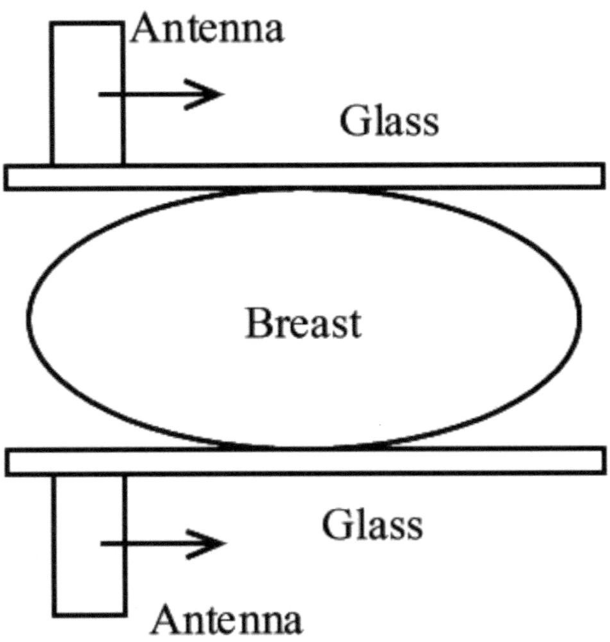

Figure 18.
Simulation model.

Frequency (GHz)		20.4 ~ 26
Scanning range (mm)	x-axis	−50 ~ 50
	y-axis	0 ~ 50
	z-axis	−10 ~ 30
Scanning step (mm)		2
CO	size(mm)	2 × 2 × 2
	permittivity	25
	Conductivity{S/m}	0.75

Table 5.
Simulation conditions.

and two antennas move on a plane at the same time. In order to obtain a resolution of 2 mm, the scattering parameters are acquired while the two antennas move in 2 mm steps on a plane of 100 × 50 mm. The frequency band used is 20.4-26GHz and the frequency step is 100 MHz. The antenna is a dipole antenna with a resonance frequency of 23.2 GHz. **Figure 19** shows the original tissue image and the reconstructed image. The reconstructed image faithfully reproduces the original image.

4.3.2 Measurement system

Figure 20 shows the appearance and system diagram of the imaging system used in the experiment. **Table 6** summarizes the measurement conditions.

The antennas are the commercially available primary feeds for Communication Satellite (CS) broadcast reception shown in **Figure 21**, and two antennas are arranged at intervals of 15 cm above and below, and can be scanned on the xy plane by an automatic stage. The imaging table is a celluloid plate with a thickness of 2 mm and 150 × 150 mm, and the height in the z-axis (vertical) direction can be adjusted by the z-axis stage. The outputs of the two CS antennas are connected to the input / output ports of the vector network analyzer, and the data of S_{11}, S_{21}, S_{12},

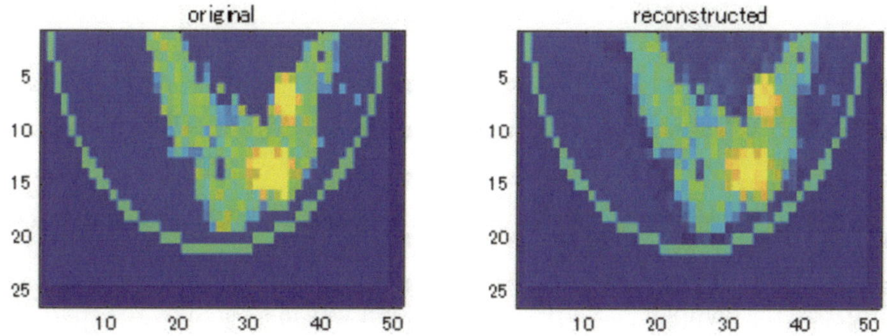

Figure 19.
Original image (left) and reconstructed image (right).

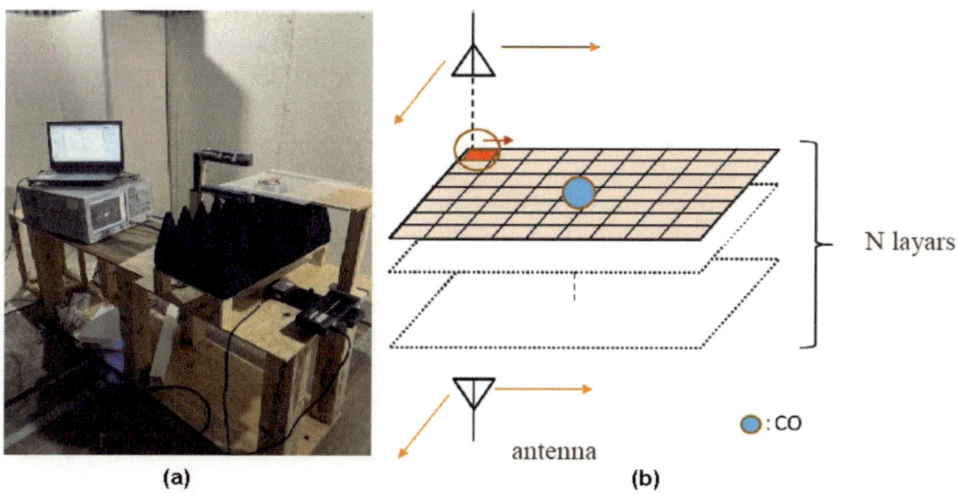

Figure 20.
(a) Overview of the NFHI system. (b) System configuration of NFHI system.

Frequency (GHz)		8.5 ~ 12.5
Scanning range (mm)	xy- plane	100 ~ 100
	z-axis	−10 ~ 30
Scanning step (mm)	xy-plane	2
	z-axis	10
CO(mm)		10 × 10 × 5

Table 6.
Measurement conditions.

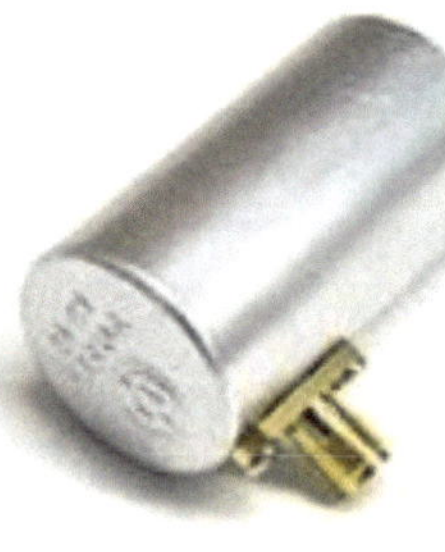

Figure 21.
Feed antenna for communication satellites broadcast.

and S_{22} are measured while changing the relative positions of the antenna and the object. The calibration object (CO) is glycerin (relative permittivity: 4.042, dielectric loss tangent: 1.021 (10 GHz)) filled with a 10×10×5 mm ABS resin container in **Figure 20a**. The complex permittivity of glycerin was measured by the equipment described in Section 2.2.

4.3.3 Measurement

The CO was placed in the center of the imaging table, and the S-parameters of the CO were measured in 10 mm steps in the range of −10 mm to 30 mm on the z-axis. Next, the pork was placed on the imaging table at the position of z = 10 mm as shown in **Figure 22b**, and the S parameter was measured. In order to acquire the scattering component, the S-parameters of the background were measured at the positions of 10 mm steps of −10 mm to 30 mm on the z-axis, and this was subtracted from the S-parameters of the object. **Figure 23** shows a reconstructed image. It can be seen that the position and shape of the pork and the contrast between the lean and white meat are reproduced.

Bright spots may appear in the reconstructed image due to measurement error. This is because the measurement data on the xy plane has a measurement error corresponding to white noise. That is, when the white noise is inverse Fourier transformed, it becomes an impulse. In this case, the median filter used in image processing is effective. Take out a part of the measurement data (for example, 9×9 data) measured at the grid points every 2 mm on the xy plane, find the median value, and use this as the measurement result of the center position of the 9×9 data. This process eliminates the bright spots caused by noise and improves the quality of the reconstructed image.

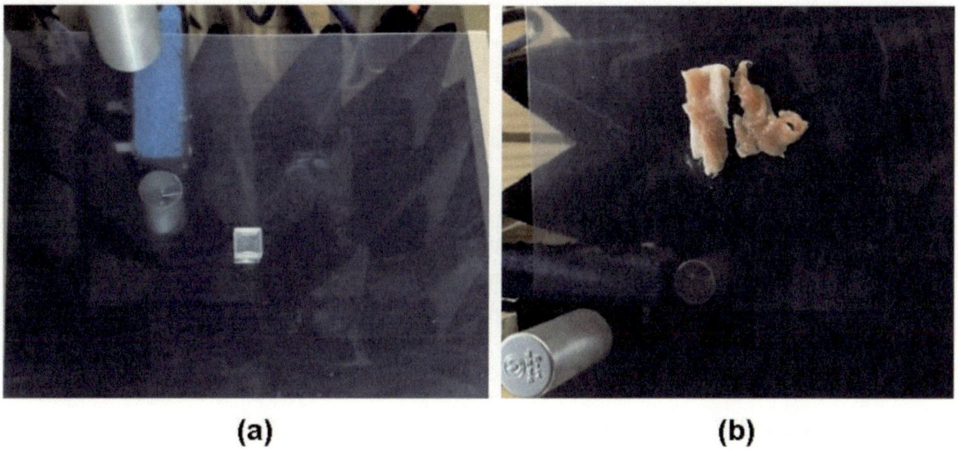

Figure 22.
(a) Calibration object (CO) on the imaging table. (b) Pork placed on the imaging table.

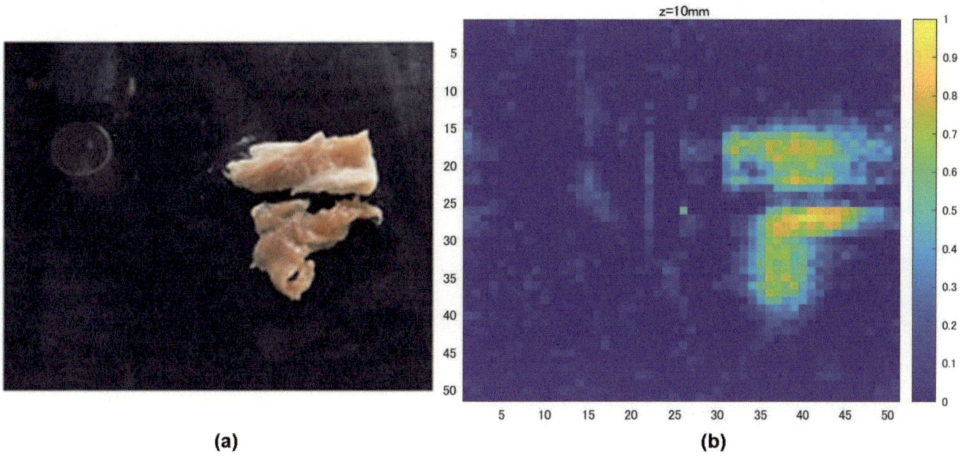

Figure 23.
(a) Original image. (b) Reconstructed image.

5. Conclusions

The breakthroughs required to put MI-based diagnostic imaging equipment into practical use are summarized below.

1. CI

   How to extract only the scattered wave of the target (lesion) in the living body?

   Reference [18] attempts to characterize breast cancer using all currently conceivable methods such as principal component analysis, independent component analysis, and kurtosis analysis. TR-MUSIC is applied to image reconstruction to improve the resolution. Clinical trial equipment has been developed and clinical trials have begun. In [19], the scattering response when the shape of the target (cancer) changes are analyzed and extraction of the characteristics of the cancer is tried. In the future, it is thought that the development of technology to determine the presence or absence of cancer by giving a response signal to artificial intelligence will progress [29].

2. ST

Improvement of simulation technology: It is required to develop a numerical analysis method that matches the experiment and the simulation result, a sensor that has a structure that easily matches the simulation result, or to establish a calibration technology. It is also expected to speed up forward analysis using cloud computing and supercomputers.

3. NFHI

It is necessary to proceed with the development of high-density sensing technology to ensure the resolution, and to find a measure in which the Born approximation can be applied in the biometric environment.

Acknowledgements

This work was supported by grants-in-aid for Scientific Research from the Ministry of Education, Culture, Sports, Science and Technology of Japan.

Author details

Yoshihiko Kuwahara
Aichi Medical University, Nagakute, Japan

*Address all correspondence to: kuwahara.yoshihiko.296@mail.aichi-med-u.ac.jp

References

[1] Lehman, C. D, Isaacs, C., Schnall, M. D., Pisano, E. D., Accher, S. M., Weatherall, P. T., Bluemke, D. A., Bowen, D. J., Marcom, P. K., Armstrong, D. K., Domchek, S. M., Tomlinson, G., Skates, S. J. and Gatsonis, C., Cancer Yield of Mammography. MR, and US in High Risk Women, Radiology, Vol.224(2), pp.381-388, Aug. 2007.

[2] M. Pasrorino, Microwave Imaging, ISBN 978-0-470-27800-0, 2010.

[3] Klemm, M., Craddock, I. J., Leenderts, J.A,. Preese. A., and Benjamin, R, Radar-based breast cancer detection using a hemispherical antenna array—experimental results. IEEE Trans. Antennas and Propag. 57(6), 1692–1704, 2009.

[4] Fear, E. C. Bourqui, J., Curtis, C., Mew, D., Docktor, C., and Romano, C., Microwave breast imaging with a monostatic radar based system: a study of application to patients, IEEE Trans. Microw. Theory Tech. 61(5), 2119-2128, 2013.

[5] Kuwahara, Y, Microwave Imaging for Early Breast Cancer Detection, DOI: 10.5772/intechopen.69562, 2017.

[6] Song, H., Sasada, S., Kadoya, T., Okada, M., Arihiro, K., Xiao, X., and Kikkawa, T., Detectability of Breast Tumor by a Hand-held Impulse-Radar Detector:Performance Evaluation and Pilot Clinical Study, Scientific Rep. 9, Article number: 16353, 2017.

[7] Solis-Nepote, M., Reimer, T., and Pistorius, S. An Air-Operated Bistatic System for Breast Microwave Radar Imaging: Pre-Clinical Validation. Int. Symp. IEEE 2019 EBMC, pp1859-1862, 2019.

[8] Kuwahara. Y. and Fujii, K., Near field microwave holography for bio-tissue imaging, open journal of medical imaging, Vol. 10, pp.143-150, 2020.

[9] Kuwahara, Y., Nozaki, A., and Fujii, K., Large Scale Analysis of Complex Permittivity of Breast Cancer in Microwave Band, advanced in breast cancer research, Vol. 9, pp.101-109, 2020.

[10] Gabriel C., Gabriel S. and Corthout E., The dielectric properties of biological tissues: I. Literature survey, Phys. Med. Biol. 41, pp.2231-2249, 1996.

[11] Popovic D., McCartney L., Beasley, C., Lazebnik, M., Okoniewski, M., Hagness, S. C., and Booske, J. H., Precision open ended coaxial probe for in vivo and ex vivo dielectric spectroscopy of biomedical tissues at microwaves frequency, IEEE trans. Microw. Theory Tech., 53, pp.1713-1722, 2005.

[12] Press, W. H., Teukolsky S. A., Vetterling, W. T., and Flannery, B. P., Numerical Recipes in C, ISBN4-87408-560-1, 1994.

[13] Sugitani, T., Kubota, S., Kuroki, S., Sogo, K., Arihiro, K., Okada, M., Kadoya, T., Hide, M., Oda, M., and Kikkawa, T., Complex permitivities of breast tumor tissues obtained from cancer surgeries, Appl. Phys. Lett. 104, 253702, 2014.

[14] Shea, J. D., Kosmas, P., Van Veen, B. D., and Hagness, S. C., Contrast-enhanced microwave imaging of breast tumors: a computational study using 3D realistic numerical phantoms, Inverse Problem 26 074009, pp. 1-22, 2010.

[15] Kuwahara, Y. Osaki, T, Nozaki, A. and Fujii, K., Utilization of preliminary knowledge in microwave tomography for breast cancer detection, IEICE Trans. Vol.J102(4), pp.86-92, 2018.

[16] Hernandez-Lopez, M. A., Martin, R. G., A rotating array antennas for confocal microwave breast imaging, Microw. Opt. Technol. Lett., vol. 39(4), pp. 307-311, 2003.

[17] Bucci, O. M., Bellizi, G., Costanzo, S., Crocco, L., DI Massa, G., and Scapaticci, R., Assessing Detection Limits in Magnetic Nanoparticle Enhanced Microwave Imaging, IEEE Access vol.6, pp. 43192 – 43202, 2018.

[18] Fasoula, A., Duchesne, L., Gil Cano, J. D., Lawrence, P., Robin, G., and Bernard, J. G., On-Site Validation of a Microwave Breast Imaging System, before First Patient Study, diagnostic 2018, 8, 53, doi:10.3390.

[19] Davis, S. K., Van Veen, G. D., Hagness, S. C., and Kelcz, F., Breast Tumor Characterization Based on Ultrawideband Microwave Backscatter, IEEE Trans. on Biomedical Eng., Vol. 55 (1), pp.237-246, 2007.

[20] Amineh, R. K., Nikolova, N. K. and Ravan, M., Real Time Three Dimensional Imaging of Dielectric Bodies Using Microwave/Millimeter Wave Holography, ISBN 9781119538868, 2019.

[21] Grzegorczyk, T. M., Meaney, P. M., Kaufman, P. A., diFlorio-Alexander, R. M., and Paulsen, K. D., Fast 3D Tomographic Imaging for Breast Cancer Detection, IEEE trans. on Med. Imag. 31 (8), pp.1584-1592, 2012.

[22] Ono, Y. and Kuwahara, Y., Microwave Tomography Assisted by Radar Imaging, Proc. EUMC2017, 10.23919/EuMC.2017.8230985.

[23] Ostadrahimi, M., Mojabi, P., Gilmore, C., Zakaria, A., Noghanian, S., Pistorius, S., and LoVetri, J., Analysis of Incident Field Modeling and Incident/ Scattered Field Calibration Technique in Microwave Tomography, IEEE Antennas and Wireless Propagat. Lett., Vol.10, pp.900-903, 2011.

[24] Poretti, S., Lanini, M., Salvade, A., Maffongeli, M. and Monleone, R., Antenna Design for microwave Tomography Imaging of High Contrast Mediums, Proc. of EUCAP2017, pp.1708-1711, 2017.

[25] Kuwahara, Y. and Nozaki, A., Effectiveness of FQSCA to Microwave Imaging, Proc. of EUCAP, 10.23919/ EuCAP48036.2020.9136049.

[26] https://www.3ds.com/products-services/simulia/products/cst-studio-suite/

[27] https://jp.mathworks.com/discovery/what-is-matlab.html

[28] Shea, J. D., Van Veen, B. D., and Hagness, S. C., A TSVD Analysis of Microwave Inverse Scattering For Breast Imaging, IEEE Tran. on Biomed. Eng., Vol. 59(4) pp.936-945, 2012.

[29] Reimer, T, Sacristan, J. and Pistrius, S., Improving the Diagnostic Capability of Microwave Radar Imaging System Using Machine Learning, Proc. of EuCAP 2019, INSPEC Accession Number: 18775801.